ORTHOTICS
CLINICAL PRACTICE AND REHABILITATION TECHNOLOGY

Books should be returned to the SDH Library on or before
the date stamped above unless a renewal has been arranged

Salisbury District Hospital Library
Telephone: Salisbury (01722) 336262 extn. 4432 / 33
Out of hours answer machine in operation

ORTHOTICS

CLINICAL PRACTICE AND REHABILITATION TECHNOLOGY

Edited by

JOHN B. REDFORD, M.D.

Distinguished Professor
Department of Rehabilitation Medicine
University of Kansas School of Medicine
Kansas City, Kansas
Chief
Physical Medicine and Rehabilitation Service
Department of Veterans Affairs Medical Center
Kansas City, Missouri

JOHN V. BASMAJIAN, M.D.

Professor Emeritus
Departments of Medicine and Anatomy
McMaster University Faculty of
Health Sciences
Hamilton, Ontario, Canada

PAUL TRAUTMAN, C.P.O.

Former Director
Department of Prosthetics and Orthotics
University of Kansas Medical Center
Kansas City, Kansas

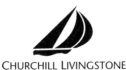

CHURCHILL LIVINGSTONE

A Division of Harcourt Brace & Company
New York, Edinburgh, London, Philadelphia, San Francisco

CHURCHILL LIVINGSTONE
A Division of Harcourt Brace & Company

The Curtis Center
Independence Square West
Philadelphia, Pennsylvania 19106

Library of Congress Cataloging-in-Publication Data

Orthotics : clinical practice and rehabilitation technology / edited by
John B. Redford, John V. Basmajian, Paul Trautman.
     p.   cm.
   Includes bibliographical references and index.
   ISBN 0-443-08992-2
   1. Orthopedic apparatus.   I. Redford, John B.   II. Basmajian,
John V., date.   III. Trautman, Paul.
   [DNLM: 1. Orthotic Devices.   WE 26 0753 1995]
RD755.O764   1995
615.3'07—dc20
DNLM/DLC   95-35492

Distributed in the United Kingdom by Churchill Livingstone, Robert Stevenson House, 1–3 Baxter's Place, Leith Walk, Edinburgh EH1 3AF, and by associated companies, branches, and representatives throughout the world.

Accurate indications, adverse reactions, and dosage schedules for drugs are provided in this book, but it is possible that they may change. The reader is urged to review the package information data of the manufacturers of the medications mentioned.

The Publishers have made every effort to trace the copyright holders for borrowed material. If they have inadvertently overlooked any, they will be pleased to make the necessary arrangements at the first opportunity.

Printed in the United States of America

Last digit is the print number: 7 6 5 4 3 2

In memory of Sidney Licht, M.D.
1907–1979
Author, Editor, Historian, Critic, Raconteur
Who inspired *Orthotics, Etcetera,*
the forerunner of this book

Contributors

Mark Agro, B.Sc., C.O.(C)

General Manager, Otto Bock Orthopedic Industry of Canada, Inc., Oakville, Ontario, Canada; President, Canadian Board for Certification of Prosthetists and Orthotists, Winnipeg, Manitoba, Canada

John V. Basmajian, M.D.

Professor Emeritus, Departments of Medicine and Anatomy, McMaster University Faculty of Health Sciences, Hamilton, Ontario, Canada

Mark Bussell, M.D., C.P.O.

Director, Amputee Rehabilitation Program, and Medical Director, Fort Worth Rehabilitation Hospital; Medical Director, ProsthetiCare Inc.; Member, Self-Assessment Examination Subcommittee, American Academy of Physical Medicine and Rehabilitation, Fort Worth, Texas

David R. Del Toro, M.D.

Assistant Professor, Department of Physical Medicine and Rehabilitation, Medical College of Wisconsin; Director, Prosthetic Clinic, Department of Physical Medicine and Rehabilitation, Curative Rehabilitation Center, Milwaukee, Wisconsin

Ruth Dickey, M.A., O.T.R.

Research Associate, Department of Rehabilitation Medicine, Mount Sinai School of Medicine of the City University of New York; Director, TEAMS (Technology and Education at Mount Sinai) Laboratory, Department of Rehabilitation Medicine, Mount Sinai Medical Center; Associate, Programs in Clinical Occupational Therapy, Columbia University College of Physicians and Surgeons, New York, New York

Laura Fenwick, C.O.

Director, Division of Orthotic Education, and Instructor, Department of Orthopaedic Surgery, Northwestern University Medical School; Orthotic Consultant, Rehabilitation Institute of Chicago, Chicago, Illinois

Ann H. Gettel, M.D.

Assistant Professor, Department of Rehabilitation Medicine, University of Kansas School of Medicine; Chief, Section of Pediatric Rehabilitation, Children's Mercy Hospital, Kansas City, Missouri

Dennis J. Janisse, C.Ped.

Consultant, Department of Orthopedics, Medical College of Wisconsin, Milwaukee, Wisconsin

Herbert Kent, M.D., F.C.C.P.

Clinical Professor, Department of Physical Medicine and Rehabilitation, University of California, Irvine, College of Medicine, Irvine, California; Professor Emeritus and Chief (retired), Rehabilitation Medicine Service, and Medical Consultant, Preservation-Amputation Care and Treatment (PACT) Program, Veterans Affairs Medical Center, Long Beach, California

Kirsten Kohlmeyer, O.T.R./L.

Adjunct Faculty, Department of Prosthetics-Orthotics, Northwestern University Medical School; Clinical Specialist, Department of Occupational Therapy, Rehabilitation Institute of Chicago, Chicago, Illinois

Arlette Loeser, M.A., O.T.R.

Clinical Specialist, TEAMS (Technology and Education at Mount Sinai) Laboratory, Department of Rehabilitation Medicine, Mount Sinai School of Medicine of the City University of New York, New York, New York

John Merritt, M.D.

Clinical Faculty, Department of Physical Medicine and Rehabilitation, University of California, Irvine, College of Medicine, Irvine, California; Medical Director, Tustin Rehabilitation Hospital, Tustin, California

Linda J. Miner, O.T.R., C.H.T.

Upper Extremity Clinical Specialist, Division of Occupational Therapy, Department of Physical Medicine and Rehabilitation, University of Michigan Medical Center, Ann Arbor, Michigan

Gabriella E. Molnar, M.D.

Clinical Professor, Department of Rehabilitation Medicine, University of California, Davis, School of Medicine, Davis, California; Director, Department of Pediatric Rehabilitation, Childrens Hospital, Oakland, California

Virginia S. Nelson, M.D. M.P.H.

Clinical Assistant Professor, Department of Physical Medicine and Rehabilitation, University of Michigan Medical School; Chief, Pediatric and Adolescent Service, Department of Physical Medicine and Rehabilitation, C.S. Mott Children's Hospital, Ann Arbor, Michigan

John B. Redford, M.D.

Distinguished Professor, Department of Rehabilitation Medicine, University of Kansas School of Medicine, Kansas City, Kansas; Chief, Physical Medicine and Rehabilitation Service, Department of Veterans Affairs Medical Center, Kansas City, Missouri

Edward Specht, B.S.

Associate Director, TEAMS (Technology and Education at Mount Sinai) Laboratory, Department of Rehabilitation Medicine, Mount Sinai School of Medicine of the City University of New York, New York, New York

Paul Trautman, C.P.O.

Former Director, Department of Prosthetics and Orthotics, University of Kansas Medical Center, Kansas City, Kansas

Jacqueline J. Wertsch, M.D.

Associate Professor, Department of Physical Medicine and Rehabilitation, Medical College of Wisconsin; Staff Physician, Department of Rehabilitation Medicine, Clement J. Zablocki Veterans Affairs Medical Center, Milwaukee, Wisconsin

Foreword

Orthotics: Clinical Practice and Rehabilitation Technology is a completely new departure from the older book, *Orthotics, Etcetera*, published a decade ago and now out of print. It is narrower in focus, and the "etcetera" of the old title has been supplanted by the term, "rehabilitation technology."

Owing to recent, dramatic developments within the field of orthotics and rehabilitation technology, an introductory foreword that looks both into the past and future seems in order. Because the amount and kinds of assistive technology now available have exceeded all predictions, a new but unofficial class of specialist, the rehabilitation technology supplier, has arisen. A rehabilitation technology supplier is a specialist who provides enabling technology in the area of wheeled mobility, seating and alternative positioning, ambulation assistance, environmental control, augmented communication, and/or activities of daily living. The rehabilitation technology supplier is employed by a company that sells durable medical equipment, offers consumers product choices along with pricing and funding information, and meets basic standards of acceptable practice in the provision of equipment, including ordering, assembling, adjusting, delivering, and providing ongoing support and service to meet individuals' rehabilitation equipment needs. The durable medical equipment industry is making available to rehabilitation technology suppliers a certification program that will enhance the expertise of these people. This will promote public and professional appreciation of the need for this new specialty. What the future holds for this group largely depends on whether the rehabilitation field becomes dominated by larger and larger medical corporations. If this occurs, the individual care and attention to detail provided by the rehabilitation technology supplier may suffer and fewer people may be available to provide expert advice.

The orthotist is the principal supplier and is responsible for most measurement and fitting of rehabilitation technology. Early editions of *Orthotics, Etcetera* described how orthotists evolved from armor and appliance makers to their present essential role in the field of rehabilitation medicine. Reflections on how the specialty of orthotics evolved in America were presented in a preface to the first edition of *Orthotics, Etcetera* by Dr. Licht:

> During the Civil War there was established in New York City an institution called the Hospital for Relief of the Ruptured and Crippled. Offhand, that sounds like a peculiar combination, and from a purely medical point of view, it was and is. The conjunctive was the appliance maker. The same artisan who made the hernia truss of metal and leather made the limb brace with metal and leather. In the twentieth century, the name of the hospital was changed, and so was that of the brace maker—he has become an orthotist. He may still make an abdominal belt, but he has progressed from a leather-and-iron craftsman to a member of the medical team that evaluates and manages disabled persons requiring functional aids—orthoses. As in most vocational and professional groups, progress has meant longer training, more research, improved technology and higher status.

Today the orthotist is no longer thought of as a mechanic, but rather as a specialist. As such, the orthotist is frequently consulted by physicians and other rehabilitation professionals for advice, particularly regarding complex fitting problems. Today, most orthotists are financially independent of hospitals and medical clinics, but work very closely with physicians and other health professionals. Unlike the past, orthotists enjoy a much less subservient role to the medical profession, although most third-party payers require a physician's signature before approving funding for durable medical equipment. The rules of this have become much more complicated in the past few years.

What is the future of orthotics and orthotists? Orthotics largely remains a cottage industry—small manufacturers who make by hand equipment and devices for individual clients. The advent of computer-assisted design and computer-assisted manufacture threatens to reduce the number of individual operators. This technology will expand the role of larger orthotic and prosthetic operations by the reduction of hands-on manufacture. Instead of the orthotist manually making a negative cast of the limb or trunk followed by a positive cast and mold, the whole process will be performed electronically. Sockets for limb prostheses are now being made by digitally recording the shape and size of a plaster negative cast. These data are fed into a computer and rectified by manually manipulating the image in the computer. The resulting template is modified to produce the desired design. The recorded information is transferred to an electronically controlled milling machine and a plaster or plastic positive mold is produced. Using a vacuum-forming thermoplastic technique, a socket is created, mounted over the foot, and fitted the usual way. The automated fabrication of mobility aids process is now operated by the Department of Veteran's Affairs in a number of Veteran's Affairs Medical Centers. The same system is about to be applied to orthotics to make body jackets and lower-limb plastic orthoses. In the near future, the cast will not be necessary; digital recordings of the shape of the trunk or the limb will be done directly by use of a laser beam to digitize the shape. The rectified computer images can be sent over telephone lines to central fabrication laboratories. Prosthetic sockets or orthoses are then made and mailed back to the orthotist or prosthetist who digitized the original shape.

The advantages of this system are as follows:

1. Hours of hands-on manual manufacture are eliminated, thus reducing cost.
2. Computer storage of models, rather than physical storage, saves storage space in orthotics and prosthetics facilities.
3. Only a few minutes are required to correct the image, rather than the hours needed to hand-carve plaster molds. If necessary, multiple modified duplicates can be made without recasting.

Although prosthetists and orthotists may fear this new development will make them obsolete, their skills will still be needed for modifying and fitting the final product. However, within five years, this process may be so widely available that a new book will be needed to describe this and other computer technology applications to the field of orthotics and assistive technology.

John B. Redford, M.D.

Preface

Like the Phoenix of mythology, this living book has risen from the ashes of the past to claim a unique place. Unlike the books it succeeds, it fulfills a role that we believe is fresh, comprehensive, and commanding in orthotics and rehabilitation. It is the first book to relate medical diagnoses directly to orthotic technology. We anticipate the book will be in great demand to those who are newly initiated in orthotics and want to understand the applicability of specific orthoses to particular medical conditions. As editors, we planned the book to be authoritative, yet readable; comprehensive, yet uncluttered; and detailed, yet pleasant to read. We were fortunate to find chapter authors who would rise to the challenge, and who succeeded with great style.

As Dr. Bruce Gans, President of the Rehabilitation Institute of Michigan, recently, wrote:

> Many of the activities the physically challenged are able to engage in are made possible by advances in engineering and technology ... Robotic technologies will continue to be applied to rehabilitation issues, allowing automation to deliver therapeutic treatments ... [and] influence practical work site modification and manipulation possibilities, especially when joined with voice recognition technology and motion detection capabilities.

A better definition of the cutting-edge developments that are the foundation for this book could not be found. However, due to the realities of today, we must balance the use of cutting-edge technology with economic considerations to provide our patients with the devices most suited to their needs. Many of the orthotic devices in use today will be just as practical in the mid-twenty-first century as they are today because their designs are based on fundamental concepts that will not change over time. As a consequence, we have described the best of today's developments while forecasting the best of tomorrow's.

Our authors are recognized experts on their respective topics and have shared their considerable knowledge and experience. As editors we have tried to provide a consistent framework for the reader. We sincerely hope this book will meet the needs of all who have an interest in providing and using practical orthotics and rehabilitation technologies now and in the future.

John B. Redford, M.D.
John V. Basmajian, M.D.
Paul Trautman, C.P.O.

Contents

Basic Principles of Orthotics and Rehabilitation Technology

John B. Redford

1

This book provides a guide for clinicians on the basic principles, indications, and usage of orthoses and other devices or equipment to improve function in persons with physical disabilities. An *orthosis* (pl., *orthoses*), according to the International Standards Organization, is an externally applied device used to modify the structural or functional characteristics of the neuromusculoskeletal system. The term *orthotics* describes the theory, practice, and manufacture of orthoses. An *orthotist* is a person skilled in the field.

The word *orthosis* is derived from the Greek "ortho," meaning straight, upright, or correct. These are all suitable descriptions of the function of most orthoses—to help maintain straight limbs or correct a spine that is not upright. Compared to the more static inference of the older term *brace,* the term *orthosis* includes devices for dynamic control of body segments. Although the terms *orthosis* and *brace* are frequently used interchangeably, orthosis is now the preferred term. Since 1960, the term has been adopted by orthotists and prosthetists in the United States in the title of their official organization, The American Orthotics and Prosthetics Association.

Orthoses are named according to the joints or spinal segments that they encompass. Most of the following medical acronyms are used in this chapter:

ADL	Activities of daily living
AFO	Ankle–foot orthosis
AO	Ankle orthosis
CO	Cervical orthosis
CTLSO	Cervicothoracolumbosacral orthosis
CTO	Cervicothoracic orthosis
EWHO	Elbow–wrist–hand orthosis
HKO	Hip–knee orthosis
HO	Hip orthosis, hand orthosis
KAFO	Knee–ankle–foot orthosis
KO	Knee orthosis
LSO	Lumbosacral orthosis
SEO	Shoulder–elbow–wrist–hand orthosis
SEWHO	Shoulder–elbow–wrist–hand orthosis
SO	Shoulder orthosis
TLSO	Thoracolumbosacral orthosis
W/C	Wheelchair
WHO	Wrist–hand orthosis

A definition of *rehabilitation technology* is also needed. The term is more recent in origin than *orthotics* but is now widely understood to mean those appliances and equipment that, unlike orthoses, do not intimately overlie parts of the body. Therefore, wheelchairs, lifting

1

devices, assistive equipment to improve self-care, and adaptive modifications of equipment to increase independence or conserve energy are all forms of rehabilitation technology. The concept includes structural changes to help disabled persons function in an adapted environment. *Assistive technology* is an equivalent term in many instances, but it is broadly understood to apply also to other devices, such as life support equipment including respirators and home dialysis units. This book concerns technology needed to rehabilitate persons who have neurologic or orthopedic impairments successfully into a home or working environment. The text omits discussion of other rehabilitation technology or equipment for physical treatment, such as diathermy, ultrasound, exercise equipment, and electrical stimulation devices.

MAJOR TRENDS

A wider understanding by health professionals and the public of orthotics and rehabilitation technology is clearly needed. The demand for a greater supply of equipment and improved assistive technology continues to grow at a rapid pace. This is in part due to the increased proportion of older people in the population, which has caused a proportionate increase in the number of physically disabled. Another factor may be that more people are surviving catastrophic disorders, such as head injury, spinal cord injury, and cerebrovascular diseases. A further trend or movement spurring growth in the United States has been the independent living or disabled rights advocacy for the Americans With Disabilities Act. This trend is described by Kirchner in an excellent review of the current social and demographic situation regarding disability in the United States.[1]

Reimbursement for the increasing costs of medical care has become one of the foremost problems in American health care. Rehabilitation, although proven effective in returning persons to employment, is an expensive process. Because orthotics and assistive technology appear inordinately expensive to the public, rehabilitative technology must be rendered in the most cost-efficient manner. If the cost of the technology cannot be shown to improve rehabilitation outcome significantly, providers will face increasing difficulty in expecting payment for their products. Decisions about paying for rehabilitation

service in the future will likely be based on outcome studies.

A great change in delivery of rehabilitation technology is occurring in America. In response to third-party payment by managed care providers, multiple locations have become an important aspect of providing orthotic and prosthetic services. It is difficult for a single-site facility to compete with larger companies, which can offer multiple locations within a city. The ability of consumers to go to the provider of their choice depends on the adoption of "Any Willing Provider" legislation. This will ensure payment to any provider of a service that is willing to accept the terms of a managed health corporation. In the case of rehabilitation services, it would enable a company to provide orthotics and prosthetics for its patients. Exclusivity would make it difficult for smaller facilities to serve such third-party payors, and competition would be reduced. Exclusivity might be more economical but might result in a decline in service and quality.

Changes from previously acceptable methods of prescribing are occurring and will certainly have a great impact on introducing new rehabilitation technologies. If innovative equipment cannot be shown to have advantages that justify improvement in function over available technology, expecting payment may become a real issue. Today, insurance carriers are questioning payment reimbursement even on small items, such as special foot and spinal orthoses. It may become very difficult to introduce new ideas under these changing circumstances.

Relatively scant attention has been paid to the issue of covering payment for assistive aids. For example, it has been reported that assistive aids provided to people rarely are used after the first month or so following discharge from a rehabilitation program. Much of this pattern of limited use arises because the disabled consumer—or whoever chooses the device on the patient's behalf—may not be fully aware of the needs for the assistive device in the long term. Only after a disabled person becomes aware of the change in his or her status can the relationships between technology and actual requirements be judged. With some consumers, this may require several repeated changes before satisfactory adaptive equipment or environmental change is evident. Chapters 9 and 10, on adaptive equipment and environmental control for persons with disabilities, respectively, discuss this problem in more detail.

An excellent source for information and sources for

assistive technology is the *Assistive Technology Source Book,* edited by Enders and Hall.[2]

ORTHOTIC AND REHABILITATIVE EQUIPMENT SERVICES

In providing orthoses or assistive equipment, four major groups are involved:

1. *Consumers:* Persons with impairments may or may not choose to buy the equipment recommended and can purchase assistive devices without intervention by a health professional.
2. *Prescribers:* In the case of orthoses, prescription is mostly done by licensed physicians, but other health professionals such as occupational therapists are often involved.
3. *Orthotists:* These are the primary suppliers of orthoses that require measurement and fitting and who are also trained to supply rehabilitation technology, particularly for custom-fitted items, such as in special seating.
4. *Manufacturers and suppliers of durable medical equipment:* Many are very knowledgeable about adaptive equipment and operate businesses exclusively devoted to rehabilitative equipment or devices.

Consumers

Consumers can be very demanding and may have unrealistic expectations about the use of orthoses or assistive equipment. The importance of education and understanding by an individual of how rehabilitation technology might affect a person's life cannot be overemphasized. Samples or pictures of proposed devices may allay concerns, because most persons have little exposure to rehabilitation technology.

Patients usually want drugs or surgery—not exercises, equipment, or "braces"—to solve their problems. Orthoses cannot be regarded as an effective substitute for surgery. However, often a trial of an orthosis before surgery will give the patient some idea of surgical expecta-

tions. In addition, an orthosis may need to be worn temporarily after surgery and in some cases forever, for example, after a heel cord lengthening for a spastic equinus foot and ankle. Orthoses can never replace active mobilizing or special strengthening exercises, and usually these are needed in conjunction with orthotic wear.

Most orthoses ultimately depend on their correct mechanical application to meet a functional need; but consumers may have other concerns, such as cosmesis. Even after a thorough discussion of orthotic expectations, the orthotist may have to reduce orthotic biomechanical effectiveness to satisfy a reluctant patient. Nevertheless, it is better to have the patient wearing an orthosis than to have it lying in a closet somewhere.

Prescribers

The prescriber of orthotic devices for the most part is the physician with the legal responsibility for patient care. In the ideal situation, the prescriber should have a clear idea of current treatment and the potentials and limitations of devices prescribed. The patient should be willing to make decisions based on full discussion with the orthotist and patient, as well as the nurse, physical therapist, occupational therapist, or whoever is treating the patient. Based on the clinical findings, the prescribing clinician should have a good understanding of the muscle strength, range of motion, skin condition, and all indications and expectations. After all, the key to using an orthosis is finding if it improves function and is safe to use, given the patient's muscle strength and sensory integration. The individual who orders the device should be sure that the patient's family understands its purpose as well as the patient and understands that it may be needed not just during recovery but lifelong. Often, more than one device may be ordered, and the interaction of two or more devices must also be considered, especially because "gadget tolerance" becomes a real issue in patients with multiple disabilities.

Clinic Team

Because of the complexity of many cases requiring orthoses or rehabilitation technology, referral is often made to an orthotic clinic team. The patient, of course, is the primary member and contributor to the team. The physician, nurse, orthotist, equipment specialist, physical therapist, occupational therapist, and social worker may all be members. Not only does the clinic team provide the evaluation and prescription and ensure delivery, but team follow-up is vital because of changes occurring in either the device or patient. Furthermore, all major devices need maintenance or replacement, and they should be evaluated periodically for proper function. Orthotic clinics for children are especially important because of changes in growth and development. Wheelchair and special seating clinics for children, for example, are now operating in many rehabilitation institutions.

The orthotist is the health professional best qualified to provide orthoses. Orthotists require a basic knowledge of anatomy, physiology, biomechanics, and functional characteristics of medical conditions affecting the neuromusculoskeletal system. To become a certified orthotist in the United States, an individual must comply with the following requirements:

1. Obtain a bachelor's degree in an accredited university or college.
2. Complete 1 year of clinical training supervised by a certified orthotist.
3. Pass a series of examinations administered by the American Board of Orthotics and Prosthetics, Inc.

In addition, to remain certified, an orthotist must obtain 75 hours of continuing education every 5 years and adhere to the American Board of Orthotics and Prosthetics canons of ethical conduct.

The orthotist not only must have a thorough understanding of the materials used and skill in their use but also should understand the psychological and social effects of disability. He may also need to train patients in the use of equipment and should anticipate problems that might occur. Some orthotists have extensive knowledge about wheelchairs and other apparatus for increasing mobility and work closely to those persons who supply such rehabilitation technology.

The orthotist must oversee fitting to ensure that the forces and pressures applied by the orthosis are at the right locations and not excessive. The orthotist may need to do some fine tuning: for example, adding pads or trimming away material after the patient has tested its function. Also, particularly with lower limb orthoses, the orthotist must ensure that the device is aligned correctly to achieve the wanted gait pattern or other function. As previously noted, follow-up with a physician and/or other members of the clinic orthotic team is most important in complex cases.

An orthotic technician is educated only in the technical or bench-level skills required in orthotics. Technicians are registered with the American Board of Orthotics and Prosthetics, as opposed to being certified.

Less complex orthoses, namely, those that can be molded directly on the patient using low-temperature thermoplastics, are often made by occupational therapists or other health professionals. The orthotist should be consulted, however, in more complex situations and fabricate any orthosis that requires manufacture following special measurements, casting, or impressions to make permanent metal or form-fitting plastic orthoses.

Suppliers

The manufacturers and suppliers of rehabilitation technology represent a fourth group with responsibility for the disabled consumer. This includes those supplying the material and manufacturers of prefabricated devices that are custom fitted by health-care professionals. Suppliers must be prepared to improve methods of production and quality control constantly, to avoid unforeseen breakdowns or risks to patient safety. The supplier to the consumer must be sufficiently knowledgeable to comprehend the function of rehabilitative equipment and to explain to the purchaser its limitations, costs, and maintenance. The patient should be warned of any problems that might occur with equipment, especially the signs of early breakdown. Materials in direct contact with the skin, for example, may cause allergic skin reactions, and poor fit may impair circulation. The patient should return the product to the supplier or orthotist for the correction of such problems as soon as they are noted.

As in any seller–buyer relationship, the dissatisfied patient should be encouraged to complain to rehabilitation technology suppliers and not simply reject equipment because it breaks down or does not fully conform to expectations. Unfortunately, it is very hard to expect suppliers of custom-manufactured equipment to return money if the device was prescribed carefully, but suppliers may be sensitive to this issue and help with reimbursement in selected cases.

BIOMECHANICS OF ORTHOTICS

The primary purpose of an orthosis is to improve function by (1) applying or subtracting forces from the body in a controlled manner to protect a body part, (2) restricting or altering motion to prevent or correct a deformity, and (3) compensating for deformity or weakness.

Because the general objective of an orthosis is to exert force on a body segment to limit or control unwanted motion, a basic understanding of biomechanics is necessary when prescribing orthoses. The human body is always subject to a system of external forces and moments, whether moving or stationary. Force has both direction and magnitude and generally is illustrated as a vector from which mathematical expressions can be derived. A majority of the applied forces on body segments affect rotation; that is, they inhibit or modify the rotary movements about the joint axes. The turning effect of the force about a joint axis is known as its *moment*. The magnitude of a moment is determined by the distance from site of force application to the axis of rotation (moment arm) and the size of that force. Units of moment are equal to force times distance and expressed as Newtons times meters (Nm). Clockwise movements are positive, counterclockwise are negative.

Stability

A joint will be at equilibrium or stable when the moments on the body segment on one side of a joint axis are equal in magnitude to those of the other. Obviously, the longer the moment arms or the greater the magnitude of the intrinsic forces, the greater must be the external forces applied to the body segment to achieve equilibrium. If these internal forces are failing because of ligamentous or muscular deficiency, an orthosis may be provided to improve stability. The concept behind such an orthosis is to provide static equilibrium by a three-point force system. The external appliance creates a balance of moments through forces applied at key points through the enclosing cuffs or plastic material (Fig. 1-1).

In a typical orthotic system designed to stabilize a joint, the moment arm should be as long as possible, and the force against the skin should be dissipated by a wide area of application. This will minimize pressure on the skin where the orthosis makes contact with the body.

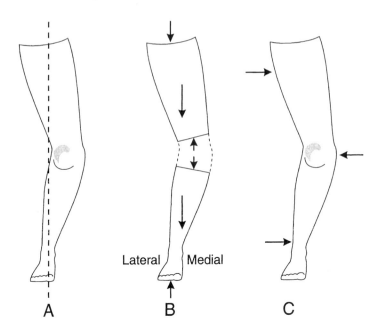

Fig. 1-1.   Three-point force system to control a valgus knee deformity. **(A)** Lower limb with a valgus knee. The dashed line shows weightbearing through the lower limb. **(B)** Free body diagram of forces showing tendency to increase knee angulation. **(C)** Corrective forces needed from an orthosis to prevent unwanted rotation into the valgus. (From Bowker,[3] with permission.)

In addition to forces producing rotation, some forces create translational motion, or motion in the same plane as the applied force. As an example, translation motion occurs when the femur glides forward on the tibia. In normal joints translational motion is minimal and insignificant; in conditions with severe ligamentous destruction, translational motion is undesirable and must be controlled to improve function. Axial forces in the longitudinal plane of the body segment also occur. These are largely generated in the lower limb by the ground reaction force counteracting the downward force from the mass of the body.

Bowker provides elegant mathematical descriptions of how orthoses may modify systems of moments and external forces acting about a joint in four different ways: (1) restricting rotation, (2) reducing shear, (3) reducing axial displacement, and (4) controlling the line of action of the ground reaction force.[3]

Rotation

First, any orthosis may act to restrict joint rotation by modifying moments using a three-point force system just described (Fig. 1-1). This system may limit motion around one or more joint axes around which rotation may occur. For example, a full-length lower limb orthosis or a knee-ankle-foot orthosis (KAFO) may be designed to limit one or more forces around the perpendicular axes of the knee joint. In fact, this system can control mediolateral, anteroposterior, and rotational forces around the knee, depending on the design.

Shear

Second, an orthosis can restrict translational motion produced by shearing forces across joints. This is always an unwanted motion that may be increased around the joint with incorrect alignment of an orthotic joint axis. Generally, translational motion occurs when ligamentous structures are unduly lax. Laxity is controlled by an orthosis designed with a rigid frame. This frame usually consists of custom-molded plastic cuffs intimately fitted to the limb.

In weightbearing, as the joint is flexed, translational forces increase proportionately to flexion. In a typical injury to the anterior cruciate ligament of the knee, liga-

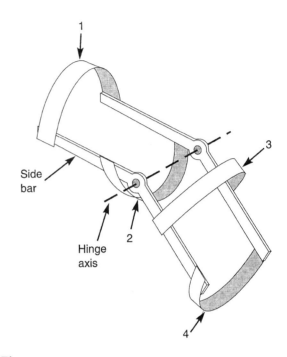

Fig. 1-2. Diagram of a four-point orthosis needed to treat anterior cruciate ligament deficiency with excessive anterior motion of the tibia. *(1)* A proximal posteriorly directed force from a rigid anterior thigh band. *(2)* A distal anteriorly directed force from a rigid posterior thigh band. *(3)* A proximal posteriorly directed force from a tibial band just below the knee. *(4)* A distal anteriorly directed force from a calf band. (From Bowker,[3] with permission.)

mentous laxity during flexion produces a marked tendency for the proximal tibia to slide forward from under the femur. Orthoses designed with rigid frameworks with firm grip between the padded cuffs and the skin surface are required to overcome this ligamentous instability at all angles of joint flexion. Four-point fixation orthoses are required to restrict this anterior shear, or "draw" (Fig. 1-2). Obviously, such orthoses must be carefully molded and padded. A double-axis hinge in the orthosis is preferred over a single-axis hinge because of its closer conformity to anatomic action.

Axial Forces

Third, an orthosis can be used to reduce axial forces developed across joints. In normal joints, axial loading along the limb or spine is created by gravitational pull of the body mass opposing a ground reaction force. This load is carried through bony structures and articular cartilages. When these tissues are intact, the loading is painless; but if they fail, as in fractures or degenerative cartilage disorders, excessive deformation may occur. This may result in pain and impaired mobility.

Axial loading in the lower limb is usually reduced by redistributing the load through the upper limbs via canes or crutches, but orthoses are sometimes used. The axial unloading requires using frictional forces produced by cuffs or intimately fitted plastic molds that suspend the limb proximally. Then, a distal component attached to the lower segment opposes the downward force in the limb.

The skin pressures resulting from frictional forces are better tolerated if the transfer of the axial load can be through a bony prominence proximally. An example of this force transfer is incorporating a quadrilateral cuff with an ''ischial seat'' into an orthosis; the ischial tuberosity rests on the proximal part of the thigh cuff. To provide the orthosis with opposing distal force, the side portions of the KAFO attach with a horizontal stirrup, caliper, or transverse piece lying under the shoe.

With the knee and ankle joint of the brace locked and the caliper lying below the shoe platform (a patten bottom), 100 percent of the weightbearing will occur through the orthosis. This can be used to completely unload the hip joint and all structures distal to it. Even without the patten bottom, axial loading can be lessened, especially in trained subjects, but partial degrees of weightbearing will still occur through the joints.[4]

Ground Reaction Forces

A fourth example of using biochemical principles in orthoses is applied exclusively to the lower limbs. It essentially involves control of the line of action of the ground reaction force. This force occurs when the foot contacts the floor and is illustrated as a line projected up through the body from the floor toward the center of mass. This ground reaction force affects all three principal body planes; the sagittal, frontal, and transverse. It changes the nature of components in these planes as the gait cycle moves from heel strike to toe-off.

The point of application on the sole of the foot of this ground reaction force moves forward progressively. The force that is very great—generally equal or greater than the body weight—at any point in time will create

moments about each lower limb joint. This is because the force constantly shifts position in relation to centers of joint rotation during gait. Therefore, applying an orthosis that will realign the ground reaction force can change considerably the moments about lower limb joints.

Practical applications of this principle are most frequently followed in shoe alterations or ankle–foot orthoses. (AFOs). Any AFO that limits ankle motion will affect to some degree the moments at the knee and hip because of the altered ground reaction force.

A simple illustration of this application is seen in shoe alterations or foot orthoses using a medial calcaneal wedge to realign a pronated hind foot. The wedge will move the center of heel pressure, which represents the ground reaction force, laterally to a more neutral position. Another example is shown in Figure 1-3 in a patient who has an unstable knee that tends to flex at heel strike. A simple heel cutoff changes the ground reaction force and reduces the moment arm, causing knee flexion. This simple measure reduces knee bending moment and thus improves knee stability; in other words, the patient requires less contraction of the quadriceps muscle to control knee flexion after heel strike.[5]

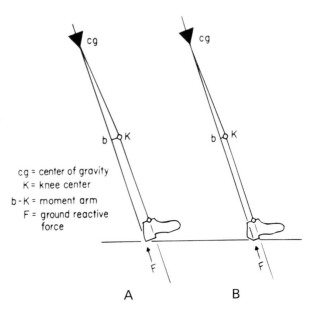

cg = center of gravity
K = knee center
b–K = moment arm
F = ground reactive force

A   B

Fig. 1-3. **(A & B)** Reduction of knee bending moment during heel strike by heel cutoff. Note that moment arm b–K on the heel cutoff side (Fig. B) is smaller than b–K without heel cutoff (Fig. A).

INTERFACE BETWEEN ORTHOSIS AND PATIENT

Whether an orthosis can be tolerated depends on its interfaces with soft tissues of the body. At the patient–orthosis interface, stability and comfort are achieved by having the force diffused by pads, leather-covered metal cuffs, molded plastic and the like. The force from an orthosis must be equal to the weight or force produced by the enclosed body in accordance to Newton's third law of motion: "When object exerts a force on a second object, then the second object exerts an equal and opposite reaction force on the first object."

Body tissues will support high levels of hydrostatic pressure if the force is equally distributed in all directions; for example, extraordinarily high hydrostatic pressure is tolerated over the entire body by deep sea divers. Hydrostatic orthoses have been developed and would be ideal because they evenly distribute pressure and cause less tissue distortion, but they are not practical.

For most orthoses, it is necessary to try to redistribute forces or pressures over wide areas by using large surface interfaces carefully contoured to provide minimal tissue distortion. Obviously, this has practical limits in reducing pressure. Bony prominences tolerate pressures much less than sites over muscle and fatty tissue and must be accommodated. Prolonged loading, even at low levels of pressure, may cause damage, especially if pressure is unevenly distributed. One such site that is repeatedly under load is the sole of the foot, which is a common site for tissue breakdown in patients with poor sensation.

Shear Stress

Two other factors that affect the patient–orthosis interface are shear stress and the local skin environment. Shear stress is formed by externally applied forces that distort tissue, typically encountered when tangential forces cause shear over weightbearing surfaces, such as under the sole of the foot. Shear-created stress under a seating surface not only will affect superficial skin tissue but will produce motion between the underlying muscle or fascia and bone. These forces distort the blood vessels beneath the skin, which in turn may restrict blood and lymph flow and damage subcutaneous tissue. This may be very hard to detect.

Undesirable shear in a limb orthosis is commonly produced by poor contouring of the orthotic surface or joint malalignment. The patient should be constantly aware of developing undue skin redness because that is the hallmark of the effects of these undesirable forces.

Local Skin

The local skin environment has a profound influence on skin integrity. Excessive heat tends to increase sweating; this in turn causes skin maceration, which promotes bacterial and fungal growth. Incontinence may also play a major role in causing tissue damage, particularly around seating surfaces.

Strategies

In orthotic design, reduction of shear and pressure is mainly achieved by the use of viscoelastic materials. At the patient–orthotic interface, polyethylene foam is widely used, as are various silicone-based materials. Shear is also reduced by slippery elastic materials, such as those commonly used in a sheath type of stump socks worn by amputees under a regular wool or cotton socks. To combat skin moisture, socks, sleeves, or undergarments made of 100 percent cotton are nearly always advocated, especially in warm environments. These wick away moisture but also cushion the body part and reduce uneven pressure or shear. Other methods to improve air circulation may be undertaken, such as ventilating limb orthoses and body jackets with multiple holes in the plastic material.

Using pressure transducers to measure pressure between the skin and externally applied devices has been the subject of extensive research. To determine variation of tissue viability under varying loads, researchers have employed various techniques to study the compression effects of orthoses or appliances on skin blood flow. Much of this experimental work has had practical applications, particularly in developing better seating systems for the disabled.

Using miniature timers and pressure transducers, the length of time an orthosis has been worn has been measured without the wearer's awareness. These devices are set at threshold levels that turn the switches on and off. Such systems have been used to study compliance in subjects wearing orthoses. Using such a system for study on scoliotic braces, Houghton et al. reported that clinicians markedly overestimate the time such braces are actually worn in adolescent girls.[6]

MATERIALS

Materials used in fabrication of orthoses have changed markedly in recent years. Orthoses must combine strength with stiffness to allow no bending and overcome the great forces on the lower limbs and spine. Steel and aluminum have been the traditional materials. However, metal uprights with limb-enclosing cuffs covered with leather and fastened with buckles or straps are becoming things of the past. Great strength and stiffness can be developed by newer plastics. They are lighter and more appealing cosmetically than metal orthoses. A survey of orthotists in 1983 revealed that almost 80 percent of practitioners are fabricating 75 percent or more of their products with plastics.[7] One suspects this percentage is even higher today.

Metal

Because adjustments can be more easily incorporated, metal is still widely used in joints instead of plastic. Joints can be made in three basic patterns to achieve the following: (1) Permit free action in one plane, but modify it in another; (2) limit range of motion, using a joint "stop"; (3) and resist or assist motion in a particular direction. Obviously, selection of a joint in a particular orthosis depends on the functional requirement. From a biomechanical standpoint, the controlling characteristics in the joint can be represented graphically by making a plot of resistance to motion exerted by the joint against the appropriate joint angle. As biomechanical principles become more widely applied in orthotics, better joint designs will be developed to mimic anatomic polycentric action.

The main disadvantage of metal compared with plastic is its greater bulk, weight, and difficulty with attachment to the body—for example, the awkward attachment of metal braces to shoes. Furthermore, the close fit of a plastic orthosis allows pressures to be better distributed over a wider area of the skin than with padded metal cuffs.

Plastic

A plastic orthosis is cosmetically more appealing; it looks better and lacks the clickity-clackity sound that is associated with some metal components. Plastic orthoses are easy to clean and are corrosion resistant. They have proven fatigue resistant with good ability to withstand frequent loading. Joints may not be needed, because flexibility can be adjusted by altering the thickness of the plastic or by increasing or decreasing its width at key areas. For example, severely trimming the plastic around the ankle in an AFO will increase its flexibility at the ankle (Fig. 1-4). If greater rigidity is needed, special graphite component pieces or composite pieces can be incorporated into the plastic for reinforcement. This is most frequently done at the ankle. Plastics for orthoses may be grouped into two major types, thermoplastics and thermosetting plastics.

Thermoplastics soften when heated and harden when cooled, so they can be molded and remolded by reheating. They can be divided into low-temperature and high-temperature types. Low-temperature thermoplastics require no more than 80°C (180°F) to become workable; thus they may be shaped directly on the body. They cannot be used effectively where high stress occurs, so they are largely used in temporary assistive or protective orthoses, mainly in the upper limbs. In contrast to low-temperature, the high-temperature thermoplastics must be shaped over a cast or model. They are much more resistant to creep, that is, changing shape with continued stress and heat. Almost all custom orthoses today are formed on models using high temperatures, and most "off the shelf" or stock plastic items are of this type.

The high-temperature thermoplastic mostly used in orthotics is an olefin plastic, polypropylene. It is applied in thicknesses of 3, 4.5, and 6 mm, depending on the stiffness required. Less rigid, but more durable is a copolymer plastic (Copoly), which is a mixture of polypropylene and polyethylene. Ionomer plastics (Surlyn and Thermavac) are transparent and in thin sheets even less rigid than the preceding types.[8] Less commonly used are acrylic plastics, mostly polymerized from methyl methacrylate monomers. They have high transparency, which makes them cosmetically attractive, and they provide good resistance to breakage.

Polyvinyl chloride (PVC) and related compounds are lighter and are available in both low-temperature and high-temperature thermoplastic forms. These com-

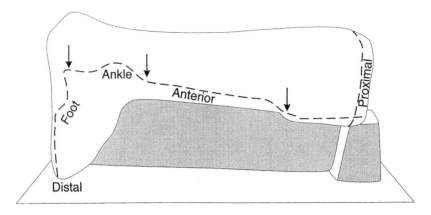

Fig. 1-4.   Thermoplastic shaped over a plaster mold showing trim lines for a plastic AFO. The dashed lines indicate where the plastic would be trimmed to create the AFO.

pounds range from very flexible to extremely rigid and are used in a wide range of applications—from making orthotic parts, coating metal orthoses or fabrics, to shoe manufacture, and providing fabric covering on wheelchairs.

Thermosetting plastics are made of liquid plastic resin such as polyester or epoxy, which sets at room temperature. They are poured over a fabric, usually nylon or fiberglass, and laminated over a model. Thermosetting plastics are very rigid and strong when set, but unlike thermoplastics, they cannot be remolded after reheating. Because thermosetting plastics are difficult to use and are somewhat more expensive, they have been replaced in most custom-molded applications by high-temperature thermoplastics. Thermosetting plastics using fiberglass fabric have strength in ratios comparable to steel. When great strength and impact resistance are required, thermosetting plastics are ideal. They are widely used in prosthetics.

Fabrics and Leather

Fabrics and leather are widely used in orthotics for fastening or for less rigid supports such as corsets, belts, and stockings. Fabrics along with plastic foam materials are widely used for padding. When a fabric must be fitted to a compliant shape, knitted forms are preferred. Hook and loop (Velcro) closures have replaced many of the buckles and multiple straps used in the past. Neoprene suspension, using a thin sheet of synthetic rubber, is now more widely used than the elasticized fabrics of the past.

INDICATIONS FOR ORTHOSES AND REHABILITATION TECHNOLOGY

Medical students and those in the health professions are familiar with the concept of learning to diagnose a disease by understanding its anatomic effects and functional manifestations. Therapeutic strategy then mainly consists of naming the disorder, followed by proposing the surgery, drugs, or physical treatment applied to control or eliminate the disordered state. Because health insurance carriers demand that a condition be named before a payment will be rendered, this text will follow the common approach to diagnosis and treatment. The name of the condition and the functional deficits it causes will be given, followed by the rehabilitative technology generally used.

In Table 1-1 a diagnosis and a generally used International Classification of Disease (ICD9) code number are given for each condition that might need physical rehabilitation. A list of appropriate orthoses and aids follows. Table 1-1 provides only an introductory outline of some clinical indications. Details of the physical effects and

Table 1-1. Diagnostic Categories for Orthoses and Devices

ICD.9.CM	Diagnosis	Orthosis or Aid
897.	Amputation, lower limb	Manual (especially weighted or designed) or electric W/C or scooter
887.	Amputation, upper limb	One-handed ADL aids for unilaterals or ADL aids for bilaterals not fitted with prostheses
724.	Back pain	LSO or TLSO; orthoses, special shoes and foot orthoses
353.	Brachial plexus injury	Shoulder orthoses; hand orthoses with dynamic features
94.9	Burns (various)	Various orthoses for positioning upper and lower extremities to prevent contractures; elastic customized garments
429.8 414.	Cardiac disorders	Lightweight manual or electric W/C and scooters
	Cerebral palsy	
343.9	1. Spastic	Special shoes, AFOs/KAFOs; W/C with adapted seating manual or electric, ADL equipment
333.7	2. Athetoid	Special shoes: special W/C; environmental control devices
436	Cerebrovascular disease	
342.9	1. Hemiplegic	Orthoses for upper limbs to support shoulder or spastic hand and wrist Orthoses for lower limbs—AFO, KAFO; W/C with one-arm drive or lower seat or specially equipped with lap boards, etc; one-handed aids for ADL
	2. Quadriplegia	Special manual or electric W/C, e.g., those with reclining back or custom seating; ADL aids; environmental control devices
	3. Ataxic or other types	Special W/C: ADL aids, weighted AFOs, environmental control devices
754. 755.	Congenital deformities	Various—depends on area affected
754.	Foot and ankle deformities	AFOs; foot orthoses: special shoes
829.	Limb fractures	Various—depends on area but primarily supportive or passive
340.	Multiple sclerosis	
	1. Ataxic type	Weighted walkers, ADL equipment
	2. Spastic	AFOs, KAFOs; special shoes; manual or electric W/Cs
359.	Muscular dystrophies (progressive)	Positioning devices and orthoses to prevent contractures; dynamic upper limb orthoses; manual or electric W/Cs; special seating, scooters
335.	Motor neuron diseases	AFOs, neck and trunk supports, special W/Cs, ADL aids and ADL equipment, electric W/Cs, environmental control devices, dynamic upper limb orthoses
723.	Neck pain	Cervical orthoses
119.	Neoplasm, malignant	Various types for spinal regions depending on cancer site, e.g., TLSOs, LSOs; for lower limb, KAFOs, AFOs; W/Cs; edema control garments for lymphedema
	Neuropathic disorders	
356. 357	1. General or polyneuropathies	WHOs, AFOs, KAFOs, special shoes, W/C, either manual or electric depending on loss
356.	2. Specific nerve loss	Local dynamic or static orthoses depending on diagnosis, e.g. WHO for carpal tunnel syndrome, dynamic WHO for radial nerve palsy, AFO for peroneal nerve palsy
733.	Osteoporosis	Various TLSOs and LSOs
715.9	Osteoarthritis	KOs; KAFOs, AFOs to reduce weight bearing or modify knee function; W/C scooter; shoe modification and foot orthoses

Continues

Table 1-1 *(Continued)*

ICD.9.CM	Diagnosis	Orthosis or Aid
332	Parkinson's disease	Orthoses for positioning to prevent contractures; manual W/Cs scooter
443.	Peripheral vascular disease	Special shoes and foot orthoses; AFOs; various supports for venous stasis
138.	Poliomyelitis (sequelae)	TLSO's, KAFO's, KOs, special shoes or foot orthoses, ADL aids, manual or electric W/C, scooters
492.	Pulmonary disorders	Lightweight manual or electric W/Cs, scooters
716.	Rheumatoid arthritis	WHOs, finger orthoses, foot orthoses and/or special custom shoes, KOs, AFOs, lightweight W/Cs, scooter
726.	Rotator cuff syndrome	Shoulder orthoses
737.	Scoliosis	Various CTLSOs, TLSOs
784.3 784.5	Speech and language disorders	Communication devices, computer-assisted speech, environmental control devices
741.9	Spinal bifida	Parapodium; AFOs, KAFOs, HKAFOs (reciprocating); spinal orthoses; W/Cs; special seating systems
344.1 336.9	Spinal cord injury or lesion	
344.	1. Quadriplegia	Supportive WHOs/dynamic WHOs, manual or electric special W/C and seating, environmental controls, ADL equipment
344.1	2. Spastic paraplegia	KAFOs, manual or electric W/Cs
344.1	3. Flaccid (various levels)	AFOs, KAFOs, manual W/Cs
737.	Spinal deformity	CTLSOs, TLSOs
726.	Tendonitis—tenosynovitis	Supportive WHOs or AFOs, special foot orthoses or shoes
800.	Traumatic head injury	
803.1	1. Early	Various static support devices for upper and lower limbs extremity, manual or electric W/C
854.	2. Later	KAFOs, AFOs, ADL aids, environmental controls, special seating, and communication devices depending on loss of function

For key to abbreviations, see p. 1.

functional purposes of the equipment are given in the chapters that follow.

ACKNOWLEDGMENT

I would like to thank Debra Mowry, D.O., who contributed significantly to this chapter, especially in relation to Table 1-1.

REFERENCES

1. Kirchner C: People with disabilities: a population in flux. p. 25 In Smith RV, Leslie JH (eds): Rehabilitation Engineering. CRC Press, Boca Raton, FL, 1990
2. Enders A, Hall M: Assistive Technology Source Book. Resna-Press, Washington, 1990
3. Bowker P: The biomechanics of orthoses. p. 27. In Bowker P, Condie DN, Bader DL, Pratt KJ (eds): Biomechanical Basis of Orthotic Management. Butterworth-Heinemann, Oxford, England, 1993
4. Lehmann JF: Lower limb orthotics. p. 331. In Redford JB (ed): Orthotics Etcetera. 3rd Ed. Williams & Wilkins, Baltimore, 1986
5. Lehmann JF: Biomechanics of ankle foot orthoses: prescription and design. Arch Phys Med Rehabil 60:200, 1979
6. Houghton GR, McInerney A, Tew A: Brace compliance in adolescent idiopathic scoliosis. J Bone Joint Surg Br 69:852, 1982
7. Pritham C: Analysis of the results from the questionnaire on metal vs. plastic orthoses. Clin Prosthet. Orthot 7:4, 1983
8. Good DC, Supan TJ: Basic principles of orthotics in neurologic disorders. p. 8. In Aisen ML (ed): Orthotics in Neurologic Rehabilitation. Demos, 1992

Lower Limb Orthoses

2

Paul Trautman

Lower limb orthoses (LLOs) are the most commonly used and prescribed orthoses in clinical practice. Most clinicians, trained to first consider a diagnosis and only then think in terms of a functional impairment, often do not know where to start in prescribing LLOs. The purpose of this chapter is to help someone familiar with a patient's diagnosis to better understand which LLO might be appropriate for that patient. Starting with a known diagnosis, such as those mentioned, and using the references mentioned in Appendix 2-1, the reader is guided to an appropriate orthosis and some of its possible modifications. This is a simplified and incomplete review, making it necessary to consult an orthotist who can explain the mechanical functions of each orthotic component and justify its efficacy for clinical purposes. Furthermore, textbooks on rehabilitation may need to be consulted for more complete descriptions of the functional disabilities listed in Appendices 2-1 to 2-4.

Knowing the patient's abilities, functions, and limitations is a critical part of selecting and/or designing an appropriate orthosis for a patient. To paraphrase: It is the patient's abilities that count, not the diagnosis, in determining which orthosis should be most appropriate for a patient. The orthosis of choice is one that effectively substitutes for lost muscles, or lost nervous control of muscles, and any resulting functional deficiency. At the same time, the orthosis should minimize any hindrance to useful remaining function. Because a particular diagnosis does not always manifest itself in the same manner and functional deficits differ, it is important that the choice of an orthosis be based on a thorough evaluation of the specific needs of the patient, as well as the implications of the diagnosis.

An important part of the orthotist's contribution to the patient's care is to identify the most effective orthosis for a patient given applicable parameters: age, sex, height and weight, muscle strength, and range of motion of joints. Level of activity, life expectancy, social setting, psychological readiness, as well as funding source must all be considered. The main consideration however, should be the goal for wearing the orthosis. The goal of a LLO is to achieve one or more of the following:

1. Relieve pain by reducing forces around joints
2. Assist locomotion
3. Maintain correction of a deformity or joint replacement after surgery
4. Influence muscle tone

It is important that an orthosis does not result in over bracing, it should not hinder remaining function any more than necessary as it compensates for a deficiency.

LLOs are effective because they apply forces that affect the manner in which the limb, bones, muscles, soft tissue, and nerves function. There is no direct correlation between a medical diagnosis and a specific orthosis, although at one time, terminology such as "polio brace" existed. Difficulties arose when the term described different braces in various parts of the country and when the brace was used for patients who did not have polio. The current system of naming orthoses by the body parts that the orthosis spans is presented in the *Atlas of Orthotics: Biomechanical Principles and Application.*[1] For example, the "short leg brace" is now called an ankle foot orthosis (AFO). Note that an AFO is any orthosis that covers the foot, spans the ankle joint, and covers the lower leg. The term does not only refer to plastic orthoses, although in common usage, an AFO is often equated with a plastic brace for the ankle.

Orthoses are mechanical devices that apply forces to the lower limb in accordance with the laws of physics. A three-point pressure system is defined as two forces applied to a body part opposed by a third force applied between the first two.[2] At least one three-point force system is required to stabilize a joint, although in the majority of orthoses, multiple three-point force systems work in combination to provide stability of one or more joints, in one or more planes, throughout the gait cycle. The forces exerted by the orthosis must be distributed in such a way that the patient can tolerate the pressure. A primary principle of orthotics is to manufacture an orthosis of carefully molded and contoured components to minimize pressures per square inch at points where the orthosis interfaces with the patient's limb.

SHOES

The shoe is an essential component of the LLO. Most metal orthoses are permanently mounted on the shoe, whereas most plastic orthoses are not physically attached to the shoe. In either case, the shoe remains a significant component of the orthotic system. Although it is true that it is easier to change shoes when one uses a plastic orthosis, it most certainly is a mistake and a disservice to patients to tell them that they can wear any shoe with the orthosis. Everyone has personal knowledge, experience, and ideas about shoes, which they bring with them when they first begin to deal with LLOs, but the orthotist must guide their choices.

For a person who must use an orthosis, shoes are not simply part of one's apparel. Even though an orthosis may be prescribed for only one limb, both shoes will have an effect on how well a patient walks. In some instances, an elevation on the contralateral shoe is required to accommodate a leg-length discrepancy.

Shoes used with an orthosis need special features that can significantly increase or decrease the ability of any orthosis to assist the patient:

1. Firmness of heel counter
2. Closure mechanism, that is, laces, or lack thereof, as in loafers
3. Heel height
4. Last or shape of the shoe
5. Flexibility of the sole
6. Size
7. Adequate room in the toe box

As long as these seven characteristics do not change—at least with plastic orthoses—the patient can use any shoe without altering the effectiveness of the orthosis.

If a patient must use the orthosis every day, 365 days a year, it is important to have more than one pair of shoes to wear so the shoes can have an opportunity to dry and air out—to say nothing about the mental health of the patient who must wear the same pair of shoes every single day until the orthosis totally fails. It is also important to note that different shoes, even though they are similar, do rub slightly differently; pressures and forces differ between shoes, and thus, alternating the wear of different shoes can aid in avoiding possible skin problems such as calluses or even skin breakdown.

The average life expectancy of quality leather shoes for a person wearing a metal orthosis is between 6 months and 1 year. This depends on the person's size, activity level, and the way the shoes are maintained. Usually after 6 to 12 months the shoe has molded to the deformities in the foot and all corrective forces are lost. This is easy to see by just looking at a pair of worn shoes in their present condition and comparing, in one's mind, what they looked like when they were new.

Condie explained the importance of adequate shoes for an orthosis this way: The footwear that is worn with an AFO is an essential and integral part of the orthotic fitting; "the upper of the footwear provides the counter pressure on the dorsum of the foot which is an essential component of the three-point force system required to resist inappropriate ankle plantar flexion."[3]

GAIT ANALYSIS

The functions of locomotion are as follows:

1. Generate a propulsion force
2. Maintain upright stability
3. Absorb the shock of the body's weight hitting the floor at each heel strike
4. Keep the amount of energy required to walk at a minimum

Before we can begin to recognize gait deficiencies, we must first be familiar with normal gait: the repetitive sequence of reciprocal motion of the legs, arms, and trunk, which advances the body while maintaining stance stability. Perry describes the basic approaches to viewing the different aspects of the gait cycle and the various body motions that occur during a single stride. The normal gait cycle has two parts: a stance phase, which begins when a heel first makes contact with the ground and continues until the toe of that foot leaves the ground to start the swing phase.[4]

A gait cycle is equivalent to a stride; it consists of the events occurring from the time the heel of one foot contacts the ground until the same heel contacts the ground the second time. This differs from a step, which is the sequence of events involved from the time the right heel contacts the ground until the left heel makes contact.

The eight different subphases of the gait cycle are often described by the percentage of time they occur during a single stride. The stance phase of the gait cycle constitutes 60 percent of the cycle; the swing phase, 40 percent. Thus, there is a period when both legs are in contact with the ground simultaneously, 20 percent of the time. This is called double stance.

The subphases of the stance phase of gait are as follows:

1. Heel strike or initial contact
2. Loading response or foot flat
3. Midstance
4. Terminal stance or heel off
5. Preswing

The subphases of swing phase are as follows:

6. Initial swing
7. Midswing
8. Terminal swing

Figure 2-1 shows the sequences of the gait cycle with the various named phases.

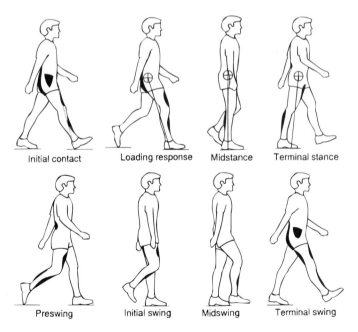

Fig. 2-1. Normal gait cycle. Muscle groups active at each stage are shown in black.

Appendix 2-2 shows the position of the joints and the action of various muscles throughout the gait cycle. For a complete discussion of gait, see Perry.[4]

The smooth, energy-efficient process of walking is determined by the laws of physics, as described by Newton, and three physical factors: skeletal design, connective tissue, and muscular functions. This chapter considers only those aspects of the skeleton (16 bones and 5 toes), connective tissue (11 articulations), and neurologic and muscular systems (57 muscles) that are relevant to the pathomechanics of gait deviations and how orthoses may be used to decrease the effects of the pathologic losses the patient has suffered.

There is no International Classification of Disease (ICD) code for every functional deviation, and a global ICD code must be used to identify a patient's deformity. In these cases, it is impossible to support the use of any type orthosis without having a descriptive, functional assessment, as well as a diagnosis. Weber has identified functional gait deviations, commonly seen in a variety of medical conditions.[2]

Ankle/foot
  Low heel strike
  Flat foot contact
  Forefoot contact (toe strike)
  Excessive plantar flexion
  Premature heel rise
  Excessive dorsiflexion
  Lack of heel rise
  Varus (inversion)
  Valgus (eversion)
  Toe drag
Knee
  Inadequate extension
  Flexion limited, absent or excessive
  Hyperextension
  Varus
  Valgus
Hip
  Inadequate flexion
  Inadequate extension
  Adduction or abduction
  External rotation
Pelvis
  Anterior tilt (symphysis down)
  Posterior tilt (symphysis up)
  Contralateral drop

  Ipsilateral drop
  Hike (ipsilateral elevation)
Trunk
  Forward lean
  Backward lean
  Rotation
  Lateral lean

Other considerations in evaluating posture and gait are:

Reflexes
  Asymmetric tonic neck reflex
  Tonic labyrinthine reflex
  Symmetric tonic neck reflex
Muscle tone classifications
  Mild, moderate, severe
  Isotonic, normal
  Hypotonic, decreased tone
  Hypertonic, increased tone
  Variable, inconsistent, or changing tone

A common type of gait not described in the above list is antalgic gait, which is that induced by a painful extremity. It is characterized by a stance time on the affected side that is shorter than that on the normal side and thus results in unequal step lengths.

In this chapter, consideration of neurologic deficits is limited to the resulting loss of control of the muscles that manipulate the skeletal system. Sensory losses may also alter gait and should be of concern when using orthoses, because sensation provides the patient's first line of defense in recognizing potential sites of excessive pressure caused by an orthosis. When lack of awareness occurs, lost sensation can lead to skin breakdown and subsequent complications.

ICD CODES AND L CODES

More than 100 diagnoses are identified in alphabetical order in Appendix 2-3 and numerical order Appendix 2-4. Seventeen lower limb orthoses and components are described and discussed. The terminology used for the orthoses is that adopted by the Committee on Prosthetics and Orthotics of the American Academy of Orthopedic Surgeons. Each orthosis is named for the joint or joints that it spans, using the first letter in capitals for the English word.

The following orthoses are discussed and illustrated in Figures 2-2 to 2-19.

Foot orthosis (FO)
AFO
    Plastic
    Metal
Knee orthosis (DO)
Knee AFO
    Metal
    Plastic
    Combination metal and plastic
    For all KAFOs
HO

HOW TO USE THIS CHAPTER

Appendix 2-3 lists diagnoses of functional deficits or of diseases that result in functional deficits. The debilitating effects caused by these deficits can sometimes be lessened by orthoses.

To use this chapter as a reference, begin by looking up the diagnosis in either the alphabetical listing of diagnoses, Appendix 2-3, or by the diagnosis ICD Code in Appendix 2-4.[5] Then proceed to Appendix 2-1, which will refer you to several orthoses that may be appropriate for the patient. The detailed information about each orthotic system in the last section of the chapter will help the reader determine an appropriate orthosis. It is important to remember that not all functional deficits have a descriptive diagnosis and not all conditions that can benefit from an orthosis are identified by an ICD Code. In patient evaluation, it is more important to understand the functional deficit than the diagnosis when selecting an orthosis.

L codes originated in 1983 when the Health Care Financing Administration (HCFA), with the cooperation of the American Orthotic and Prosthetic Association developed HCPCS, a Common Procedure Coding System. This was the beginning of a national coding system, which is required when reporting services provided to Medicare and Medicaid beneficiaries.[6] Each base orthosis has an identifying L code, and each base procedure is modified so it reflects the service provided to the patient.[7]

An addition (designated as ADD) to a basic L-code procedure is a substantive modification to the basic orthotic service that materially affects the manner in which the orthosis functions. The use of ADD represents a significantly increased professional or material input by the orthotist and thus merits its own L code.

In addition to the L code, common ADD on items to various orthoses such as dual-action ankle joints, T straps, femoral condyle pads, knee cap straps, and knee joint locks must be identified. The use of each additional modifier, like the orthosis itself, should be identified with a specific patient need. Not all of the orthoses or the modifications identified in Appendix 2-1 are illustrated or discussed in detail in this chapter.

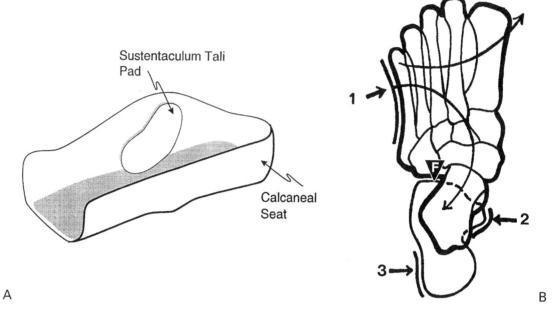

Fig. 2-2. **(A)** Three-quarter view of a left UCBL-ST foot orthosis with sustentaculum tali pad. **(B)** Arrows indicate force system in the transverse plane to control forefoot abduction.

Name/Description

The UCBL-ST (University of California Berkeley Laboratory FO) with sustentaculum tali support (Fig. 2-2)

L Code

L3000

Function

To position the entire foot into as neutral a position as possible and thereby maintain a more functional and comfortable foot

While controlling the motion of the subtalar joint, affects rotational forces applied to the entire leg during stance phase

Force Systems

The first force system affects the transverse plane in stance phase: it limits forefoot abduction.

1. A medially directed force on the shaft of the fifth metatarsal
2. A laterosuperiorly directed force at the sustentaculum tali[8]
3. A medially directed force along the lateral side of the calcaneus

The second force system affects the coronal plane and controls calcaneovalgus, midfoot collapsing, and pronation.

1. A medially directed force at the lateral base of the calcaneus
2. A laterosuperiorly directed force at the sustentaculum tali.[8]
3. The body's center of gravity: a laterally directed force

Common ICD Codes

343	Cerebral palsy
45.1	Poliomyelitis, acute
714	Rheumatoid arthritis
138	Poliomyelitis, late effects
357	Guillain-Barré syndrome
716.7	Foot and ankle disorders: forefoot adduction, pronation
716.7	Foot and ankle disorders: forefoot abduction, supination
736.79	Pronation or supination
734	Pes planus
736.76	Calcaneovarus
736.76	Calcaneovalgus

Comments

A UCBL-ST-style footplate design may be molded into any custom-molded plastic AFO.

It is most common to have the orthosis span the joint or joints it is affecting. In some orthoses, however, one of the primary forces is applied superiorly to the orthosis. The person's center of gravity (CG) becomes the third point of a three-point force system. The velocity and direction of the CG can have a significant effect on the orthotic system and how it affects gait.

Because the CG is so high in the body, relative to the lower limbs, it has a significant mechanical advantage in relationship to the other two parts of the force system in providing control of the lower limb. The effects of the CG, and the mechanical advantage it has in an orthotic system, is most graphically seen in the second force sys-

tem of the UCBL-ST FO, shown in Figure 2-3 and described by Inman.[9] The importance of well-molded and -contoured components in an orthosis, to minimize pressures per square inch at points where the orthosis interfaces with the patient's limb, cannot be overemphasized.

The UCBL, as originally presented by Inman, has obtained poor clinical results and has often ended up duplicating the foot deformity rather than providing correction or skeletal realignment. As a result, it is not prescribed as often as it once was. Carlson and Nielsen's work has shown that modifications to the original UCBL design have increased its effectiveness. To distinguish between the designs, it has been suggested that the latter design, shown in Figure 2-2, be referred to as a rotational foot control orthosis rather than a UCBL.[8]

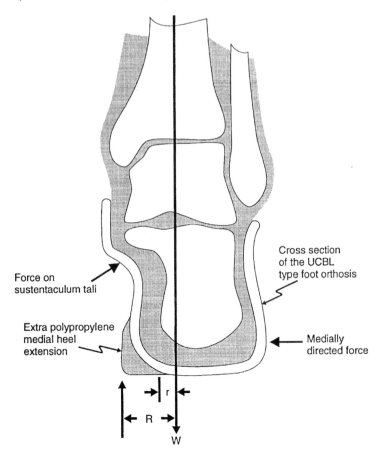

Fig. 2-3. Coronal section through ankle and a UCBL orthosis. Arrows on medial and lateral side indicate primary location of forces produced by orthosis for control in the coronal plane. Correcting movement *WR* created by sustentaculum tali support and medial heel extension is greater than moment *WR* as featured in standard foot orthosis.[10]

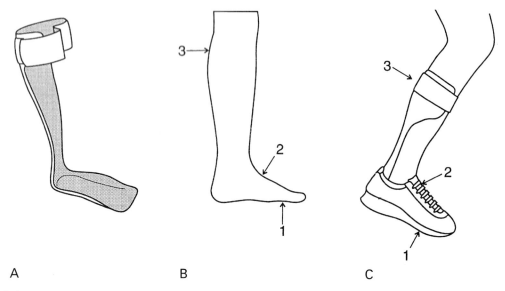

Fig. 2-4.   Posterior leaf spring design AFO. Forces applied to the leg by the brace are indicated by the arrows.

Name/Description
AFOvposterior leaf spring design (Fig. 2-4)

L Code
L1930

Function
Limits foot drop in swing phase of gait, preventing toe drag

Force System
There is one three-point force system in swing phase:

1. A superiorly directed force on the sole of the foot.
2. A posteriorly directed force on the dorsum of the foot. The closure mechanism of the shoe is laces or hook and pile strap.
3. An anteriorly directed force on the back of the calf.

Common ICD Codes
436	Stroke, CVA
736.72	Pes equinus
342	Hemiplegia and hemiparesis
342.00	Flaccid hemiplegia
331.89	CVD, ataxia
357.0	Guillain-Barré syndrome
138	Polio, late effects

Comments
There are two methods of dispensing this type of AFO. The first method, called *custom fitted,* involves taking a prefabricated AFO out of stock and adjusting it to fit the patient. It can be done rapidly, less expensively than a custom-molded AFO, and it is a good way for evaluating the design and applicability of an AFO for a patient. The second is custom molded and results in a better fitting, more functional orthosis that is more likely to meet the patient's needs for a longer period of time.

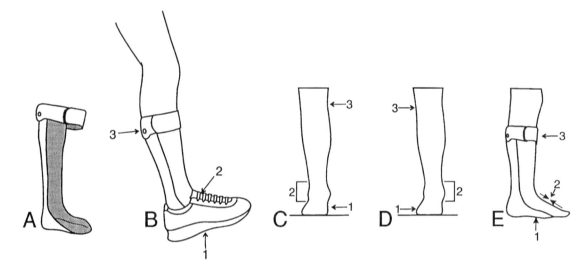

Fig. 2-5.   Solid ankle design AFO. **(A)** Oblique view; **(B)** theoretic force system during swing (system 1); **(C)** varus control (system 2); **(D)** valgus control (system 3); **(E)** dorsiflexion control (system 4). Note compression force.

Name/Description
Plastic AFOvsolid ankle design (Fig. 2-5)

L Code
L1960

Function
Limits foot drop

Controls inversion or eversion of foot, as well as dorsiflexion of the ankle joint in stance phase

Force Systems
There are four force systems:

The first force system controls plantar flexion. See L1930, Posterior Leaf Spring AFO for description.

The second force system controls varus/inversion.

1. A laterally directed force on the medial side of the foot
2. A medially directed force on the distal fibula and calcaneous (bridging lateral malleolus)
3. A laterally directed force on the medial, proximal tibia

The third force system controls valgus/eversion.

1. A medially directed force on the lateral side of the foot
2. A laterally directed force on the distal-medial tibia and calcaneous (bridging the medial malleolus)
3. A medially directed force on the lateral side of the lateral side of the proximal fibula, distal to the peroneal nerve

The fourth force system controls dorsiflexion in stance phase.

1. An upwardly directed force on the sole of the foot during and after midstance
2. A compression force in the plastic at the ankle joint from midstance to toe-off
3. A posteriorly directed force on the proximal tibia

Common ICD Codes
436	Stroke, CVA
342.9	Hemiplegia and hemiparesis
333.7	Cerebral palsy, athetoid and dystonic
343.0	Cerebral palsy, diplegic
343.9	Cerebral palsy, spastic mild to moderate
344.0	Quadriplegia, quadriparesis
340	Multiple sclerosis
355.356	Peripheral neuropathic disorders
138	Polio, late effects
357	Guillain-Barré syndrome
359.1	Muscular dystrophy

736.72	Pes equinus
736.71	Equinovarus
736.72	Equinovalgus
714	Rheumatoid arthritis
718.47	Ankle joint contracture
727.81	Short Achilles tendon
741.9	Spina bifida: L1 to L4 level
845.09	Achilles tendon torn or surgically repaired

Comments

The effectiveness of these force systems depends on a number of variables including the type and thickness of the plastic and the trim lines, that is, how far the plastic is trimmed away from the anterior portion in relation to the ankle position.

This orthosis can be custom fitted or custom fabri-cated, but the former is seldom effective. The inability to control the shape, type, and thickness of the plastic in a custom-fitted AFO makes it less suitable to meet a patient's needs than a custom-fabricated one.

Rheumatoid arthritic involvement at the ankle and subtalar joints can lead to decreased walking velocity and single limb support time. Application of rigid orthoses for these cases has been shown to reduce pain and allow greater walking velocity and a more normal single limb support time.[10] Also, the use of a custom-fabricated orthosis might be helpful in an evaluation process if surgical correction is being considered.

"Taking into consideration bilateral knee and ankle motion for 19 patients with ankle arthrodesis, the ideal position for fusion of the ankle was found to be neutral flexion, that is, 0 to 5 degrees valgus angulation of the hindfoot, and 5 to 10 degrees of external rotation."[11]

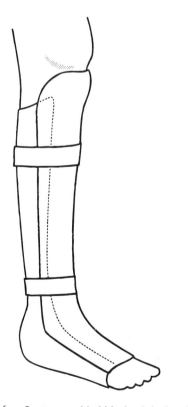

Fig. 2-6.   Custom-molded bivalved design AFO.

Name/Description
Custom-molded bivalved AFO (Fig. 2-6)

L Code
L1960

Function
Provides total contact support of the foot and ankle joint, which can stabilize a fracture.

Immobilizes the joint and aid in healing some wounds through compression

Force Systems
The force systems are essentially the same as those described for the solid ankle AFO. The effectiveness of the force systems depends on the rigidity of the plastic, which is determined by a number of variables including the trim lines, type and thickness of plastic. The value of a total-contact AFO is to distribute pressure equally over the entire surface of the foot, ankle, and lower leg, thus avoiding concentrated areas of pressure.

The first force system controls plantar flexion. See L1930, posterior leaf spring AFO for a description.

The second force system controls varus/inversion. See L1960, solid ankle AFO for a description.

The third force system controls valgus/eversion. See L1960, solid ankle AFO for a description.

The fourth force system limits dorsiflexion. See L1960, solid ankle AFO for a description.

Possible Additional L Codes
L2341	anterior shell
L2820	soft interface—below knee

Common ICD Codes
250.8	Ulcers, diabetic mellitus, lower limb
454.0	Venous stasis ulcers
454.2	Venous stasis ulcers with inflammation
707.1	Ulcers, foot

733.8	Malunion/nonunion of fracture
733.82	Pseudoarthosis in lower leg
713.16	Osteomyelitis tibia/fibula
823.2	Fracture tibia and fibula

Comments
Crepe soles can be added directly to the sole of the AFO to avoid the necessity of obtaining a shoe large enough to fit over this type of AFO. Total-contact AFOs have been used with diabetic patients to aid wound healing. They may be extended proximally with a patelar tendon-bearing modification and thus reduce weight bearing through the tibia, ankle, and foot.

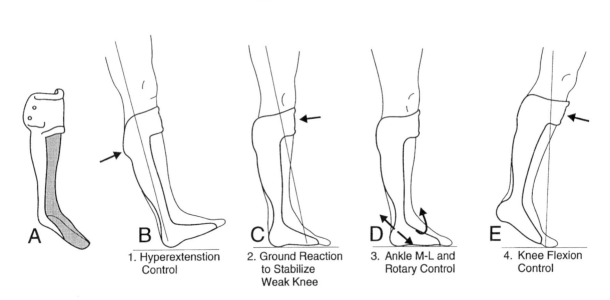

1. Hyperextenstion Control

2. Ground Reaction to Stabilize Weak Knee

3. Ankle M-L and Rotary Control

4. Knee Flexion Control

Fig. 2-7. **(A–E)** Floor reaction design AFO. Arrows indicate primary control force during different phases of the gait cycle. ML,

Name/Description
Custom-molded plastic ground reaction AFO (Fig. 2-7)

L Code
L1945

Function
Often used to create an extension moment at the knee joint by locking the ankle joint in plantar flexion
Other functions similar to that of the solid ankle AFO

Force Systems
The first force system controls plantar flexion. See L1930, leaf spring AFO for a description.
The second force system controls inversion. See L1960, solid ankle AFO for a description.
The third force system controls eversion. See L1960, solid ankle AFO for a description.
The fourth force system controls dorsiflexion.

1. A posteriorly directed force on the proximal tibia or preferably on the patellar tendon

2. A compression force in the plastic at the ankle joint from midstance to toe-off.
3. An upwardly directed force on the sole of the foot during and after midstance.

Possible Additional L Codes
L2220   Dorsiflexion–plantar flexion assist/resist ankle joint, times two (one medial, one lateral)

L2820   Soft interface—below knee

Common ICD Codes
436   Stroke, CVA
438   Hemiplegia, late effects
342   Hemiplegia and hemiparesis
342.00   Flaccid hemiplegia
736.72   Pes equinus
736.71   Equino varus

333.7   Cerebral palsy, athetoid/dystonic
736.72   Equino valgus
343.9   Cerebral palsy, spastic: mild to moderate
437.8   Cerebral palsy, diplegic
340.0   Multiple sclerosis
736.5   Genu recurvatum
344.0   Quadriplegia and quadreparesis
138   Polio
357   Guillain-Barré syndrome
854.6   Head trauma
718.46   Knee contracture
718.47   Ankle contracture

Comments
To maximize function, it is often advisable to use dual adjustable ankle joints to achieve the most advantageous angle of the ankle joint.

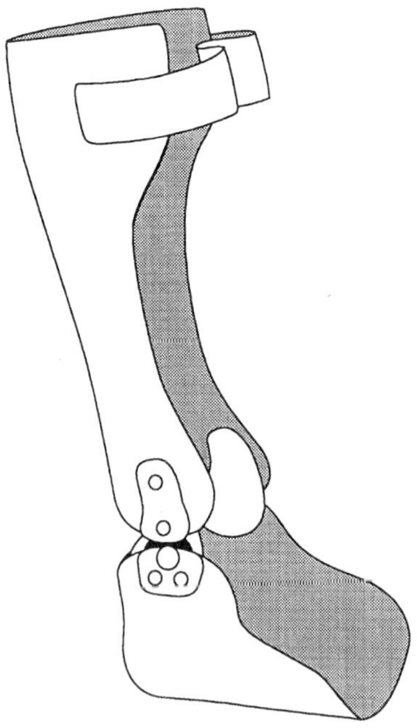

Fig. 2-8.   Plastic AFO with ankle joints.

Name/Description
Plastic AFO with ankle joints (Fig. 2-8)

L Code
L1970

Function
Depends on the type of ankle joint and how it is set; most often used with a plantar flexion stop

Force Systems
The first force system controls plantar flexion. See L1930, Apring leaf AFO for a description.

The second force system controls inversion/varus. See L1960, solid ankle AFO for a description.

The third force system controls eversion/valgus. See L1960, solid ankle AFO for a description.

The fourth force system limits dorsiflexion if a dorsiflexion stop is in place. See L1960, solid ankle AFO for a description

Common ICD Codes
436   Stroke, CVA
342.00   Flaccid hemiplegia and hemiparesis
342   Hemiplegia and hemiparesis

331.89	Cerebral vascular disease, ataxia
333.7	Cerebral palsy, athetoid and dystonic
343.0	Cerebral palsy, paraplegic, diplegic
343.9	Cerebral palsy, spastic: mild to moderate
344.0	Quadriplegia, quadriparesis
344.1	Paraplegia
344.3	Monoplegia, paralysis, lower extremity
340	Multiple sclerosis
355.356	Peripheral neuropathic disorders
359.1	Muscular dystrophy, Duchenne's, Becker's
138	Polio, late effects
357	Gullain-Barré syndrome
359.1	Muscular dystrophy
437.8	CVD—quadriplegia
438	Hemiplegia, late effect
736.72	Pes equinus
736.71	Equinovarus
736.72	Equinovalgus
736.5	Genu recurvatum
718.47	Ankle joint contracture
727.81	Short achilles tendon
741.9	Spina bifida: L1 to L4 level
782	Paresthesia, lower limb, Berger's
845.09	Achilles tendon, torn or surgically repaired

Comments

Numerous ankle joints may be used, each with its own advantages. Selection of the specific ankle joint is determined by the functions it will be required to perform, taking into account the patient's size, activity level, and personal preference. See Figure 2-9 for further details on types of ankle joints.

Articulated AFOs can be used when the patient has passive range of motion of at least 5 degrees of dorsiflexion (preferably, 10 degrees without compromising the neutral position of the subtalar and midtarsal joints). Plantar flexion is used to control genu recurvatum and encourage progression of the lower extremity over the foot. Allows stretch of the calf muscles during stance.[2] The forward movement of the tibia, in relationship to the foot, creates a stretching force on the Achilles tendon.

The effectiveness of the force systems depends on the rigidity of the plastic, which is affected by a number of variables including the trim lines, type and thickness of plastic, and type of ankle joint used.

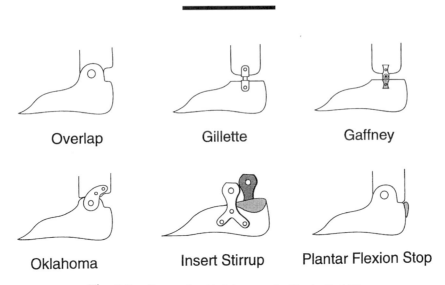

Overlap Gillette Gaffney

Oklahoma Insert Stirrup Plantar Flexion Stop

Fig. 2-9. Types of ankle joints used with plastic AFOs.

Name/Description

Overlap, Gillette, Gaffney, Oklahoma, variable motion/dual action metal stirrup, plantar flexion stop (Fig. 2-9)

Not illustrated: Scott, Select, Appalachian, Wafer

L Code

L1970

Functions

To approximate the axis of rotation of the patient's anatomical ankle joint and to provide control of the range of motion of the ankle joint

By controlling the range of motion, provides control of a variety of gait deviations ranging from foot drop in swing phase to knee instability in stance phase

Scott, Gafney, Oklahoma, and Gillette ankle joints are free motion joints that are used in custom-molded plastic orthoses. By themselves, they do not limit the range of motion of the ankle but are used in conjunction with a number of mechanisms that do limit the range of motion to obtain desired results.

Because of their rigidity in the coronal plane, the Scott, Gaffney, and Oklahoma ankle joints may be used to control calcaneal valgus or varus.

Comments

Plantar flexion assist/dorsiflexion assist joints (also called dual-action joints) are the best when the exact angle of the ankle joint is critical in obtaining the type of gait pattern desired because they are the easiest to adjust and are the most versatile. They also are very adaptable to alterations, making it easy to change the orthosis when the patient's condition changes. The additional bulk, weight, and cost of these orthoses are possible contraindications.

Any joint that limits dorsiflexion in stance will have a greater tendency for mechanical failure because of the great amount of stress placed on it at heel-off.

If the ankle joint is rigid, compensatory movement at other joints will occur; for example, subtalar joint pronation and midfoot may collapse into a rocker midfoot. Severe spasticity usually is a contraindication for articulated AFOs. A hinged AFO is contraindicated if the midfoot is unstable, contracted, and is not correctable.[2]

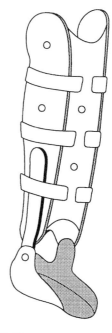

Fig. 2-10. Tibial fracture brace.

Name/Description

Tibial fracture brace (Fig. 2-10)

L Code

Only one of the following different ways of fabricating this orthosis can be used at one time:

L2102	Tibial fracture orthosis, plaster material
L2104	Tibial fracture orthosis, synthetic casting material
L2106	Tibial fracture orthosis, thermoplastic casting material
L2108	Tibial fracture orthosis, lightweight plastic, molded to patient model
L2112	Tibial fracture orthosis, soft custom fitted
L2114	Tibial fracture orthosis, semirigid, rigid, custom fitted

Function

To stabilize fracture of the tibia and/or fibula while allowing ambulation with articulation of the ankle and knee joints to minimize possible loss of range of motion and muscle atrophy following healing of the fracture

Force Systems

One force system applies force around the entire circumference of the leg, extending from the knee joint to the ankle joint. By containing and compressing the soft tissue, hydrostatic pressure is created, which provides stabilization of the fracture.

Common ICD Codes

823.0	Tibial fracture
823.2	Tibial and Fibula fracture

Comments

Because this orthosis is removable, patient compliance plays a significant role in successful outcome.

Indications for fracture bracing include the following:

Diaphyseal fractures of the tibia, fibula, and distal one-third of the femur

A subsiding of initial pain and swelling

Intact sensation

Adequate reduction with acceptable alignment and minimal shortening

The contraindications include the following:

Intra-articular fractures

Excessive pain or swelling

Failure to maintain alignment of fracture

Wound drainage (a rule of thumb is not more than can be absorbed by a single four-by-four bandage in 24 hours)

Spastic or insensate limbs or excessive shortening (more than $\frac{3}{8}$ inch)[12]

Name/Description

Single upright AFO—a single metal bar on either medial or lateral side of the leg with calf cuff, metal ankle joint, and shoe attachment (not illustrated)

L Code

L1980

Functions

To control foot drop and/or calcaneovalgus/varus

Force Systems

The force systems vary depending on the deformity that the orthosis is designed to control. The three most common force systems are as follows:

The first force system is in swing phase and controls foot drop:

1. A superiorly directed force on the sole of the foot by the sole of the shoe and stirrup
2. A posteriorly directed force on the dorsum of the foot by the closure mechanism of the shoe
3. An anteriorly directed force on the back of the calf by the calf band and cuff

The second force system is in stance phase to control calcaneovalgus and requires the upright to be lateral:

1. A medially directed force along the lateral side of the foot
2. A laterally directed force at the medial maleolus
3. A medially directed force at the lateral side of the calf cuff

The alternative second force system in stance phase controls calcaneovarus and requires the upright to be on the medial side of the leg:

1. A laterally directed force along the medial side of the foot
2. A medially directed force at the lateral maleolus
3. A laterally directed force at the medial side of the calf cuff

Possible Additional L Codes

L2200	Limits ankle joint range of motion
L2210	Dorsiflexion assist or resist plantarflexion
L2220	Dual-action resists both plantar and dorsiflexion
L2230	Split stirrup allows easy removal of upright from the shoe
L2250	Custom-molded footplate allows better control of the foot
L2270	Correction strap for calcaneal valgus or varus
L2360	An extended steel shank inserted into the inner sole of the shoe, increases the rigidity of the sole of the shoe
L2750	Chrome or nickel plating

L2770	Stainless steel bar		718.47	Ankle joint contracture
L2780	Noncorrosive finish to retard corrosion		727.81	Short achilles tendon
L3201 to L3250	Orthopedic shoes		741.9	Spina bifida: L1 to L4 level
			845.09	Achilles tendon, torn or surgically repaired

Common ICD Codes

436.0	Stroke, CVA
342.9	Hemiplegia and hemiparesis
333.7	Cerebral palsy, athetoid and dystonic
343.9	Cerebral palsy, spastic: mild to moderate
340	Multiple sclerosis
355.356	Peripheral neuropathic disorders
138	Polio, late effects
736.72	Pes equinus
736.71	Equinovarus
736.72	Equinovalgus
343.0	Cerebral palsy, diplegic
344.0	Quadriplegia, quadriparesis
357	Guillain-Barré syndrome
359.1	Muscular dystrophy
736.72	Equinovalgus
714	Rheumatoid arthritis

Comments

Patients do not accept cosmesis of this orthosis as well as they do plastic AFOs. When this orthosis is used with an L2230, a split stirrup, the patient can wear the shoe without the brace on some occasions. Edema and volume changes in the leg are indications for using this design rather than a plastic molded AFOs. Because of its flexibility, the single upright AFO is used mainly in children and light-weight, older adults.

The quality and condition of the shoe are of great significance. A supportive counter and stiff sole are required, and the condition of the shoe must be maintained if the orthosis is to be effective. This requires replacing the shoe and transferring the brace to a new shoe as often as every 6 months or at least annually if this is the only shoe the person wears every day.

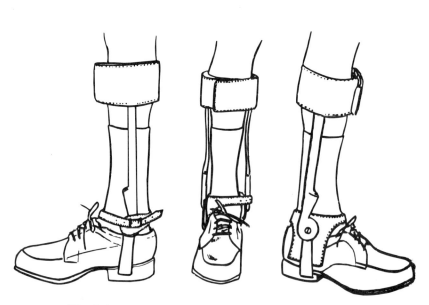

Fig. 2-11. Double metal upright AFO with lateral T strap.

Name/Description
Double metal upright AFO (Fig. 2-11)

L Code
L1990

Functions
The functions are the same as for a single upright AFO, L1980. The second upright makes it more rigid and gives it additional strength, which makes it more effective in applying forces to the foot and leg. Uprights are most commonly aluminum but may be steel for increased strength and durability. The determining factors in going from a single upright to dual upright, or from aluminum to steel include weight, height, excessive spasticity, or an abusive, rough working environment. The advantages of increased durability most often offset the increased weight compared to a single upright AFO. Leather valgus or varus control (T-straps) may be added to control calcaneovalgus/varus.

Force Systems
The first force system controls plantar flexion. See L1930, spring leaf AFO for a description.

The second force system controls inversion. See L1960, solid ankle AFO for a description.

The third force system controls eversion. See L1960, solid ankle AFO for a description.

The fourth force system is created when dorsiflexion in stance phase is inhibited by a stop and an extension moment is created at the knee joint. See L1945, floor reaction AFO for a description.

Possible Additional L Codes
See single upright AFO, L1980.

Common ICD Codes
436.0	Stroke, CVA
342.9	Hemiplegia and hemiparesis
333.7	Cerebral palsy, athetoid and dystonic
343.9	Cerebral palsy, spastic: mild to moderate
340	Multiple sclerosis
355.356	Peripheral neuropathic disorders
138	Polio, late effects
736.72	Pes Equinus
736.71	Equinovarus
736.72	Equinovalgus
343.0	Cerebral palsy, diplegic
344.0	Quadriplegia, quadriparesis
357	Guillain-Barré syndrome
359.1	Muscular dystrophy
736.72	Equinovalgus
714	Rheumatoid arthritis
718.47	Ankle joint contracture
727.81	Short Achilles tendon
741.9	Spina bifida: L1 to L4 level
845.09	Achilles tendon, torn or surgically repaired

Comments
The double metal upright AFO has mostly been replaced by the lightweight, custom-molded, plastic AFOs but is the orthosis of choice when the following conditions exist: (1) The volume of the leg varies greatly, usually as a result of edema. (2) The patient considers the plastic too hot to wear. (3) Loss of sensation with lack of ability to care for the skin of the leg and prevent possible skin breakdown.

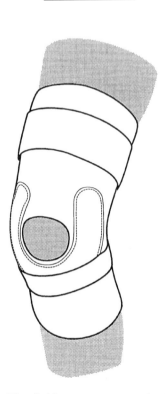

Fig. 2-12. Elastic knee orthosis.

Name/Description

Flexible knee braces are made with either an elastic material or rubber. They are available in a variety of configurations with assorted features: hinged metal knee joints, patellar pads, stays to keep the material from rolling, and adjustable straps to change the tension. They may have an anterior cutout to relieve pressure on the patella when the knee is flexed (Fig. 2-12).

L Code

L1800	Elastic with stays
L1810	Elastic with joints
L1815	Elastic with condylar pads
L1820	Elastic with condylar pads and joints
L1825	Elastic kneecap

Function

To provide comfort for patients with osteoarthritis of the knee, minor knee sprains, and mild edema

To provide proprioceptive feedback as well as minimal mechanical support and can retain body heat

Force Systems

Flexible knee braces provide compression and mild valgus, varus, and extension control.

Common ICD Codes

736.41	Genu valgum
736.42	Genu varum
844	Knee sprains and strains
717.89	Knee sprain, old
728.4	Ligament laxity
736.6	Patella deformity, acquired
714.0	Rheumatoid arthritis
717.7	Chondromalacia, patella

Comments

Flexible knee braces are low-cost, easily available, and user friendly. They can be used as an evaluation device to determine the patient's tolerance of wearing an orthosis.

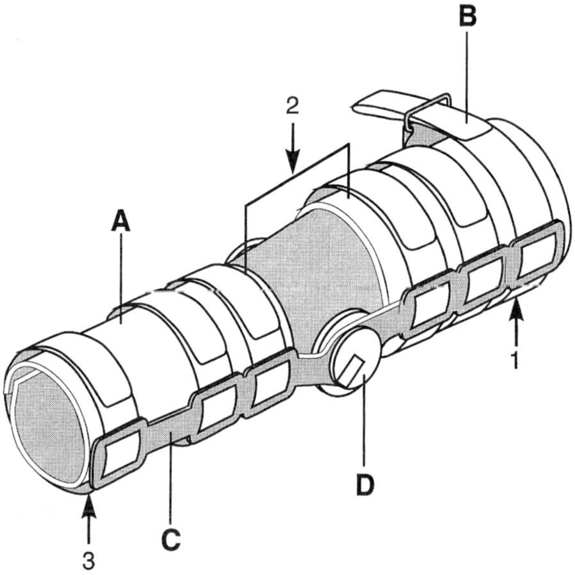

Fig. 2-13. Rehabilitative knee orthosis. *A,* Open cell foam interface; *B,* nonelastic Vellcro straps; *C,* aluminum side bar; *D,* single pivot hinge.

Name/Description

Knee immobilizer, canvas or equal

Knee orthosis with adjustable knee joints for positioning the knee (Fig. 2-13)

L Code

L1830

L1832

Function

To limit the range of motion of the knee joint following an injury or surgery on the knee, especially when the anterior cruciate ligament is involved

The first keeps the knee at 0 degrees, while the latter allows for a controlled range of motion. Both styles are custom fitted.

Force Systems

To limit flexion:

1. An anteriorly directed force on the posterior proximal thigh.
2. A posteriorly directed force on the anterior surface of the knee. This can be directly over the patella,

or a combination of support just proximal and just distal to the patella

3. An anteriorly directed force on the posterior aspect of the calf.

To limit extension, the forces are the reverse of those just described. Stresses that generate genu valgum and varum are also limited.

Possible Additional L Codes

L2180   Plastic shoe insert with ankle joints may be used to control distal migration of the orthosis.

Common ICD Codes

718.86   Knee instability
718.36   Displacement within the knee that is due to ligament or structural deficiency
717.83   ACL deficiency

Comments

Knee orthoses are relatively simple to apply. However, one must be careful to thoroughly instruct the patient on how to don or doff it, because it is likely the first time they have used such a device. The patient must also be compliant, because it is easily removed, and as with all orthoses, it is a bother to wear.

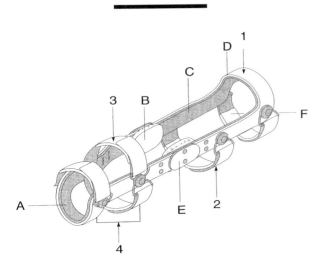

Fig. 2-14. Functional knee orthosis. Numbered arrows indicate force systems described in text. Components: *A*, calf section; *B*, medial/lateral condylar pads; *C*, thigh section; *D*, carbon composite frame; *E*, adjustable knee hinge; *F*, thigh strap.

Name/Description

Knee orthosis with derotation and mediolateral, anterior cruciate ligament control, custom fabricated
Knee orthosis of molded plastic, polycentric knee joints and pneumatic knee pads (Fig. 2-14)
A rigid KO to limit knee extension

L Code

L1840
L1858

Function

To limit knee extension to slightly less than 0 degrees to protect the anterior cruciate ligament
Distribute forces directed at the side, usually the lateral side, of the knee joint to the femur and tibia to protect the knee joint capsule

Force Systems

A combination three-point force system is at work in a functional KO to limit the tibia shifting anteriorly in relation to the femur. The components of the force systems follow:

1. A posteriorly directed force on the anterior, proximal portion of the thigh
2. An anteriorly directed force on the posterior, distal femur
3. A posteriorly directed force at the proximal third of the tibia
4. An anteriorly directed force aimed at the posterior tibia midshaft

Two other sets of force systems protect the knee from valgus and varus stresses. These are similar to the force system described for the single upright KAFO, Figure 2-15.

L Codes

L1840   Custom fabricated to patient model
L1845   Adjustable flexion and extension control and mediolateral control; fitted
L1846   Adjustable flexion and extension control and mediolateral control; custom fabricate
L1855   Molded plastic thigh and calf sections with knee joints

L1858   KO, Polycentric knee joints, pneumatic knee pads, molded to model of patient.

L1870   KO, double upright with knee joints, thigh and calf lacers, molded to model

L1880   KO, double upright with knee joints, thigh and calf cuffs nonmolded

Possible Additional L Codes

L2405   Addition to knee joint drop lock, each joint

Common ICD Codes

718.86   Knee instability
717.83   ACL deficiency

Comments

One of the goals of L codes is to be as generic as possible and describe a function or service rather than a specific orthosis. However, in the case of KOs, several of the L codes have become so identified with specific orthoses that these codes are used in the description function above, as well as in the L code identification section.

These types of knee braces are more effective in controlling translatory movement than rotary movement between the femur and the tibia.[13]

Loomer concluded, "Valgus bracing can be a useful treatment modality for the patient with medial gonarthrosis to replace or delay surgery, and should be considered in the young, the elderly, the infirm, and the reluctant."[14]

Marans observed, "An interesting point that has not been discussed in any of previous studies is that of the need for a double-hinged brace compared with a laterally hinged brace. Throughout the study it can be seen that the laterally hinged braces were found to be at least as effective as their potentially more cumbersome double-hinged counterparts and also had the least effect on performance during straight-ahead running."[15]

Name/Description

Prophylactic KO. This is not necessarily a specific brace so much as it is the manner in which a functional knee brace is used. Some braces, however, are designed for prophylactic use only. (Not illustrated.)

L Code

L1840   KO with derotation and mediolateral, anterior cruciate ligament control, custom fabricated

L1858   KO of molded plastic, with polycentric knee joints and pneumatic knee pads; a rigid KO to limit knee extension

Function

Theoretically designed to prevent injury to the knee, or at least reduce the degree to which the knee is injured, in athletic activities

Force Systems

The force systems are the same as for L1840 and L1858.

Common ICD Codes

Knee orthoses have no ICD codes because their function is preventive.

Comments

Concluding from presently available clinical, epidemiologic, and statistical studies pertaining to prophylactic brace efficacy, the majority of devices are inadequate for protecting the medial collateral ligament from a direct lateral impact. A few, however, appear to protect the anterior cruciate ligament preferentially.[16]

"Though prophylactic braces continue to be manufactured and used, their efficacy has yet to be resolved in the minds of many clinicians."[17]

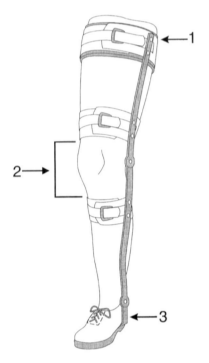

Fig. 2-15. Single lateral metal upright KAFO.

Name/Description
Single upright KAFO with free knee and ankle joints (Fig. 2-15). The upright may be on the medial or lateral side of the leg, depending on the deformity to be controlled.

L Code
L2000

Function
Most often, single lateral upright KAFOs are used to control genu valgum or varum. For the former, the upright is on the lateral side of the leg, while it is on the medial side to control genu varum. A ring lock may be used to control knee flexion for some smaller, lightweight patients. Ankle varus/valgus can be controlled with the addition of a T strap. Free, limited motion, dorsiflexion assist, or dorsiflexion and plantar flexion assist ankle joints may be incorporated. See the ankle joints in Figure 2-9.

Force Systems
The first force system to control genu valgum consists of the following:

1. A medially directed force on the lateral, proximal thigh band and cuff
2. A laterally directed force on the medial aspect of the knee joint (i.e., femoral condyles)
3. A medially directed force on the lateral side of the calcanous by the counter of the shoe

The force system to control genu varus is the opposite of that just described for valgum control.

Possible Additional L Codes
See L2036, double upright KAFO.

Common ICD Codes
436	Stroke, CVA
736.72	Pes equinus
736.71	Equinovarus
736.41	Genu valgum
736.42	Genu varum
342.9	Hemiplegia and hemiparesis
736.72	Equinovalgus

Comments
This KAFO has limited use due to the lack of rigidity resulting from having only a single upright. It can be useful, however, in working with children and small elderly patients, among whom mass and forces are smaller.

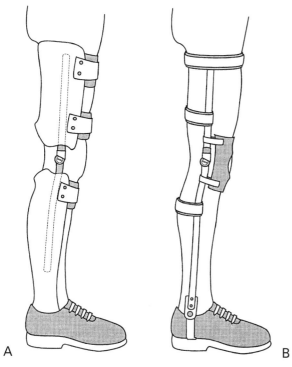

Fig. 2-16. **(A)** Custom-molded, plastic KAFO with drop lock knee joints, and rigid ankle joint. **(B)** Double metal upright KAFO with drop lock knee joints, full kneecap pad, and dual-action ankle joints.

Name/Description

Full plastic KAFO with double uprights, ring lock knee and solid ankle joints, molded to patient model (Fig. 2-16A)

L Code

L2036 plastic, custom molded to patient model

Name/Description

Double upright KAFO with ring knee lock, full kneecap pad and double adjustable ankle joints additions (Fig. 2-16B)

L Code

L2020	KAFO
L2405	Add: drop lock, each
L2795	Add: full kneecap pad
L2220	Add: dual-action ankle joint, assists, resists both plantar and dorsiflexion, each

Functions

To control genu valgum or varus and/or hyperextension of the knee.

With modifications to the knee joint, knee flexion is controlled.

Dorsiflexion and plantar flexion are unrestricted unless a modifying ankle joint is installed or the plastic is rigid enough to affect either ankle joint motion or subtalar joint motion.

Force Systems

For genu valgum and varus, see single upright KAFO, L2000.

For flexion and extension of the knee, see knee joint locks L2405, L2415 (see Fig. 2-17).

For ankle joint, see single upright AFO, L1980

Possible Additional L Codes

For ankle joint options see L1980, single upright AFO.

L2320	Nonmolded thigh lacer
L2330	Molded to model thigh lacer
L2335	Anterior tibial swing away band
L2340	Pretibial shell, molded to patient model
L2370	Patton bottom
L2385	Heavy-duty knee joint, each joint
L2390	Offset knee joint, each joint
L2395	Heavy-duty offset knee joint
L2405	Drop lock, each joint
L2415	Cam, bail, Swiss or French lock, each joint
L2425	Disc or dial knee joint for adjustable knee flexion to accommodate flexion contractures
L2492	Lift loop for drop lock ring
L2795	Full kneecap control pad
L2800	Kneecap pad, medial or lateral pull
L2500	Gluteal ischial weightbearing ring
L2510	Quadrilateral weightbearing brim, molded to patient model
L2520	Quadrilateral weightbearing brim, custom fitted
L2525	Ischial containment, narrow M/L brim, custom molded to patient model
L2550	Weightbearing high-roll cuff
L2795	Full kneecap pad
L2800	Kneecap pad with medial or lateral pull
L2810	Condylar pad

Common ICD Codes

436	Stroke, CVA
342.9	Hemiplegia and hemiparesis
138	Poliomyelitis, late effects
357	Guillain-Barré syndrome
340	Multiple sclerosis
344.0	Quadriplegia and quadriparesis
344.1	Paraplegia
344.3	Monoplegia
344.89	Brown-Séquard syndrome
952	Spinal cord injury
359.1	Muscular dystrophy, Duchenne syndrome, Becker's nevus
741.9	Spina bifida
730.15	Osteomyelitis femur
736.71	Equinovarus
736.72	Equinovalgus
736.72	Pes equinus
741.9	Spina bifida

Comments

The most commonly used plastics for KAFOs are thermomolded plastics such as polypropylene and its numerous derivatives. Major advantages include a more acceptable appearance to most patients; patients can use multiple shoes of similar style; less weight is at the distal end because a steel stirrup is not needed for shoe attachment; and the orthosis can be cleaned and does not absorb perspiration or urine.

Thermosetting, laminated plastics are also used, and though more expensive, they provide increased rigidity along the length of the leg to control rotational forces commonly seen in lower limb pathologies. They are also heavier than the thermomolded plastics.

Condie identified three principal impairments for which KAFOs are indicated:

1. Weakness of the muscles that control the knee joint
2. Upper motor neuron lesions resulting in hypertonicity in the lower limbs
3. Loss of structural integrity of the hip or knee joint[18]

To control subtalar inversion or eversion, the foot section of the orthosis can include designs like those previously described for the UCB-ST, L3000. By controlling the forces that start in the subtalar joint and are transmitted through the talocrural joint as rotational forces to the tibia and fibula, rotational forces being applied to the knee joint can be affected with plastic KAFOs.

Name/Description

KAFO, to include a custom molded to patient AFO section with metal bands and leather thigh cuffs
Not illustrated

L Codes

L2020	Double upright KAFO with the addition of L2280 molded inner boot

Functions

The same as L2020 and L2036, double upright KAFOs (see Fig. 2-16)

Force Systems

See L2036, double upright KAFO, Figure 2-16A.

Possible Additional L Codes

See L2036, double upright KAFO, Figure 2-16B.

Common ICD Codes

See double upright KAFO, Figure 2-16.

Comments

This KAFO is a good design combination that takes advantages of the best benefits of an all-plastic KAFO and the KAFO with metal bands and leather cuffs or thigh lacer. Plastic thigh sections tend to be warmer, causing significant perspiration and can result in chafing and pinching of soft tissue between the plastic and a sitting surface or, in the case of bilateral orthoses, between the two orthoses. Hosiery must be worn to interface between the plastic and the skin. Leather thigh cuffs are tolerated better by the skin and are cooler.

The custom-molded plastic AFO portion of the KAFO allows for a more intimate fitting and thus control of the foot and ankle complex, resulting in better correction of deformities and anatomic alignment. Two other advantages are that the patient can use more than one pair of shoes and that a significant amount of weight is eliminated at the distal end of the limb. This makes it much easier for the patient to control the limb during swing phase. Many patients also prefer this type of orthosis because it goes inside of the shoe and is less visible than a metal stirrup.

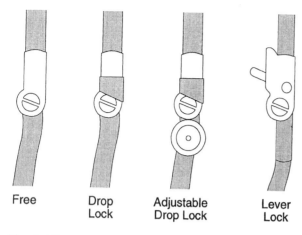

Fig. 2-17.   Four types of knee locks used in custom-made KAFOs.

Name/Description

1. Free offset knee joint
2. Ring or drop locks (one per upright)
3. Adjustable for flexion contracture
4. Bail, Swiss, cam or French locks (all are a type of lever lock) (Fig. 2-17)

L Code

L2405	Addition to knee joint drop lock
L2415	Addition to knee joint cam lock, each joint
L2425	Addition to knee joint disc or dial joint for adjustable knee flexion to accommodate knee flexion contracture, each joint
L2435	Addition to knee joint polycentric joint, each

Common ICD Codes

045.1	Poliomyelitis, acute
342.9	Hemiplegia
138	Poliomyelitis, late effects
357.0	Guillain-Barré syndrome
344.0	Quadriplegia and quadriparesis
344.1	Paraplegia
344.3	Monoplegia, lower limb
344.89	Brown-Séquard syndrome
952	Spinal cord injury
359.1	Muscular dystrophy, Duchenne syndrome, Becker's nevus
730.15	Osteomyelitis femur
741.9	Spina bifida
718.46	Knee flexion contracture

Function

To keep the knee extended during gait while allowing the knee to flex for sitting.

Force Systems

1. An anteriorly directed force on the posterior proximal thigh.
2. A posteriorly directed force on the anterior surface of the knee. This can be a kneecap pad directly over the patella, a patella-tendon strap or a combination of the distal thigh and calf straps.
3. An anteriorly directed force on the posterior aspect of the calf.

Possible Additional L Codes

The L codes for these devices are both add-on codes for knee joints, thus these devices do not have additional codes. Some other additional codes can be used in conjunction with these; some of the more common are as follows:

L2385	Heavy-duty knee joint, each joint
L2390	Offset knee joint, each joint
L2395	Offset, heavy duty, each joint
L2425	Disc or dial lock for adjustable knee flexion, (flexion contractures), each joint
L2492	Lift loop for drop lock ring
L2785	Drop lock retainer, each
L2795	Full kneecap pad
L2800	Kneecap pad with medial or lateral pull
L2810	Condylar pad (in place of L2800)

Comments

Ring locks are the most durable, lowest maintenance, and therefore the safest of the knee joint locks. The various cam-locking mechanisms can be quickly worn because of the size of the moment involved in knee flexion and the small surface area of the locking mechanism. Cam locks have a strong clinical appeal because they make it easier for patient to unlock the knee and sit down.

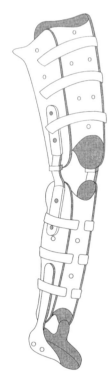

Fig. 2-18. Fracture orthosis KAFO.

Name/Description

KAFO fracture orthosis, molded to patient, or may be custom fitted (Fig. 2-18)

L Codes

L2122	Uses plaster material
L2124	Uses synthetic casting material
L2126	Uses low-temperature thermoplastic
L2132	Custom-fitted soft material
L2134	Custom-fitted, semirigid material
L2136	Custom-fitted, rigid material

Function

To provide stability for fractured long bones in the thigh and lower leg, if there is also a tibial fracture

Force Systems

Force systems to control genu varum and valgum are the same as those described for single upright KAFO, L2000, Figure 2-15. If knee joints are used, and they usually are not, the force systems are as described under knee joint locks, Figure 2-17.

More importantly, what distinguishes fracture orthoses from others is the hydrostatic pressure that is created inside the circumferential shell that surrounds the fractured bone and extends from the joint at one end of the long bone to the joint at the opposite end. As the shell is tightened, the soft tissue is compressed and a 360 degree circumferential, hydrostatic pressure is created, which stabilizes the new callus at the fracture site.

Possible Additional L Codes

L2850	Femoral length fracture sock
L2180	Plastic shoe insert with ankle joints
L2182	Drop lock, each joint
L2184	Limited motion knee joint, each joint
L2186	Adjustable range of motion knee joint
L2188	Quadrilateral brim
L2190	Waist belt, for suspension, in place of L2180
L2192	Hip joint with pelvic band and belt

Common ICD Codes

821.01	Fracture, femur, shaft

Comments

Fracture braces are used to provide support for a fracture site while at the same time allowing the use of joints at each end of the fractured bone, thus resulting in less loss of muscle strength and range of movement (ROM) of joints caused by lack of use. Other benefits are improved circulation in the limb as a result of increased patient use. Stimulation of the bone also promotes healing.

Orthotic femoral fracture management must be delayed until there is intrinsic stability at the fracture site, usually between the fourth and sixth week after injury.[19]

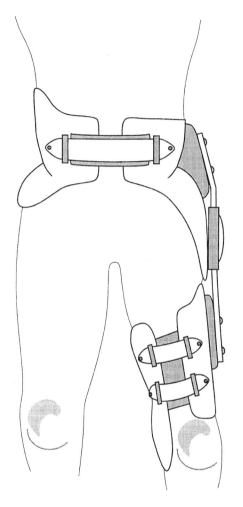

Fig. 2-19.   Postoperative hip abduction orthosis.

Name/Description
Postoperative hip abduction orthosis (Fig. 2-19)

L Codes
L1685	Custom fabricated
L1686	Custom fitted

Function
To limit adduction and flexion of the hip joint following total hip replacement

Force Systems
Adduction control is provided by the portion of the pelvic belt on the contralateral side. As adduction forces are applied to the femur, resistive force is applied to the contralateral iliac crest.

To limit hip flexion, posteriorly directed forces are applied to the anterior portion of the thigh and to the anterior portion of the pelvis or abdomen.

Common ICD Codes
996.4	Complications of hip prosthesis

Comments
At times, control of rotation at the hip joint is also needed to prevent dislocation of the hip prosthesis. In these situations, it is desirable to convert the hip orthosis into a hip KAFO so that the below knee section can help control rotation of the hip joint.

Patients using this orthosis often lack understanding of its purpose. It is designed to limit flexion of the hip joint; if the limitation is less than 90 degrees of flexion, they will not be able to sit up straight in a chair. When they try, the orthosis will irritate their abdomen. Patients should position themselves properly within the limits of the orthosis and not try to exceed the motion it allows. The same is true for adduction. Patients with their hips restricted in an abducted position by an orthosis should not sit in a wheelchair that forces their legs into neutral or adduction. This results in patient discomfort and putting unnecessary strain on the total hip replacement.

Lima reported, "This hip orthosis is used routinely as a prophylactic device to prevent dislocation after surgery by restricting motion that could lead to dislocation, providing a favorable environment for graft incorporation, training patients in total hip precautions and reducing the tendency of stronger hip adductors to override hip abductors."[20]

REFERENCES

1. Bunch WH, Keagy RD, Kritter AE, et al: Atlas of Orthotics: Biomechanical Principles and Application. 2nd Ed. C.V. Mosby, St. Louis, 1985
2. Weber D: Clinical Aspects of Lower Extremity Orthotics. Elegan Enterprises, Oakville, Ontario, 1990
3. Condie DN, Meadows CB: Ankle-foot orthoses. p. 99. In Bowker P (ed): Biomechanical Basis of Orthotic Management. Butterworth-Heinemann, Oxford, England, 1993

4. Perry J: Gait Analysis Normal and Pathological Function. Slack, Thorofare, NJ, 1992

5. Puckett CD: The Educational Annotation of ICD-9-CM. 4th Ed. Channel Publishing, Reno, NV, 1994

6. Jones MK, Boulware C, Falconer C, Hall DC: 1994 HCPCS Level II Codes, St. Anthony Publishing, Alexandria, 1993

7. The Illustrated Guide to Orthotics and Prosthetics. O & P's Comprehensive Guide to Medicare Codes and Reimbursement. National Office of Orthotics and Prosthetics, Alexandria, VA, 1992

8. Nielsen JP, Fish DJ: OOS-1 basic seminar on lower extremity rotational control orthotics, course manual. Oregon Orthotic Systems. 2nd Ed. 1993

9. Inman VT: Dual axis ankle control system and UC-BL shoe insert: biomechanical considerations. Bull Prosthet Res BPR 10–11:130, 1968

10. Carlson JM, [in error Colson JM] Berglund C: An effective orthotic design for controling the unstable subtalar joint. Orthot Prosthet 33:1, 1979

11. Smidt GL (ed): Gait in Rehabilitation. Churchill Livingstone, New York, 1990

12. Conry MA: Orthomedics fracture bracing at LA county USC Medical Center. J Prosthet Orthot 4:151, 1992

13. Bowker P, Pratt D: Knee orthoses. p. 124, Bowker P, Condie DN, Bader DL et al: Biomechanical Basis of Orthotic Management. Butterworth-Heinemann, Oxford, England, 1993

14. Loomer R, Horlick S: Valgus knee bracing for the osteoarthritic knee. Paper presented at the meeting of the International Society of the Knee, Toronto, 1991

15. Marans HJ, Jackson RW, Piccinin J et al: Functional testing of braces for anterior cruciate ligament deficient knees. Can J Surg 34:2, 1991

16. Marks PH, Freddie HF: Status of Prophylactic Knee Braces, Bone and Joint Diseases: Index and Reviews. Vol. 1, No. 6, 1993

17. Cawley PW: Is knee bracing really necessary? A review of current research on brace function, the natural history of graft remodeling, and physiologic implications. Smith & Nephew Donjoy Biomechanics Research Laboratory, Carlsbad, CA

18. Condie D, Lamb J: Knee-ankle-foot orthoses. p. 146. In Bowker P, Condie DN, Bader DL et al: Biomechanical Basis of Orthotic Management. Butterworth-Heinemann, Oxford, England, 1993

19. Sarmiento A, Ross, Steven DK, Racette WL: Functional fracture bracing. In Bunch, (ed): Atlas of Orthotics. 2nd Ed. CV Mosby, St. Louis, 1985

20. Lima D, Magnus R, Paprosky WG: Team management of hip revision patients using a post-op hip orthosis. J Prosthet Orthot 6:20, 1994

SUGGESTED READINGS

Buckland AE, Brouch KL, Jones MK, Aaron WS (eds): St. Anthony's Color-Coded Illustrated ICD 9-CM Code Book. St. Anthony Publishing, Alexandria, VA, 1993

Lohman M, Goldstein H: Alternative strategies in tone-reducing AFO design. J Prosthet Orthot, 5:1, 1993

Appendix 2-1

Conversion Table From Diagnosis to Orthosis[a]

ICD Code	Diagnosis	Functional Deficit(s)	Likely Orthotic Recommendations	Figure No.
736.81	Leg length discrepancy	Side bending, back pain Shoulders uneven	L3300 Heel elevation tapered to metatarsals L3310 Heel and sole elevation, neoprene L3320 Heel and sole elevation, cork L3332 Heel elevation inside of shoe up to ½ inch L3334 Heel elevation, rubber heel	

45.1
138
 	
357.0
	Poliomyelitis, acute
	Poliomyelitis, late effects
	
	Guillain-Barré syndrome
		Functional deformities in hip, pelvis and/or trunk
		In the Hip
		  1. Inadequate extension
		  2. Excessive internal or external rotation
		  3. Excessive adduction or abduction
		In the pelvis
		  1. Contralateral drop
		  2. Ipsilateral drop
		  3. Ipsilateral hike or elevation
		In the trunk
		  1. Lateral Leaning
		In the knee
		  1. Flexion, to the point of falling
		  2. Genu varus
		  3. Genu valgus
		In the ankle and foot
		  1. Foot drop; equinus
		  2. Calcaneovarus
		  3. Calcaneovalgus
		  4. Excessive dorsiflexion of ankle joint
		  5. Hypermobility of midfoot
			L2020 KAFO, double upright, metal with leather cuffs
			L2036 KAFO, double upright, plastic molded to patient model
			L1940 AFO, plastic custom molded to patient model, spring leaf design
			L1945 AFO, floor reaction design, limits plantar flexion and assists knee extension
			L1960 AFO, custom molded to patient model, plastic, solid ankle design
			L1970 AFO, custom molded to patient model, plastic, with ankle joints
			L3000 FO, UCBL-ST
			L1990 AFO, metal, double upright
			L1945 AFO, floor reaction design, can be used to affect knee joint position as well as position of the ankle and foot
			L3300 Heel elevation tapered to metatarsals
			L3310 Heel and sole elevation neoprene
			L3320 Heel and sole elevation cork
			L3332 Heel and elevation inside of shoe up to ½ inch
			L3334 Heel elevation rubber heel
				16B
				16A
				4
				7
				5
				8
				2
				11
				7

[a] Only those orthoses listed in boldface are described in the text.

Continues

41

Appendix 2-1 *(Continued)*

ICD Code	Diagnosis	Functional Deficit(s)	Likely Orthotic Recommendations	Figure No.
331.89	Cerebral vascular disease—ataxia	Knee	L1850 Knee orthosis, Swedish style to control genu recurvatum	
342	Hemiplegia and hemiparesis	Recurvatum and excessive flexion	L1990 AFO, spring wire, dorsiflexion assist to prevent toe dragging	
342.00	Flaccid hemiplegia			
436	Stroke, CVA	Foot and ankle	L1910 AFO, single posterior upright, clasps to counter of shoe	
		Seen in swing phase		
436	Hemiplegia, cerebrovascular lesion	Foot drop and toe drag	**L-1930 AFO, custom-fitted plastic**	4
438	Hemiplegia, late effects	Calcaneovarus, supination and forefoot adduction	L-1940 AFO, plastic, custom molded to patient model, spring leaf design	4
		Seen in stance phase		
		Calcaneovalgus resulting in medial maleolus moving medially relative to the AFO, resulting in pressure if it makes contact with the orthosis.	**L-1945 AFO, floor reaction design, limits plantar flexion and assists knee extension**	7
			L1950 AFO, spiral design, limits plantar flexion	
			L1960 AFO, custom molded to patient model, plastic, solid ankle design	5
			L1970 AFO, custom molded to patient model, plastic, with ankle joints	8
			L1980 AFO, metal, single upright	
			L1990 AFO, metal, double upright	11
333.7	Cerebral palsy athetoid/dystonic	Most effectively used in conjunction with other modalities such as surgery, medications or physical therapy	**L1945 AFO, floor reaction design, can be used to affect knee joint position as well as position of the ankle and foot**	7
343.0	Cerebral palsy-diplegia/paraplegia			
343.1	Cerebral palsy-hemiplegia			
343.9	Cerebral palsy-spastic	Used postsurgically to maintain correction	**L1960 AFO, custom molded, solid ankle design**	5
437.8	Cerebral vascular disease—quadriplegia	With inhibitive footplate modifications, may reduce tone	**L1970 AFO, custom molded with ankle joints**	8
		With fixed ankle joint, can increase or decrease knee flexion	**L1980 AFO, metal, single upright**	
		Instabilities within the foot can be controlled by molding UCBL-ST design into footplate of AFO or KAFO	**L1990 AFO, metal, double upright**	11
			L3000 FO, UCBL-ST	2

Continues

ICD Code	Diagnosis	Functional Deficit(s)	Likely Orthotic Recommendations	Figure No.

340	Multiple sclerosis	Seen in swing phase
		   Foot drop, toe dragging
		Seen in stance phase
		   Genu recurvatum, or
		     hyperextension
		Orthoses may be used
		   prophylactically to avoid
		   contractures
			L1945 AFO, floor reaction design, can be used to affect knee joint position as well as position of the ankle and foot
			L1960 AFO, custom molded, solid ankle design
			L1970 AFO, custom molded with ankle joints
			L1980 AFO, metal, single upright
				7
				
				5
				
				8

344.0
344
344.09
 	
344.89
952
344.1
344.3
355.8
	Quadriplegia and quadreparesis
	SCI—spastic paraplegia
	Other quadriplegia
	
	Brown-Séquard syndrome
	Spinal cord injury without
	  evidence
	Paraplegia
	Monoplegia of lower limb
	Paralysis, thigh
		Patients with lesions between T6
		  and L1 may use KAFOs
		Upper body strength and
		  motivation are primary
		  considerations
		AFOs for T6–T11 level may help
		  prevent contractures of ankle
		  and foot that makes it
		  impossible to keep the foot on
		  the footrest of a wheelchair or is
		  prone to pressure sores while
		  lying in bed
		Lesions below L2 are likely to be
		  functional with AFOs.
			L2020 KAFO, double upright, metal with leather cuffs
			L2036 KAFO, double upright, plastic, molded to patient model
			
			L1945 AFO, floor reaction design
			L1960 AFO, custom molded, solid ankle design
			L1970 AFO, custom molded with ankle joints
			
			L1990 AFO, metal, double upright
				16B
				
				16A
				
				7
				
				5
				
				8
				
				11

355.356
 	
356.1
250.0
 	
443.9
	Peripheral neuropathic disorders
	Charcot joint
	Diabetes mellitus
	
	Peripheral vascular disease
		Skeletal deformities: pes planus,
		  calcaneal valgus or varus
		Weakening of muscles inervated
		  by the peroneal nerve, burning
		  pains, paresthesia, numbness,
		  hyperesthesia, and reduced
		  sensation
		Pressure ulcers on foot
		Goal to prevent amputation
			L1960 AFO, custom molded, solid ankle design
			L1970 AFO, custom molded with ankle joints
			L3001 FO, removable insole, molded to patient model, Spenco-type material
			L3002 FO, removable insole, molded to patient model, Plastazote-type material
			L3216 Orthopedic footwear, ladies' depth inlay shoes
			L3217 Orthopedic footwear, ladies' hightop, depth inlay shoes
			L3221 Orthopedic footwear, men's depth inlay shoes
			L3222 Orthopedic footwear, men's hightop, depth inlay shoes
			L2330 Orthopedic footwear, custom, molded to patient model, depth inlay
			L3252 Foot, shoe molded to patient model, Plastazote or equal
			L3253 Foot, shoe, custom fitted, Plastazote or equal
				5
				
				8

Continues

Appendix 2-1 *(Continued)*

ICD Code	Diagnosis	Functional Deficit(s)	Likely Orthotic Recommendations	Figure No.
359.1 718.47 718.40 718.46	Muscular dystrophy Ankle joint contraction Contraction of a joint Knee contraction	Plantar flexion and inversion result from weak quadriceps Ankle, knee, and hip flexion contractures	**L1960 AFO, custom molded, solid ankle design** **L1970 AFO, custom molded with ankle joints** **L2036 KAFO, double upright, plastic, molded to patient model**	5 8 16A
714 734 715.7 715.5 715.6	Rheumatoid arthritis Pes planus Osteoarthritis, ankle, foot, tarsals or metatarsals Osteoarthritis, femur, and hip Osteoarthritis, tibia, fibula, knee, or patella	Pain in foot and or ankle, pes planus, pronation, calcaneovalgus Collapse of longitudinal arch Pain while weightbearing or ambulating Pain in hip or knee joint while ambulating Pain while weightbearing or ambulating	L3001 FO, removable insole, molded to patient model, Spenco-type material L3002 FO, removable insole, molded to patient model, Plastazote-type material L3216 Orthopedic footwear, ladies' depth inlay shoes L3221 Orthopedic footwear, men's depth inlay shoes L2330 Orthopedic footwear, custom, molded to patient model, depth inlay **L-3000 FO, UCBL-ST** **L1960 AFO, custom molded, solid ankle design** L3450 heel, SACH cushion, rocker sole **L1800 KO, elastic with stays** **L1810 KO, elastic with knee joints** **L1855 KO, custom molded to patient model, with joints**	 2 5 12 12 14
734 736.79 736.76 736.79	Pes planus Pronation or supination, Calcaneal valgus/varus, Foot deformity valgus/varus	Forefoot abduction, adduction, supination or pronation, or calcaneovalgus or varus	**L3000 UCBL with emphasis or sustentaculum tali support**	2
717 717.7 717.89 714.0	Knee disorders Chondromalacia, patella Knee sprain Rheumatoid arthritis	Hypermobility of patella Pain while weightbearing	**L1815 Flexible knee orthosis with condylar pads or Palumbo design**	12
717.83 717	ACL deficiency Internal derangement of knee, not result of acute injury	Pain, knee instability while walking or participating in physical activities like sports or working Loss of stability in the plane	**L1840 Knee orthosis with derotational, mediolateral control** **L1858 Knee orthosis, custom molded to model of the patient**	14 14

Continues

Appendix 2-1 *(Continued)*

ICD Code	Diagnosis	Functional Deficit(s)	Likely Orthotic Recommendations	Figure No.
718.36	Displacement in knee joint that is due to ligament structural deficiency	Loss of stability in the anteroposterior and/or mediolateral plane	**L1840 Knee orthosis with derotational, mediolateral control** **L1858 Knee orthosis, custom molded to model of the patient**	14 14
718.86	Knee instability	Inability to control flexion	**L1840 Knee orthosis with derotational, mediolateral control** **L1858 Knee orthosis, custom molded to model of the patient**	14 14
730.15	Osteomyelitis femur	Pain when weightbearing	**L2036 KAFO, double upright, plastic, molded to patient model** **L2020 KAFO, double upright, metal with leather cuffs** Ischial weightbearing added to both to reduce weight through the femur	16A 16B
730.16 730.17 733.82 733.8	Osteomyelitis tibial/fibula Osteomyelitis ankle/foot Pseudoarthrosis Malunion/nonunion of fracture	Pain when weightbearing Pain when weightbearing	**L1960 AFO, custom molded to patient model, plastic, solid ankle design** **L1970 AFO, custom molded to patient model, plastic, with ankle joints** **L1990 AFO, metal, double upright** Patella tendon weight bearing can be added to reduce weight through the tibia or ankle	6 8 11
734	Pes planus	Loss of longitudinal arch	**L3000 UCBL with emphasis on sustentaculum tali support**	2
736.41 736.42 736.5	Genu valgum Genu varum Genu recurvatum	Knee pain Knee pain, antalgic gait Hypertension	**L2020 KAFO, double upright, metal with leather cuffs** **L2036 KAFO, double upright, plastic, molded to patient model** **L2000 KAFO, Single upright** L1850 Knee orthosis, Swedish style to control genu recurvatum	16A 16B 15
736.2	Pes equinus	Lack of heel strike, weightbearing starts at metatarsals, leg length discrepancy	Shoe modifications can be used to accommodate this deformity, heel wedge tapered to midfoot	

Continues

Appendix 2-1 *(Continued)*

ICD Code	Diagnosis	Functional Deficit(s)	Likely Orthotic Recommendations	Figure No.
736.73	Pes cavus	Pain in longitudinal arch, difficulty finding a shoe to fit and not irritate dorsum of foot	Custom molded foot orthosis	
736.76	Calcaneal foot or calcaneal valgus or varus	Uneven wear pattern or shoe, pain in hindfoot, poor balance	**L3000 UCBL with emphasis or sustentaculum talus support for valgus control of the calcanous**	**2**

741.9	Spina bifida	Level of lesion S2–S5
		  Pes cavus, calcaneovalgus
		Lesion L5–S1
		  Equinovalgus or equinovarus, calcaneal heel
			L3000 UCBL	2

		Lesion L4
		  Knee extension or hyperextension
		  Foot, calcaneal heel
		  Spasticity in lower limbs
			L2036 KAFO, double upright, plastic, molded to patient model
			
			L1960 AFO, custom molded, solid ankle design
				16A
				
				5

		Lesion L1–L3	**L2036 KAFO, double upright, plastic, molded to patient model** **L1960 AFO, custom molded, solid ankle design** HKAFOs	16A 5
821.01	Fracture, femoral shaft	Pain and skeletal instability Unable to bear weight	L2122 KAFO, femoral fracture orthosis, plaster L2124 KAFO, femoral fracture orthosis, synthetic casting material L2126 KAFO, femoral fracture orthosis, thermoplastic material L2128 KAFO, femoral fracture orthosis, molded to patient model L2132 KAFO, femoral fracture orthosis, soft material, custom fitted **L2134 KAFO, femoral fracture orthosis, semirigid, custom fitted** L2136 KAFO, femoral fracture orthosis, rigid material, custom fitted	18

Continues

Appendix 2-1 *(Continued)*

ICD Code	Diagnosis	Functional Deficit(s)	Likely Orthotic Recommendations	Figure No.
823.2 823.0	Fracture, Tibia and fibula Fracture, tibia	Pain and skeletal instability Unable to bear weight Pain with skeletal instability Unable to bear weight	L2102 AFO, tibial fracture orthosis, plaster L2104 AFO, tibial fracture orthosis, synthetic casting material L2106 AFO, tibial fracture orthosis, thermoplastic material L2108 AFO, tibial fracture orthosis, molded to patient model L2112 AFO, tibial fracture orthosis, soft material, custom fitted **L2114 AFO, tibial fracture orthosis, semirigid, custom fitted** L2116 AFO, tibial fracture orthosis, rigid material, custom fitted **L1960 AFO, custom molded bivalved AFO**	 10 6
845.09 727.81	Achilles tendon, torn or surgically repaired Short achilles tendon, acquired	Pain, inability to push off when running or jumping prior to repair Postsurgically, goal is to protect tendon while healing Plantar flexion deformity	**L1960 AFO, custom molded, solid ankle design** **L1970 AFO, custom molded with ankle joints**	5 8
854.6	Head trauma	Extention pattern, equinus, hyperextended knee, internal rotational hip joint	**L1945 AFO, floor reaction design**	7
718.46	Knee contracture	Relative leg length discrepancy, side bending gait, possible inability to stand or walk depending on the degree of contracture	**L1945 AFO, floor reaction design** **L1858 Knee orthosis, custom molded to model of the patient** **L2020 KAFO, double upright, metal with leather cuffs** **L2036 KAFO, double upright, plastic, molded to patient model**	7 16A 16B

Continues

Appendix 2-1 (Continued)

ICD Code	Diagnosis	Functional Deficit(s)	Likely Orthotic Recommendations	Figure No.
718.47	Ankle contracture	Equinas	**L1945 AFO, floor reaction design**	7
			L1945 AFO, floor reaction design, limits plantar flexion and assists knee extension	7
			L1960 AFO, custom molded to patient model, plastic, solid ankle design	5
			L1970 AFO, custom molded to patient model, plastic, with ankle joints	8
			L1990 AFO, metal, double upright	11
996.4	Complications of hip prosthesis	Dislocated hip prosthesis, pain	L1685 HO, hip abduction orthosis, custom fabricated	
			L1686 HO, hip abduction orthosis, custom fitted	19
707.1 250.8	Ulcers, foot Ulcers, diabetes mellitus, lower limb	Open ulcers and possible infection, possibly leading to amputation	**L1960 AFO, custom molded bivalved**	**6**

Appendix 2-2

Appendix 2-2. Normal Gait

	A	Distance from Initial Contact at Point "A" to the End of Terminal Swing at Z is One Stride						Z
		Stance Phase (60% of One Stride)				Swing Phase (40% of One Stride)		
	Initial Contact	Loading Response	Midstance	Terminal Stance	Preswing	Initial Swing	Midswing	Terminal Swing
Stage of gait cycle (%)[a]	0–2%	0–10%	10–30%	30–50%	50–60%	60–73%	73–87%	87–100%
Hip point Position	Flex 30 degrees	20 degrees	Extension starts	Neutral at 38% of GC Extension 10 degrees at 50% of GC	Neutral at 60%	Flexion to 10 degrees	Flexion to 25 degrees	Maintains 25 degrees flexion
Muscle activity	Extensors (lower gluteus maximus, adductor magnus) Hip abductors			Anterior portion of tensor fascia lata	Hip flexors start rectus femoris	Hip flexors and adductors: gracilis, sartorius	Hip flexors end early Passive flexion	Hip extensors in late mids wing; semimembranosis, semitendinosis, and biceps femoris

		Col 1	Col 2	Col 3	Col 4	Col 5	Col 6	Col 7	Col 8
Knee joint	Position	From 2 degrees extension to 5 degrees flexion	Flexed from 12–18 degrees	Flexion from 12 to 5 degrees	Zero to 5 degrees flexion	Flexes 0–40 degrees	Flexion 40–60 degrees	Flexion 60–65 degrees	From 2 degrees extension to 5 degrees flexion
	Active muscles	Vasti Upper gluteus maximus and iliotibial band Lower hamstrings	Hamstrings Quadriceps Biceps femoris Tensor fascis lata	Quadriceps Vasti Hip abductors Iliotibial band	Popliteus Gastrocnemius	Gastrocnemius Popliteus	Gracilis Sartorius	Passively	Vasti extend the knee Hamstrings temper extension moment
Ankle joint	Position	Neutral to plantar flexion of 3–5 degrees	Plantar-flex up to 7 degrees	Dorsiflexion degrees starts from 8 degrees plantar flexion to 5 degrees dorsiflexion	Dorsiflexion up to 10 degrees Plantar flexion starts at 48% of GC	Plantar flexion to 20 degrees continues to 62% of GC	Dorsiflexion to neutral 62–100% of GC	0–2 degrees dorsiflexion	Neutral to 3–5 degrees plantar flexion
	Active muscles	Pretibial muscles	Pretibial muscles to decelerate plantar flexion: tibialis anterior and long toe extensors	Soleus, gastrocnemius	Soleus and gastrocnemius, triceps surae	Soleus and gastrocnemius Extensor hallucis longus tibialis anterior	Pretibial muscles, toe extensors, and tibialis anterior	Tibialis anterior and extensor hallucis longus	Tibialis anterior
Subtalar joint	Position	Eversion	Eversion	Maximum eversion at 14% of GC. 4–6 degrees 7 degrees calcaneal valgus		Maximum inversion at 52% of GC	Neutral at midswing	Neutral at midswing	Neutral at midswing
	Active muscles		Tibialis posterior	Soleus Flexor digitorum and hallicus longus	Tibialis posterior at 30% of GC, soleus				

Abbreviation: GC, gait cycle.

[a] One stride equals the distance from initial contact at point A to the end of terminal swing at point Z. Two strides equal one gait cycle.

(Data from Perry.[4])

Appendix 2-3
Diagnoses in Alphabetical Order

ICD Code	Description
781.2	Abnormal gait: ataxi, patalytic, spastic
845.09	Achilles tendon, torn or surgically repaired
717.83	Anterior cruciate ligament deficiency
718.47	Ankle contraction
845	Ankle sprains and strains of ankle and foot
344.89	Brown-Séquards syndrome
736.76	Calcaneal foot
736.76	Calcaneal valgus/varus
343.9	Cerebral palsy—spastic
333.7	Cerebral palsy—athetoid or dystonic
343	Cerebral palsy—diplegic, paraplegic
343.1	Cerebral palsy—hemiplegic
331.89	Cerebral vascular disease—ataxia
437.8	Cerebral vascular disease—quadriplegia
356.1	Charcot-Marie-Tooth dystrophy
717.7	Chondromalacia, patella
736.71	Clubfoot
736.71	Clubfoot, acquired
754.7	Clubfoot, congenital
736.71	Clubfoot, paralytic
996.4	Complications of hip prosthesis
754.3	Congenital dislocation of hip
718.4	Contraction of a joint
742.3	Dandy-Walker
736.7	Deformity ankle, acquired

ICD Code	Description
718.47	Deformity, ankle joint contraction, contracture
718.47	Deformity, ankle joint, abduction
736.9	Deformity, lower extremity, acquired
835	Dislocation of hip
836	Dislocation of knee
718.36	Displacement in knee joint that is due to ligament or structural deficiency
728.3	Edema
823.2	Fibula with tibia
342	Flaccid hemiplegia and hemiparesis
342	Flaccid hemiplegia and hemiparesis, unspecified side
718.47	Foot contraction
736.7	Foot deformity, acquired
736.75	Foot deformity, cavovarus
736.79	Foot deformity, valgus, acquired
736.79	Foot deformity, varus, acquired
824	Fracture, ankle
825	Fracture, calcaneus, closed
821.01	Fracture, femur, shaft
823.1	Fracture, fibula alone
825.2	Fracture, foot
822	Fracture, patella
823	Fracture, tibia alone
823	Fracture, tibia and fibula
736.5	Genu recurvatum

ICD Code	Description
736.41	Genu valgum
736.42	Genu varum
357	Guillan-Barré syndrome
854.6	Head trauma with loss of consciousness
342	Hemiplegia and hemiparesis
436	Hemiplegia, cerebrovascular accident
438	Hemiplegia, late effect
718.45	Hip contraction
V43.64	Hip joint replacement status
718.87	Hyperextension of midfoot
717	Internal derangement of knee
718.46	Knee contraction
718.86	Knee instability, inability to control flexion
V43.65	Knee joint replacement status
717.89	Knee sprain, old
844	Knee sprains and strains
736.89	Leg deformity, upper, lower, acquired
732.1	Legg-Calvé-Perthes disease
728.4	Ligament laxity
733.8	Malunion and nonunion of fracture
344.3	Monoplegia of lower limb
340	Multiple sclerosis
359.1	Muscular dystrophy, Duchenne syndrome, Becker's nevus
717	Old bucket handle tear of medial meniscus
715.7	Osteoarthritis, ankle, foot, tarsals, and metatarsals
715.5	Osteoarthritis, femur and hip
715.6	Osteoarthritis, tibia, fibula, knee, or patella
730.17	Osteomyelitis—ankle/foot
730.15	Osteomyelitis—femur
730.16	Osteomyelitis—tibia/fibula
733	Osteoporosis
344.09	Other quadriplegia
342.8	Other specified hemiplegia/paresis
355.8	Paralysis, thigh
344.1	Paraplegia

ICD Code	Description
782	Paresthesia, lower limb, Berger's disease
443.9	Peripheral vascular disease
355.356	Peripheral neuropathic disorders
V12.02	Personal history of poliomyelitis
736.73	Pes cavus
736.72	Pes equinua
734	Pes planus
138	Poliomyelitis (sequelae), late effects
45.1	Poliomyelitis, acute
736.79	Pronation, excessive or maltimed
733.82	Pseudo arthrosis
344	Quadriplegia and quadriparesis
344.01	Quadriplegia, C1–C4, complete
344.02	Quadriplegia, C1–C4, incomplete
344.03	Quadriplegia, C5–C7, complete
344.04	Quadriplegia, C5–C7, incomplete
344	Quadriplegia, unspecified
714	Rheumatoid arthritis
727.81	Short achilles tendon, acquired
342.1	Spastic hemiplegia and hemiparesis
741.9	Spina bifida
952	Spinal cord injury
736.79	Supination, excessive or maltimed
754.51	Talipes equiovarus, congenital
750.5	Talipes varus, congenital
726	Tendonitis—tenosynovitis
785.4	Ulcer with gangrene
250.8	Ulcer, diabetes mellitus, lower limb
707.1	Ulcer, foot
707.9	Ulcers, with gangrene
736.81	Unequal leg length, acquired, unspecified duration
342.91	Unspecified hemiplegia/paresis, dominant side
342.92	Unspecified hemiplegia/paresis, nondominant side
342.9	Unspecified hemiplegia/paresis, unspecified side
V49.60	Unspecified level upper limb amputation
754.5	Varus deformities of feet, congenital

Foot Orthoses and Prescription Shoes

3

Dennis J. Janisse
Jacqueline J. Wertsch
David R. Del Toro

The foot is a key element in aligning the joints of the lower limb to achieve a normal gait pattern. Shoes and foot orthoses can affect many aspects of gait, such as the pattern of plantar weight loading, stride length, knee flexion, and degree of lumbar lordosis. Shoes and foot orthoses therefore play a major role by modifying or correcting pathologic foot conditions that may affect gait.

Foot disorders can affect all the more proximal joints of the lower limb. Unlike orthoses that apply forces and moments directly to proximal joints, corrective shoes and foot orthoses work by realigning the ground reaction force. If the patient has a mobile foot with malalignment or correctable deformity, the foot should be placed in its optimal functioning position. Fundamentally, this requires holding the subtalar and midtarsal joints in neutral position with rigid or semirigid materials. This principle is mainly applied in children's footwear. In contrast, a rigid foot with fixed deformities requires realignment of a shoe's plantar surface to achieve an effective foot rollover during stance. An additional aim with the rigid foot must be to mold the shoe and the orthosis to allow for deformity, to redistribute plantar pressure, and to relieve dorsal pressure.[1]

Foot disorders are generally poorly understood by health professionals. Unfortunately, practitioners who have little understanding of the functions of the foot usually order "shoe inserts" for patients. Often only by trial and error does the person suffering from a foot disorder arrive at a reasonably satisfactory solution.

The aim of this chapter is to improve the prescription of shoes and foot orthoses. First we summarize information on the biomechanics of the foot. This is followed by a description of shoes and foot orthoses in common use. Finally, Table 3-1 lists choices of shoes, shoe modifications, and orthoses with comments on their functional effects for specific clinical conditions.

PRINCIPLES OF FOOT BIOMECHANICS

Foot biomechanics is defined as the study of the forces acting on the various anatomic structures of the foot, including bones, joints, ligaments, tendons, and muscles and the effects of these forces.[2] The anatomic components of the foot must act in a coordinated manner because the foot is the body's primary direct mechanism for weightbearing, shock absorption, and propulsion. In addition, the foot provides traction during movement, adapts to uneven surfaces, and helps to maintain balance.

Biomechanically, a normal foot should adequately distribute and absorb multiple forces (including compressive, shear, tensile, and rotatory) in standing and during the stance phase of gait.[2] If the force distribution or shock absorption is inadequate, then skin breakdown can occur over those areas of the foot subject to excessive forces.

Knowledge of the basic anatomy of the foot is a prerequisite before one can understand biomechanics of the foot in standing and during gait. Anatomically and func-

tionally, the foot is divided into three parts: hindfoot, midfoot, and forefoot. The hindfoot consists of the talus and calcaneus, and one of its primary functions is to convert the torque of the lower leg.[3] Specifically, the subtalar joint, which is the joint between the talus and the calcaneus, converts transverse rotatory forces of the lower leg and then dictates subsequent movements of the midfoot and forefoot.[2] The subtalar joint acts as a hinge by functionally connecting the lower leg to the midfoot and forefoot (Fig. 3-1).[4] Thus, the movements and functions of the midfoot and forefoot to a large degree depend on the biomechanics of the hindfoot. The midfoot consists of the navicular, cuboid, and three cu-

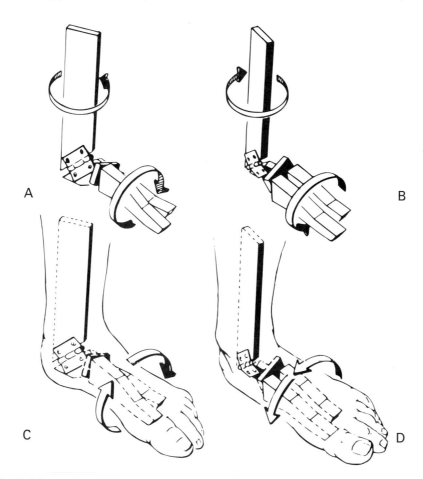

Fig. 3-1. **(A–D)** Schema of the mechanism by which rotation of tibia is transmitted through the subtalar joint into the foot. In Fig. A, the outward rotation of the upper stick results in inward rotation of the lower stick; thus, outward rotation of the tibia causes inward rotation of calcaneus and subsequent elevation of the medial border of the foot and depression of the lateral border of the foot, as seen in Fig. C. In Fig. B, inward rotation of the upper stick results in outward rotation of calcaneus and depression of medial side of border of foot and elevation of lateral border of foot, as seen in Fig. D. (From Mann,[4] with permission.)

neiform bones; it transmits movement from the hindfoot to the forefoot and is involved with promoting stability of the foot.[2] The forefoot includes the metatarsals and phalanges. Its primary functions include helping the foot adjust to uneven surfaces and adapting to uneven terrain.[2]

Examining both the static force distribution of the plantar surface of the foot during stance and the dynamic changes that occur during gait is important when trying to understand the biomechanics of the foot. In one study of weight distribution during barefoot standing, the heel accounted for approximately 60 percent, the toes less than 4 percent, the midfoot 8 percent, and the metatarsals 28 percent.[5] Forefoot peak pressures were most often found under the heads of the second or third metatarsals (not the first metatarsal), and no significant relationship between body weight and peak plantar pressure was noted.[5] During gait, plantar weight distribution changes throughout stance phase and depends on many factors including stride length, cadence, and whether the subject is wearing shoes.[6–10]

At the beginning of stance phase of the gait cycle, the tibia internally rotates, which then causes eversion of the hindfoot with eventual translation of this rotational force into pronation of the foot. Pronation is a complex triplanar movement of the foot consisting of abduction (transverse plane), dorsiflexion (saggital plane), and eversion (frontal plane) with the force conversion occurring at the subtalar joint of the hindfoot.[2] Pronation of the subtalar joint gives flexibility to the foot.[3] Thus, this suppleness of the foot during early stance phase allows for shock absorption, torque conversion, adjustment to various terrains, and maintaining balance.[2] During the end of stance phase when the tibia is externally rotating, inversion of the hindfoot with subsequent supination of the foot occur. This supination is a complex triplanar movement of the foot combining adduction, plantar flexion, and inversion with conversion of the rotational forces occurring at the subtalar joint.[2] Supination of the foot at the subtalar joint allows the foot to function as a rigid lever at the end of stance phase near toe-off.[2] This rigid lever function of the foot allows for propulsion and for muscle pulleys to be established around the tarsal bones, which by changing the direction of muscle pull, can increase the efficiency of muscle function across the foot and ankle.[2] This rigid lever function, also called the "windlass" effect, is created by the plantar fascia (origin at the medial aspect of the calcaneus and insertion into the base of the proximal phalanges) because the collagen fibers within the plantar fascia tend to resist tensile forces and progressively stiffen with increasing loads. This increased loading occurs when the metatarsophalangeal joints are dorsiflexed during toe-off at the end of stance phase.

In summary, the subtalar joint transmits rotational forces from the lower leg to the foot with the foot being flexible at the beginning of stance phase but converting to a rigid body near the end of stance. Another feature of foot biomechanics during gait is that the midfoot essentially moves as one unit, and its rotational movements allow the forefoot to rotate on the hindfoot. In the forefoot during gait, normal motion and stability depend on good mobility of the metatarsophalangeal and interphalangeal joints and stable metatarsals.

An understanding of the above basic principles of foot biomechanics is necessary when considering various types of prescription shoes and foot orthoses. The primary concepts behind foot orthotic prescription are that rigid feet need less control but more shock-absorbing materials, whereas feet that are relatively flexible need materials that provide more rigid control to improve stability and function.

Many professionals are knowledgeable in shoe fitting and foot orthoses. However, complex problems are best managed by a certified pedorthist. Pedorthics is the field that encompasses the knowledge and expertise in shoe fitting and shoe corrections including external shoe modifications and foot orthoses.[11,12] The Board for Certification in Pedorthics (BCP) tests and certifies the pedorthic profession.[11] The Pedorthic Footwear Association's (PFA) primary goal is education provided though university courses, regional seminars, and topic-specific annual symposiums and is open to anyone interested in footwear and footcare. The two organizations (BCP and PFA) work together to expand and share the conservative footcare knowledge of pedorthics.

SHOES

Shoe Components

The upper of the shoe is divided into the toe box, the vamp (the part of the upper that covers the instep), the throat (where the vamp meets the tongue at the begin-

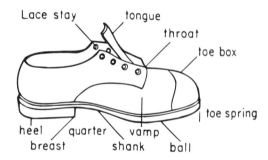

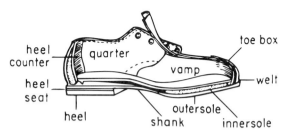

Fig. 3-2. Shoe components. (From Ragnarsson,[13] with permission.)

The Last

The shape of a shoe depends primarily on the *last*, which is the three-dimensional wooden or plastic form or mold over which the shoe is made. Lasts are created by and specific to each manufacturer.[14,15,19–21] No national standards have been established for shoe sizes. As a result, a size can vary greatly from manufacturer to manufacturer even with a similar last (Fig. 3-3). A standard last is used for many mass-produced shoes and usually comes in only limited sizes and two standard widths. In contrast, orthopedic lasts come in many sizes, widths, and shapes (inflare, outflare, short toed, and long toed).[14,19,20] The inflare last has an inward curvature of the anterior quarter and vamp sections and thus provides more medial forefoot surface area.[15,16] The outflare last has an outward curvature and thus would accommodate a more abducted foot. A combination last, which has the heel narrower than the forefoot is used in some mass-produced shoes and thus enhances heel fit. There is also the in-depth last, used for the so-called extra-depth shoes, which allows extra volume to accommodate generic or custom inserts. Extra-depth shoes are now very widely used for foot deformities. With improvements in materials and fitting of foot orthoses such shoes have largely replaced custom-molded varieties.

ning of the laces), and the counter (the part behind and around the heel)[13–17] (Fig. 3-2). The toe box needs to provide sufficient room for the metatarsal heads and the toes. The vamp is the part of the shoe that covers the instep. It needs to be high enough to accommodate the foot dorsum without pressure but tight enough to hold the shoe on. Laces provide day-to-day adjustability of the vamp. Pumps and slip-ons have very little vamp and thus require a snug fit to help keep the shoe on. The throat is the area at end of the lace stay. There are two types of throat opening; the balmoral, which is dressy but is not adjustable, and the blucher, which is the most common and usually preferred because it has greater adjustability, allows easy entry, and conforms more to foot shape.[16,18] The counter controls the heel and needs to be strong enough to control the foot within the shoe. If more medial support is needed, the counter may extend more distally on the medial aspect of the shoe (long medial counter). Soles are basically of two types: wedge or with a separate heel. To maintain the shape of the shoe, shoes with separate heels usually have a steel shank placed between the sole, and the shoe upper and extends from the heel to the midarch.

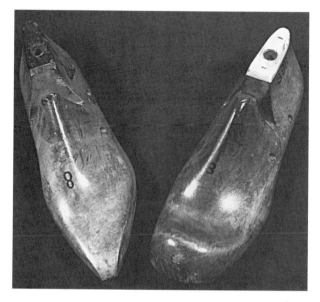

Fig. 3-3. Two lasts of the same size (size 8) that would produce shoes with dramatically different shapes.

Shoe Construction

Several methods are used to attach the upper parts of the shoe to the lower part. Common construction methods are Goodyear welt, cement lasted, slip lasted, stitch down, Little/McKay, and injection molded.[17] Athletic shoes often use cement-lasted construction, where glue is used to attach the outsole to the insole and upper with a thin layer of filler between the outsole and insole. For moccasins or deck shoes, the upper is fastened to the insole with staples, while the outsole is attached with either lock stitches (Littleway) or chain stitches (McKay). With injection molding, the outsole is a thermoplastic material, which is heat sealed to the upper and cools to become the shoe bottom. Injection molding, which uses no stitches, is probably the least expensive construction technique but is generally more difficult to modify. The Goodyear welt is the easiest type of shoe to use in attaching an ankle–foot orthosis (AFO). In the Goodyear welt, a flat narrow strip of leather (the welt) is chain stitched to the insole and upper. The outsole is then lock stitched to the welt, forming a strong, sturdy, but somewhat inflexible shoe. This type of construction usually provides less cushion in the sole compared to many of the cement- or injection-molded constructions.

Shoe Fitting

Shoe size can be very misleading and certainly does not ensure an adequate shoe fit. Early measurement systems used anatomic parts as standards: The "foot" was the length of a man's foot, the "inch" was the width of a thumb, the width of the hand across the knuckles was "4 inches," the span of the hand was "9 inches," and the "yard" was the length from shoulder to fingertips.[21] The legendary beginning of shoe sizes was in 1324, when King Edward II decreed that three barleycorns placed end to end equaled 1 inch and that each barleycorn (about $\frac{1}{3}$inch) would represent one full shoe size.[14,21] In 1688 Randle Holme published a shoe-sizing system in England that used $\frac{1}{4}$inch per size.[21] Then in 1856, a $\frac{1}{3}$-inch size scale was again introduced and reported in the British text, *The Illustrated Handbook of the Foot* by Robert Gardiner.[21] Edwin B. Simpson introduced a system in America in 1880 that added half sizes ($\frac{1}{6}$ inch) and proportional measurements that included length, ball width, waist, instep, and heel.[21] He also set up individual

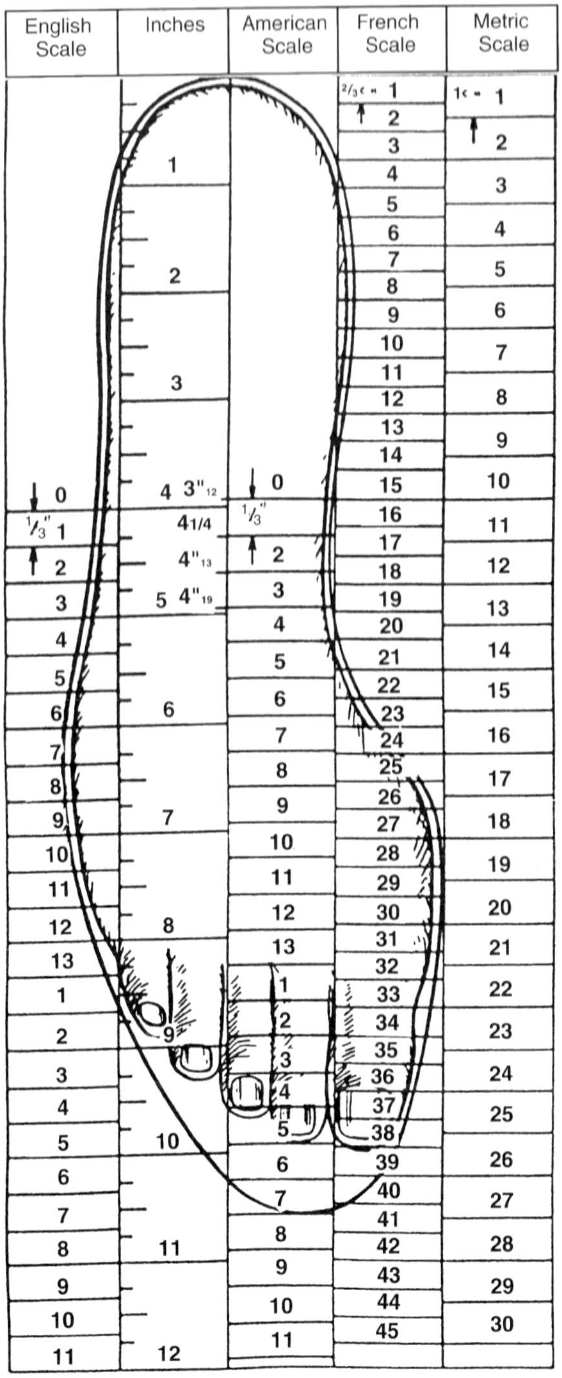

Fig. 3-4. American versus European shoe size scales. (From Rossi and Tennant,[21] with permission.)

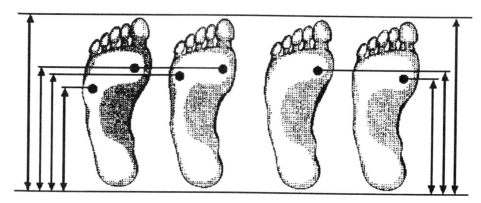

Fig. 3-5.   Four feet that are of the same length from heel to toe. Note that the two feet on the left have different lateral side and fifth metatarsal head measurements. The two feet on the right have different longitudinal arch and first metatarsal head measurements. Extreme care must be taken to choose a last that will accommodate each of these points. (From Prescription Footwear Association,[11] with permission.)

sizing systems for infants, children, women, and men. Simpson's system is still widely used today in America. In Great Britain, the English system is similar to the American system except each size is $\frac{1}{16}$ inch longer.[21] The Continental metric system uses 2/3 cm or 1 cm per size, and there are no half sizes (Fig. 3-4).[21] Widths and last shapes are not similar. Thus, translation in sizes is difficult, but a foot 10 inches long would approximately take a size 8 American and a size 41 Continental.[21]

Proper shoe fit is not defined by just length and width.[22] Fifteen key test points for fit have been defined: overall length, heel-to-ball, ball-to-toe, heel-to-outer-ball, ball width, heel fit, back of heel, quarter top edges, top lines, vamp room, tip of little toe, instep and waist, throat and throat line, arch fit, and tread.[21] Shoe shape is a key factor in fit; the shape not only of the sole but also of the upper.[14,18] Determination of the shoe length needs to consider arch length as much as foot length.[16] The arch length (heel to ball) measured from the heel to the first metatarsal represents where the foot is widest, but the location of the fifth metatarsal also needs to be considered.[11] The importance of accurate measurement of the location of the fifth metatarsal is illustrated in Figure 3-5. The Brannock device measures overall foot length, heel-to-ball length, and ball width.[18] The Brannock has a separate measurement scale and device for children, women, and men. The Ritz stick is a measuring device that generally only gives heel to toe length.

Foot measuring and shoe fitting should be done both nonweightbearing and weightbearing. Feet with greater flexibility can increase in size and width with weightbearing. Nonweightbearing measurements are also important to consider, especially in the patient with a flexible foot. In such a patient, functional foot orthoses would give a fit closer to the nonweightbearing measurement. The average foot will increase by a full size by the end of the day.[21] Vigorous exercise can result in an 8 percent increase in foot volume (which can represent as much as a 1½-size increase). Thus, it is important to consider the time of day and prior activity level when fitting a shoe. Both feet need to be measured, because most people have mismatched feet with one foot a half to a full size longer (70 percent of people), and with a difference in medial heel-to-ball length (75 percent), width across the metatarsal heads (60 percent), and heel width (66 percent).[22]

SHOE MODIFICATIONS

Upper Modifications

Possible modifications of the upper include lace stay extension, counter modification, toe box modification, and Velcro closure. Upper modifications are done to accommodate a variety of deformities such as hammer toes, Charcot joint deformities, severe hallux valgus, and severe edema. Such modifications may allow the patient to use less expensive extra-depth shoes rather than requiring custom shoes.

Modifying Shoes for Brace Attachment

Traditionally, leather sole with rubber heel shoes have been used for attaching metal orthoses. Many other types of shoes can be used, however, if the shoe is modified by adding a steel shank (either regular or extended) and an additional layer of sole (Fig. 3-6).

Extended Steel Shank

An extended steel shank is a strip of steel inserted between the layers of the sole all the way from the heel to the toe. Extended steel shanks are used to prevent the shoe from bending, to limit toe and midfoot motion, to aid propulsion on toe-off, and to strengthen the sole.[16,17,23] Specific indications for extended steel shanks may include painful hallux limitus or rigidus, limited ankle motion, midfoot arthritis, Charcot foot and partial foot amputations.[24,25] An extended steel shank is commonly used with a rocker sole when it is desired to minimize motion in joints of the foot.

Rocker Soles

The rocker sole is the most commonly prescribed external shoe modification.[16] The basic function of the rocker sole is to rock the foot from heel-strike to toe-off without bending the shoe.[26] If motion is lost in the foot and/or

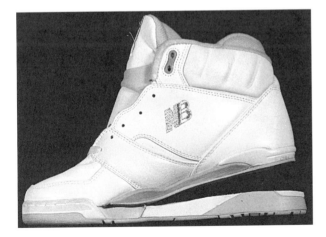

Fig. 3-6. A standard athletic shoe prepared for addition of a steel shank and attachment of an AFO.

ankle from stiffness, deformity, or pain, a rocker sole can be used to help biomechanically or functionally restore the lost motion. Rocker soles can also be used to help relieve plantar pressure on a specific area.[16] The shape of the rocker needs to be individualized to the patient's needs. Types of rockers soles include the mild rocker, toe-only, heel-to-toe, negative heel, and double rocker (Fig. 3-7).

The most widely used rocker sole has a mild rocker at both the heel and the toe (Fig. 3-7A) and is often used in athletic walking shoes. The mild rocker sole can relieve metatarsal pressure and may assist gait by increasing propulsion and reducing energy expenditure.[16] The toe-only rocker (Fig. 3-7B) is designed to increase the weight bearing proximal to the metatarsal heads, to provide stable midstance, and to reduce the need for toe dorsiflexion on toe-off. The toe-only rocker sole would be indicated in hallux rigidus, callus, ulcer on the distal portion of a claw toe, hammer toe, or mallet toe, and metatarsal ulcers.[16] The heel-to-toe rocker sole (Fig. 3-7C) is designed to aid propulsion at toe-off, decrease heel-strike forces on the calcaneus, and reduce the need for ankle motion.[16] The heel-to-toe rocker sole would be considered for patients with fixed claw toe or rigid hammertoe, midfoot amputation, or calcaneal ulcers. The negative heel rocker (Fig. 3-7D) is used to relieve forefoot pressure by shifting it to the midfoot and hindfoot.[16] It can also be used to accommodate a foot fixed in dorsiflexion. Caution is needed with negative heel rockers because sufficient ankle dorsiflexion range is needed to ensure that the desired biomechanical effect is achieved.[16] Some type of negative heel rocker may be used on "healing" shoes with the goal to virtually eliminate weight bearing on the metatarsal and toe areas. The double rocker sole (Fig. 3-7E) is similar to the mild rocker except that a section of sole is removed from the midfoot. This midfoot relief may be desired in patients with midfoot arthritis nodules, Charcot foot deformity, or a rocker bottom foot.[16]

Toe-only rocker sole (Fig. 3-7B)

Definition	This rocker sole has minimal rock on the heel but a very significant rock on the toe. When standing, the patient has a very broad stable base.
Function	Used to relieve metatarsal heads, joints and the toes.
L code	L3410
A code	A5503

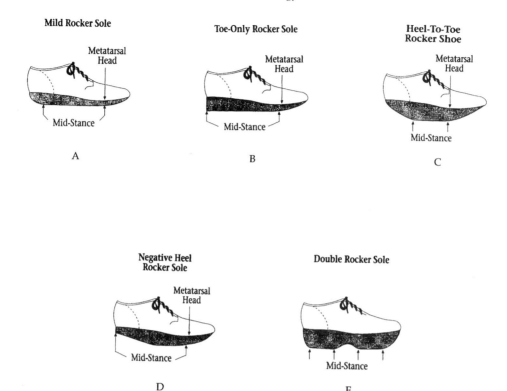

Fig. 3-7. **(A–E)** Types of rocker soles. (Adapted from Prescription Footwear Association,[11] with permission.)

Heel-to-toe rocker sole (Fig. 3-7C)

Definition — This rocker sole has a very significant rock on both the heel and the toe. When fabricating this rocker, some midstance is possible for stability while standing.

Function — Provides a very stable gait, aids in propulsion, and replaces lost or painful motion.

L code — L3410

A code — A5503

Negative heel rocker (Fig. 3-7D)

Definition — This rocker has a decreased heel height or no heel at all. Sometimes there may even be less thickness under the heel. Usually, rock is significant on the toe and minimal on the heel.

Function — Very effective for metatarsal relief as well as distal toe pressure relief.

It is also helpful when the patient feels unstable because of the height added to the shoe with the other types of rockers. A significant forefoot rock can be achieved without adding a lot of height. Because this rocker puts the foot into dorsiflexion, caution must be taken to check if there is sufficient range to accept the modification.

L code — L3410

A code — A5503

Double rocker sole (Fig. 3-7E)

Definition — This rocker sole has a moderate rock on the heel and the toe, but unlike the others, this modification has two rockers distal and proximal, creating a type of relief in the midfoot portion of the shoe.

Function | This rocker sole is useful in relieving pressure on midfoot prominences while still providing a smooth comfortable gait. Indications may include midfoot arthritis nodules and prominences or rocker-bottom Charcot feet.

L code | L3410

A code | A5503

Flares[16] (Fig. 3-8)

Definition | A flare is a medial or lateral extension of either the heel and or the sole. Flares broaden the plantar surface of the foot.

Function | Flares can be used for stabilization and support of the hindfoot, midfoot, or forefoot.

L code | L3390

A code | A5507

Wedges (Fig. 3-9)

Definition | A wedge is a strip of leather or other material thicker on one side than the other. It can be either inserted between the heel or sole and the upper or attached externally on the shoe.

Function | Wedges are used to redistribute weight or change alignment. Wedges are ineffective on rigid deformities.

L code | Heel L3340, sole L3360

A code | Heel A5504, sole A5504

Extensions

Definition | An addition of material to the sole and heel, also called *lifts* or *elevations.*

Function | Extensions compensate for a leg length discrepancy. Because adding material increases the rigidity of the shoe, some motion must be built in by use of rocker sole.

L code | L3310

A code | No designated code

Extended steel shanks

Definition | A piece of spring steel extending from the heel to the toe inserted between the sole and the shoe or imbedded in the sole.

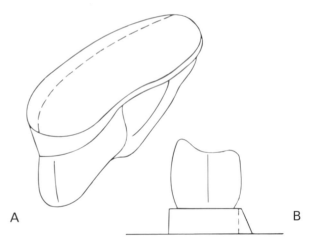

Fig. 3-8. Lateral flare viewed from **(A)** plantar view and **(B)** posterior view. (From Janisse,[16] with permission.)

Function | Limits toe and midfoot motion and prevents the shoe from bending. It is most commonly used with rocker soles.

L code | L2360

A code | No designated code

Cushion Heels (Fig. 3-10)

Definition | A wedge of solid ankle cushion heel (SACH) or similar material placed in the heel of the shoe. It can be placed in any type of sole

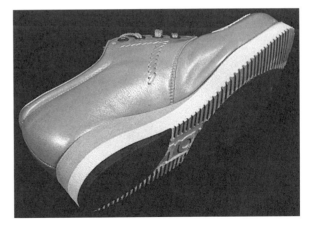

Fig. 3-9. Wedges can be added to the heel and/or the sole.

	and heel (i.e., leather, rubber, crepe, eva, etc.)
Function	Absorbs shock on heel strike during gait yet maintains stability when standing.
L code	L3450
A code	No designated code

CUSTOM-MADE SHOES

A custom-made shoe is constructed from a cast or model of the patient's foot and is used when a standard shoe cannot accommodate one or both feet for various reasons. A primary indication for fitting a custom-made shoe is when a severe bony foot deformity prohibits the use of an in-depth shoe despite extensive shoe modifications. Clinical conditions that might require custom-made shoes include severe Charcot or rheumatoid foot deformities and some partial foot amputations. Another example is when a patient requires a muscle flap to cover a large or unusual soft tissue foot defect, which then would be too bulky to be accommodated by an in-depth shoe. Also, for cosmetic purposes, custom-made shoes are sometimes used to incorporate an extensive modification. For instance, in a patient with significant leg length discrepancy, the custom-made shoe can have a built-in large shoe extension rather than simply adding it on the bottom of an in-depth shoe, which would be more noticeable.

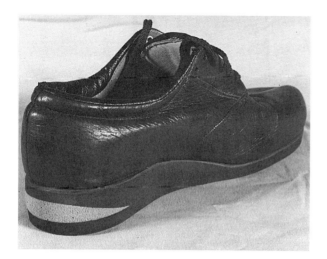

Fig. 3-10.   Solid ankle cushion heel (SACH).

FOOT ORTHOTICS

By definition, *foot orthotics* is the measurement and fabrication of devices inserted into shoes to modify foot alignment or pressure. *Foot orthoses* are the devices that insert into the shoes. The distinction is important because many sports trainers, advertisers, and even some allied health personnel call all shoe inserts "orthotics" instead of "foot orthoses."

Many types of foot orthoses are not custom fitted, including various pads of cushioning material such as Spenco. However, this chapter reviews only those that are shaped or molded to the foot in the same way that most limb orthoses are now fabricated.

Total Contact Concept

Total contact orthotic insoles assist the impaired foot in a number of ways but ultimately must help in shock absorption and force dissipation or distribution by controlling excessive movements of the foot. The total contact foot orthosis (FO), sometimes referred to as a total-contact insert, employs the same principle as the total contact cast and is manufactured over a positive model of the foot. There are several components to the total contact concept. First, areas of excessive plantar pressure can be relieved by evenly distributing the pressure over the entire plantar surface.[27] This is done to reduce the possibility of ulceration occurring over high-pressure areas. Second, shock absorbing materials are often used in a total contact FO to decrease the overall amount of pressure on the entire plantar aspect of the foot, especially in a foot with a Charcot joint or a bony prominence on the plantar surface. A third way a total contact FO minimizes ulceration, callus formation, or pain is to decrease the amount of horizontal movement within the shoe that results in reduction of shear forces.

The total contact or functional FO made with soft or semirigid materials can be used to accommodate a fixed deformity, such as a rheumatoid arthritic foot of Charcot joint. In addition, a relatively fixed or rigid deformity can be stabilized with a functional FO through the use of more rigid and supportive materials. A functional FO may assist in controlling a flexible deformity by supporting and stabilizing the deformed foot, thus decreasing progression of the deformity. Finally, through the use of rigid supportive materials a functional FO can limit joint motion in the foot, adding further stability, decreasing inflammation, and relieving pain.

Types of Foot Orthoses

Total contact FOs are made of materials with varying densities depending on whether they are soft, semirigid, or rigid FOs. Most total contact FOs are custom made for each foot, and there are several basic types. Many FOs can be fit in conventional shoes, especially the sports and running shoes widely worn today, but many are designed to fit inside an extra-depth shoe when the deformity is too severe to fit in conventional shoes. A full-length FO, which extends from the posterior end of the heel to the end of the toes, allows the foot to be more plantigrade and supports the entire plantar aspect of the foot.[11] A three-quarter FO extends from the posterior end of the heel and ends distal to the metatarsal heads or at the sulcus of the foot.[28] A metatarsal-length FO ends immediately proximal to the metatarsal heads.[28]

The UCBL orthosis, named for the University of California at Berkeley Laboratory, is made of rigid materials and is used for a flexible (or mobile) foot to stabilize hindfoot in a neutral position between inversion and eversion.[11] This type of FO functions by changing the line of action of the ground reaction force to realign anatomic joints into their optimum functioning positions.[29] In adults, the UCBL orthosis is used to support or maintain the position of the foot to decrease pain in conditions such as posterior tibial tendinitis or midfoot arthritis. In children, especially those with spastic cerebral palsy, the UCBL orthosis is used to maintain stability of the midfoot and hindfoot. For more discussion of its function, see Chapter 2 and Figure 2-2.

Materials

The materials used for the FO can be either soft (accommodative) or rigid (functional). Accommodative inserts can be made from either heat-moldable or nonmoldable materials. Most of the heat-moldable foot orthoses are cross-linked polyethylene foams; the nonmoldable materials are either microcellular rubber or polyurethane foams. The ideal would be a combination of both because the heat-moldable materials provide the full contact but will "bottom out" over time, whereas the nonmoldable materials will maintain the shock absorption and provide support.[30] Functional FOs require more rigid materials such as leather, cork, acrylic plastics, and thermoplastic polymers to control foot positioning.

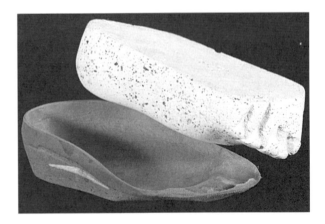

Fig. 3-11. Casting insert. A positive plaster model of the foot is made from an impression.

Casting and Fabrication Techniques

The total contact FO is made from a model (or positive mold) of the patient's foot. Initially, an impression of the foot is made; then the impression is filled with plaster to create a positive model or cast. The orthotic materials are then molded over the model with a vacuum-forming technique (Fig. 3-11). The impression can be either weightbearing or semiweightbearing. Weightbearing is used when the desired FO is to be an accommodative device or when the patient has a rigid-type deformity. The FO is created with semiweightbearing when there is a flexible foot or a flexible deformity and the FO needs to supply either support or stability.

Four different techniques are employed when taking the impression: plaster bandages, foam boxes, wax, and sand/wax. Although each practitioner may have personal preferences, some general guidelines indicate which technique might be preferred. Plaster casts are often used if many details are desired, such as a custom shoe cast and for complicated fractures or amputations. Plaster is often used for nonweightbearing prone casting, which may be the impression technique preferred for rigid functional devices. The foam box is technically the easiest, but has a disadvantage because the practitioner lacks control. The practitioner has less control of further manual custom molding of the orthosis because the patient's foot impression is fairly complete after their foot is removed from the foam box. Thus, the foam box technique might be preferred when manufacturing an accommodative FO for a more rigid deformity as compared to a functional FO, which is indicated for a flexible deformity. The wax technique is often used when correction is necessary, because there is better control of the foot while taking the impression. Thus, the wax technique is often preferred for a flexible, mobile foot. A sand/wax technique uses a softened piece of wax on top of a bed of silica sand. The wax on top of the sand allows compression of fatty tissues and makes it easier to identify the bony prominences. The sand/wax technique is used for intricate plantar surface deformities such as rheumatoid arthritis, diabetic deformities, plantar fibromatosis, and so on.

After the impression is taken, it is filled with molding plaster to create the positive mold of the foot. Modifications of the positive mold may be done for specific objectives such as metatarsal relief, relief for bony prominences, or for forefoot or hindfoot posting, which is wedging of the orthoses to change alignment of the foot in its frontal plane. A post is a wedge on the medial or lateral side of the FO that is designed to support or control movement.[2] The heat moldable materials are vacuum formed over the positive mold in numerous layers. Nonmoldable materials are incorporated as prescribed.

Metatarsal Pad Versus Metatarsal Bar

Metatarsal pads are available in a variety of sizes, shapes, and materials and can accommodate a number of foot disorders. A metatarsal pad is fitted inside the shoe just proximal to the metatarsal head and helps to realign the

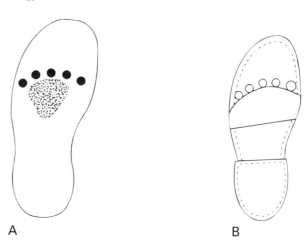

Fig. 3-12. **(A)** Metatarsal pad. **(B)** Metatarsal bar. Note that both are placed proximal to the metatarsal heads.

prominent metatarsal head by applying a corrective force under the affected metatarsal shaft.[29] Thus, the metatarsal pad redistributes the weight from the metatarsal head to the shaft[11] and functions to reduce pain and pressure under the affected metatarsal head. A metatarsal bar is a piece of material, usually leather or rubber, that is attached transversely across the outer sole of a shoe immediately proximal to the metatarsal heads to relieve pressure and reduce pain.[13] A metatarsal bar is used when pressure relief and/or pain reduction is needed below more than one metatarsal head as compared to a metatarsal pad, which is used for just one metatarsal head. Both a metatarsal pad and a metatarsal bar are shown in Figure 3-12.

Table 3-1. The Most Common Foot Disorders and Prescription Choices

Clinical Condition/ ICD No.	Shoes	Shoe Modifications	Orthotic Considerations	Comments
Achilles tendinitis 726.71	Shoe with removable insert and extended medial counter	Cushion heel Heel extension	Total contact FO	Heel extension may be added to total contact FO or may be removable Gradually decrease heel extension as tendinitis improves

Continues

Table 3-1 *(Continued)*

Clinical Condition/ ICD No.	Shoes	Shoe Modifications	Orthotic Considerations	Comments
Ankle Fusion 718.57	Shoe with removable insert and cushioned sole	Rocker sole Extended steel shank Medial and/or lateral flares Cushion heel	Total contact FO	Evaluate degree of ankle fusion before shoe prescription to determine correct heel height
Charcot deformities 713.5 Diabetic 250.6	Extra-depth shoe Possibly use a heat-moldable shoe May need custom-made shoe or sandal Stretching for pressure relief	Rocker sole Extended steel shank Possible SACH heel Medial or lateral flares Upper modifications may be needed	Total contact FO	Flexible vs. fixed deformities need to be managed differently Very important to educate patient to observe for areas of increased pressure
Diabetic foot at risk 250.6	Type of shoe not as important as the proper fit	Stretching for pressure relief	Protective FO	Very important to educate patient about proper shoe selection and to watch for pressure areas
Diabetic foot with active ulcer 250.8	Negative-heel shoe Total contact sandal			Total contact casting often preferred Frequent monitoring of healing because modifications may be needed
Diabetic foot with healed ulcer 250.6	Extra-depth shoe Possibly use a heat-moldable shoe Custom total-contact sandal	Rocker sole Extended steel shank Possible SACH heel	Total contact FO	Initial weekly monitoring because modifications may be needed
Diabetic foot with autonomic deficits	Socks that breathe			
Diabetic partial foot amputation or partial foot amputation 896	May need high-top shoe Possibly use a heat-moldable shoe	Rocker sole Extended steel shank Possible SACH heel Medial or lateral flares	Partial foot FO	Changes in plantar loading and kinetics Remaining foot needs to be protected
Hallux rigidus 735	Shoe with removable insert	Rocker sole Extended steel shank	Total contact FO Metatarsal pad or bar	Total contact FO could be made of rigid polymer to eliminate need for extended steel shank
Hallux valgus 735	Extra-depth shoe Stretching for pressure relief Last with prominent medial flare	Upper modifications may be needed Rocker sole Extended steel shank Medial heel wedge	Total contact FO Metatarsal pad or bar	Total contact FO to decrease pressure, reduce pronation, and deformity

Continues

Table 3-1 *(Continued)*

Clinical Condition/ ICD No.	Shoes	Shoe Modifications	Orthotic Considerations	Comments
Hallux varus 735.1	Extra-depth shoe with oblique toe Stretching for pressure relief Heat-moldable shoe	Upper modifications may be needed Rocker sole Extended steel shank	Total contact FO Metatarsal pad or bar	May need custom shoe if deformity is extremely prominent or too rigid
Hammer toes/claw toes 735.4 735.5	Extra-depth shoe Stretching for pressure relief Heat-moldable shoe	Upper modifications may be needed Rocker sole Extended steel shank	Total contact FO Metatarsal pad or bar	Must determine whether flexible vs. rigid deformity (orthosis may be different) Evaluate plantar pressures on ends of toes
Heel pain syndrome (central) Spur 726.73	Extra-depth shoe with removable insert and cushioned sole	Cushion heel	Total contact FO Heel cup ± cushion	
Interdigital neuroma 355.6	Last that accommodates width of forefoot	Rocker sole Extended steel shank	Total contact FO Metatarsal pad or bar	Metatarsal relief should be provided only for MT heads adjacent to neuroma
Metatarsalgia 726.7	Shoe with removable insert	Rocker sole Extended steel shank	Total contact or ¾-length FO Metatarsal pad or bar	May not need extra depth shoe if ¾-length FO used
MTP hyperextension injury or "turf toe" 735.8	Shoe with removable insert	Rocker sole Extended steel shank	Total contact FO	Total contact FO could be made of rigid polymer to eliminate need for extended steel shank
Paraplegia 344.1	Extra-depth shoe with extended blucher opening	Upper modifications may be needed May need to modify shoe for brace attachment Extended steel shank	Tone-reducing total contact FO	Total contact FO also provides plantar pressure relief
Pes cavus 736.73	Proper shoe fit Strong counter Shoe with removable insert	Lateral heel wedge Lateral flare Rocker sole SACH heel	Total contact FO Metatarsal pad or bar	Further shoe considerations if hammer/claw toes present Need to distinguish three types of pes cavus: global, calcaneal cavus, forefoot valgus
Pes planus 734	Proper shoe fit Long medial counter Shoe with removable insert	Medial heel wedge Medial flare	Total contact FO	Important to distinguish flexible vs. rigid pes planus Accommodate rigid deformity Control flexible deformity
Plantar fasciitis 728.71	Extra-depth shoe with extended medial counter	Medial heel wedge Cushion heel	Total contact FO UCBL orthosis Heel cup	May need to modify shoe or FO to provide pressure relief for plantar fascia attachment

Continues

Table 3-1 *(Continued)*

Clinical Condition/ ICD No.	Shoes	Shoe Modifications	Orthotic Considerations	Comments
Posterior tibialis tendon rupture or tendinitis 726.72	Extra-depth shoe with extended medial counter	Medial heel wedge Medial heel flare	Total contact FO UCBL orthosis	May need to modify medial aspect of orthosis to provide pressure relief for posterior tibial nerve
Rheumatoid arthritic foot 714	Extra-depth shoe Possibly use a heat-moldable shoe Stretching for pressure relief	Rocker sole Extended steel shank Possible SACH heel Medial or lateral flares Upper modifications may be needed Wedges	Total contact FO MT pads or bar Viscoelastic polymer relief	Weekly monitoring may be needed initially to ensure that relief is in correct place Due to the ongoing changes of the foot, adjustments may be needed periodically Very important to educate patient to observe for areas of increased pressure
Subtalar arthritis 716.7	Extra-depth shoe with extended medial counter	Rocker sole Extended steel shank Medial and/or lateral flares Cushion heel	Total contact FO UCBL orthosis	
Posterior tarsal tunnel syndrome	Extra-depth shoe with extended medial counter	Medial heel wedge Medial heel flare	Total contact FO UCBL orthosis	May need to modify medial aspect of orthosis to provide pressure relief for tendon

Abbreviations: ICD, International Classification of Disease; FO, foot orthosis; MT, metatarsal; MTP, metatarsophalangeal; SACH, solid ankle cushion heel; UCBL, University of California at Berkeley Laboratory orthosis.

INDICATIONS FOR PRESCRIPTION OF SHOES AND FOOT ORTHOSES

In Table 3-1, the most common disorders of the foot are listed, followed by choices for prescription.

REFERENCES

1. Pratt D, Tollafield D, Johnson G, Peacock C: Foot orthoses: p. 25. In Bowker P, Condie DN, Bader DL, Pratt DJ (eds): Biomechanical Basis of Orthotic Management. Butterworth-Heinemann, Oxford, England, 1993
2. Donatelli R: Normal anatomy and biomechanics. p. 3. In: The Biomechanics of the Foot and Ankle. FA Davis, Philadelphia, 1990
3. Chan CW, Rudins A: Foot biomechanics during walking and running. Mayo Clinic Proc 69:448, 1994
4. Mann RA: Biomechanics of the foot. p. 257. In: American Academy of Orthopaedic Surgeons: Atlas of Orthotics: Biomechanical Principles and Applications. Mosby, St. Louis, 1975
5. Cavanaugh PR, Rodgers MM, Iiboshi A: Pressure distribution under symptom-free feet during barefoot standing. Foot Ankle 7:262, 1987
6. Soames RW: Foot pressure patterns during gait. J Biomed Eng 7:120, 1985
7. Soames RW, Richardson RPS: Stride length and cadences: their influence on ground reaction forces during gait. p. 406. In Winter DA, Norman RW, Wells RP et al (eds): Biomechanics IX-A, 5A. Human Kinetics, Champaign, IL, 1985
8. Jansen EC, Jansen KF: Vis-velocitas-via: alteration of foot-to-ground forces during increasing speed of gait. p. 267. In Asmussen E, Jorgensen K (eds): Biomechanics VI-A. University Park Press, Baltimore, 1978
9. Zhu H, Wertsch JJ, Harris GF et al: Foot pressure distribution during walking and shuffling. Arch Phys Med Rehabil 72: 390, 1991

10. Zhu H, Wertsch JJ, Harris GF et al: Sensate and insensate in-shoe plantar pressures. Arch Phys Med Rehabil 74:1362, 1993

11. Prescription Footwear Association: Directory of Pedorthics. Prescription Footwear Association/Board for Certification in Pedorthics, Columbia, MD, 1994–1995

12. Rossi WA: The high incidence of mismatched feet in the population. Foot Ankle 4:105, 1983

13. Ragnarsson KT: Orthotics and shoes. p. 494. In DeLisa JA (ed): Rehabilitation Medicine Principles and Practice. 2nd Ed. JB Lippincott, Philadelphia, 1993

14. Janisse DJ: The art and science of fitting shoes. Foot Ankle 13:257, 1992

15. McPoil TG: Footwear. Phys Ther 68:1857, 1988

16. Janisse DJ: Pedorthic care of the diabetic foot. p. 551. In Levin ME, O'Neal LW, Bowker JH (eds): The Diabetic Foot. 5th Ed. Mosby Yearbook, St. Louis, 1993

17. Janisse DJ: The shoe in rehabilitation of the foot and ankle. p. 4. In Sammarco GJ (ed): Rehabilitation of the Foot and Ankle. Mosby Yearbook, St. Louis, 1995

18. Zamosky I, Redford JB: Shoes and their modifications. p. 394. In Redford JB (ed): Orthotics Etcetera. 3rd Ed. Williams & Wilkins, Baltimore, 1986

19. Edwards CA: A Manual of Orthopedic Shoe Technology. Precision Printing, Muncie, IN, 1981

20. Steele R: History of shoe making. p. 1c. In Edwards CA (ed): Manual for Proprietors, Managers, and Assistants of Stores Dealing in Functional and Prescription Footwear. Ball State University, Muncie, IN, 1981

21. Rossi WA, Tennant R: Professional Shoe Fitting. National Shoe Retailers Association, New York, 1984

22. Rossi WA: The enigma of shoe sizes. J Am Podiatr Med Assoc 73:272, 1983

23. Bordelon RL: Orthotics, shoes, and braces. Orthop Clin North Am 20:751, 1989

24. Gould JS: Metatarsalgia. Orthop Clin North Am 20:553, 1989

25. Johnson JE, Janisse DJ, Kaczmarowski J: Modern pedorthic and orthotic management of complications of foot and ankle surgery. In Johnson JE, Gould JS, Brennan MJ (eds): Complications of Foot and Ankle Surgery. Williams & Wilkins, Baltimore, 1995

26. Janisse DJ: Indications and prescriptions for orthoses in sports. Orthop Clin North Am 25:95, 1994

27. Janisse DJ: A scientific approach to insole design for the diabetic foot. Foot 3:105, 1993

28. Wu KK: General considerations of foot orthoses. p. 99. In: Foot Orthoses: Principles and Clinical Applications. Williams & Wilkins, Baltimore, 1990

29. Pratt D, Tollafield D, Johnson G, Peacock C: Foot orthoses. p. 70. In Bowker P, Condie DN, Bader DL, Pratt DJ (eds): Biomechanical Basis of Orthotic Management. Butterworth-Heinemann, Oxford, England, 1993

30. Brodsky JW, Kourash S, Stills M et al: Objective evaluation of insert material for diabetic and athletic footwear. Foot Ankle 9:111, 1988

Spinal Orthoses

4

Mark Bussel
John Merritt
Laura Fenwick

Spinal orthoses have the longest history of any device applied to the body to protect or correct a musculoskeletal disorder. The main purpose of spinal orthoses is to immobilize the spine. A spinal orthosis may be employed for pain management, substitution for absent or weakened muscles or ligaments, fracture management, and reduction of deformity such as scoliosis. This chapter describes commonly used orthoses and includes the following information:

1. Nomenclature including generic names and eponyms
2. The L code for the orthosis
3. Indications and contraindications for use
4. Biomechanical function, or efficacy
5. Component parts
6. Measurements and/or impression techniques for fabrication and fitting parameters

Spinal and cervical orthoses are used for stable spinal injuries. The only exception to this rule is the halo cervicothoracic orthosis. Even the halo is rarely used without preceding traction or cervical fusion. A contraindication for all orthoses except the halo therefore is the presence of unstable spinal fractures. For such fractures, surgical stabilization is the only safe solution. A spinal orthosis is frequently used in addition to surgical stabilization.

Most orthoses are fabricated of metal or plastic. For any orthosis fabricated in metal, the common materials are aluminum or steel alloys. Where aluminum or steel contacts the body, it is padded and covered with leather or vinyl. Exposed bars that do not contact the body remain uncovered but should be rounded or beveled on their edges to avoid injury. Aluminum is chosen for its radiolucency and light weight. Steel is generally chosen when an orthosis will be subject to high external forces as in a lower limb orthosis or a scoliosis orthosis such as the Milwaukee-style cervicothoracolumbosacral orthosis (CTLSO).[1] Today, high-temperature thermoplastics are most commonly employed for the fabrication of all orthoses. Some orthoses are hybrids of metal and plastics. Thermoplastics are chosen, because they can be readily fabricated to effect an intimately fitting orthosis that is most comfortable, most cosmetic, and most functional from the standpoint of motion control. The Milwaukee-style CTLSO is a hybrid fabricated of aluminum, steel, and thermoplastics. When the materials are listed for the orthosis in the following descriptions, the reader is encouraged to consider the biomechanical rationale for the design.

BIOMECHANICAL FUNCTIONS

Biomechanical functions of spinal orthoses include the following:

1. Kinesthetic reminder
2. Increased intracavitary pressure
3. Three-point pressure systems
4. Counterpressures
5. End-point control
6. Distraction.[2,3]

These are defined as follows:

Kinesthetic reminder: The orthosis provides feedback through the sensory system that consciously or in some instances subconsciously causes the patient to adopt a more corrective or more appropriate position of the spine.

Increased intracavitary pressure: The orthosis assists the activity of trunk muscles. During forward flexion and in lifting, total contact orthoses increase pressure inside the body's interior cavities. This increased intracavity pressure transfers load from the intervertebral discs to the surrounding soft tissues and thus reduces the load borne on the involved spinal segments.

Three-point force system: The orthosis provides a force in one direction that is opposed but in equilibrium with two forces in the opposite direction at either end of the spinal segment. The opposing forces can be corrective or simply increase immobility in the segment involved.

Counter pressure: A term sometimes used to denote opposing forces that are necessary for motion control in the transverse plane.

End-point control: Applying spinal orthoses in such a way that collapse of the spinal column between opposite end points is resisted.

Distraction: Orthotic generation of longitudinal forces along the spine to distract underlying segments.

In the discussion of representative orthoses, the appropriate principles are further described and then simply listed when appropriate for other orthoses.

Unless otherwise specified, spinal orthoses are available as custom-fitted or custom-fabricated designs. Custom-fabricated designs require specific measurements or a plaster impression of the patient to make a system unique for that individual. A custom-fitted design is prefabricated in a limited number of choices designed to adequately fit a variety of body sizes. An orthotist certified by the American Board for Certification in Orthotics and Prosthetics is the professional best suited to custom fit or custom fabricate any orthosis. These practitioners have appropriate education and undergo a rigorous certification process that make them uniquely qualified to evaluate patients for, fabricate, fit, and modify orthoses for the spine and upper and lower limbs. No health professional works alone, however, and rehabilitation patients are best served by a well-coordinated team of professionals.

NOMENCLATURE

Nomenclature is of primary importance when discussing orthoses. The following listing is extracted from the Health Care Financing Administration Common Procedure Coding System.[4] The names used are those that are in that directory. However, more correct and descriptive terminology is available and will be included for each orthosis. The most scientific nomenclature uses the American Academy of Orthopedic Surgeons (AAOS) technical analysis form terminology. The AAOS created a task force in 1970 to investigate orthotics terminology, and the system they created is a generic rationale that considers two basic characteristics of any orthosis. These characteristics are (1) the area of the body encompassed by the orthosis and (2) the mechanical motion control the orthosis provides. This system was published in the *Atlas of Orthotics* in 1975.[5] The generic names available for spinal systems based on the area of the body encompassed are as follows:

CO	Cervical orthoses
CTO	Cervicothoracic orthoses
CTLSO	Cervicothoracolumbosacral orthoses
TLSO	Thoracolumbosacral orthoses
LSO	Lumbosacral orthoses
SO	Sacral orthoses
SIO	Sacroiliac orthoses

The motion control an orthosis provides is named by cardinal reference plane. For example, an orthosis appropriate for multiple traumatic fractures of the low thoracic and lumbar spine is a T L S O, Triplanar control because it limits motion in the sagittal, coronal, and transverse planes. If only a portion of the plane is controlled, that portion is listed. For example, the eponym Jewett Brace[6] is most scientifically named a TLSO, flexion control. For each orthosis, the plane of control and the control provided in that plane will be discussed using terms from the technical analysis form originally printed in the *Atlas of Orthotics.*[5]

Free: Free motion.
Assist: Application of an external force for the purpose of increasing the range, velocity, or force of a motion.
Resist: Application of an external force for the purpose of decreasing the velocity or force of a motion.
Stop: Inclusion of a static unit to deter an undesired motion in one direction.
Hold: Elimination of all motion in prescribed plane.
Variable: A unit that can be adjusted without making a structural change.[7]

To recommend a spinal orthosis, one must keep in mind the objectives for that orthosis. If the practitioner has clear knowledge of the patient's disability and clear knowledge of the biomechanics of orthoses, then the recommendation is a matter of matching the correct orthosis to the disability needing relief. Musculoskeletal disability encompasses the decrease in function resulting from osteologic, ligamentous, neurologic, or myologic injury. Functional assessment of a patient's disability is mandatory for appropriate spinal orthotic prescription. This functional assessment, completed by a physician, often in consultation with other rehabilitation professionals, is requisite to appropriate orthotic recommendation.

CRANIAL ORTHOSES

Helmet—Custom (L0100)
Helmet—Prefabricated (L0110)
Function
Helmets, or cranial orthoses, are used ultimately for protection of the brain. Protective helmets act as a rigid covering for the head to prevent injury. Cranial molding helmets serve as modeling devices for the head.

Indications
Protective helmets have commonly been used when a patient has an absent or surgically repaired portion of the skull.[8] A helmet might also be indicated when a patient shows massive uncontrolled movements or head banging[9,10] or has a history of head injury from such movements. When a child is born with a misshapen skull, helmets have been used to encourage normal modeling of the skull with growth.[11]

Fabrication and Fitting Parameters
To create a custom-fabricated helmet (L0100), an impression of the patient's head is required, the impression typically bounded by the patient's hairline. The orthosis is then fitted in this area. If necessary, the orthosis may not be total contact, as in cranial molding. Protective helmets can be prefabricated and available in a number of sizes based on the circumference of the head at the equator.

Materials
The orthosis is fabricated from a high-temperature polymer. The orthosis is typically fully lined with foam padding to cushion any blows received while wearing the helmet.

Contraindications
Psychosocial issues have been raised from the long-term use of helmets.[8] Further, dermatologic conditions or conditions of the scalp may be irritated by the heat caused from wearing a helmet.

CERVICAL/CERVICOTHORACIC

Soft Foam Cervical Collar (L0120)
Biomechanical Efficacy
The soft collar provides no-control of motion in the cervical spine[12] but does provide a kinesthetic reminder to limit motion.[13] Increasing a patient's awareness of an injured area through contact on the skin may remind the patient to self-restrict motion of the involved area. This increased kinesthetic awareness is thought to contribute to the comfort felt by patients wearing the soft collar as well as many soft spinal orthoses. The orthosis

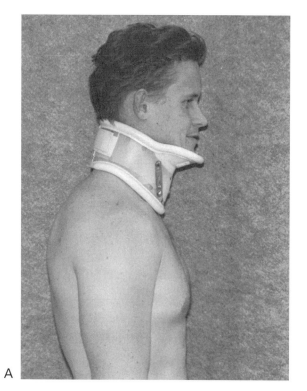
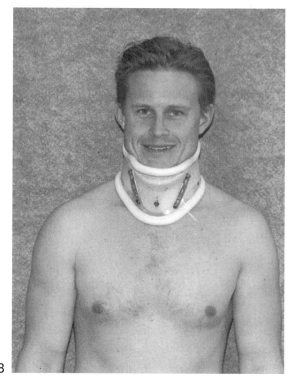

A   B

Fig. 4-1. **(A & B)** Plastic collar with height adjustability.

also provides warmth to the injured area, which may further contribute to the comfort felt when it is worn.

Indications
A soft cervical orthosis is indicated for soft tissue injuries of the neck, such as muscle strain that is due to whiplash-type injuries.

Contraindications
Because this orthosis provides no control of motion, it is contraindicated in the presence of ligamentous or bony injury to the neck.

Fitting Parameters
The orthosis is sized using circumference of the neck. The height is standard at 3 inches, but orthoses are also available from $2\frac{1}{2}$ to $4\frac{1}{2}$ inches in height in $\frac{1}{2}$-inch increments.

Materials
Polyurethane foam with cotton stockinet covering and Velcro closure. This orthosis is prefabricated, readily available, and rarely requires adjustment.

Plastic Collar (L0130)
Adjustable Plastic Collar (Fig. 4-1) (L0140)
Wire Frame Collar (L0160)
Biomechanical Efficacy
These orthoses purportedly limit motion control to the midcervical spine in flexion only.[14–16] The short leverage of these devices makes them inadequate to control extension, lateral flexion, or rotation of the cervical spine.

Indications
Soft tissue disorders of the cervical spine are indications for these orthoses.

Contraindications
Any bony or ligamentous injury of the cervical spine is a contraindication for these orthoses.

Fitting Parameters
These orthoses are fitted by neck circumference and are available in a variety of heights or, for L0140, can be adjusted for length from sternal notch or clavicle to chin.

Materials

L0130 and L0140 are prefabricated from polyethylene with foam edges. L0140 is adjustable because it has two overlapping layers. L0160 is prefabricated from (steel wire).

SemiRigid Plastic Collar With Chin and Occipital Piece (L0150)
Biomechanical Efficacy

This orthosis affords better purchase on the chin and occiput for cervical control than the adjustable plastic collar L0140. As such, it may provide better sagittal plane immobilization than the previously described orthoses. It still has inadequate leverage to truly immobilize the cervical spine and offers only minimal control of lateral flexion and rotation.

Indications

The L0150 is indicated for soft tissue injuries of the cervical spine, more severe sprains, and arthritis.

Contraindications

This orthosis is contraindicated for bony or ligamentous injury to the spine.

Fitting Parameters

The fitting parameters for the L0150 are the same as those for the L0130, L0140, and L0160. The L0150, however, may be more difficult to fit because of the skin contact on the mandible. This orthosis may require heat adjustment or padding to increase wearing comfort.

Materials

The L0150 is constructed of polyethylene with foam edging.

Custom Cervical Bivalve (L0170) (Fig. 4-2)
Biomechanical Efficacy

The custom cervical bivalve is a total contact device that is used for motion control in the sagittal plane of the midcervical spine only. It can be custom modified to a Minerva-style cervicothoracic orthosis, encompassing more of the head and thorax. These modifications can significantly improve motion control in the sagittal, coronal, and transverse planes.[17,18] This orthosis functions through end-point control. End-point control has been described as fixing the end points of a mobile segment, which renders the segment better capable of accepting

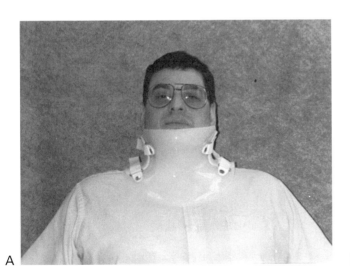
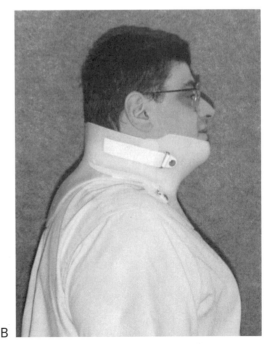

A   B

Fig. 4-2. **(A & B)** Cervical orthosis—custom bivalve.

external forces. The end points fixed in this orthosis are the head and the thorax. The mobile segment affected is the cervical spine.

Indications

The custom cervical bivalve can be used for stable bone or ligamentous midcervical spinal injury, as well as severe sprains.

Contraindications

This orthosis is contraindicated for conditions of the neck in which total contact cannot be tolerated, as in open wounds or coexisting injuries of the occiput or chin.

Fitting Parameters

The L0170 is fabricated from a molded impression of the neck and inferior head. The chin and occiput are incorporated into the impression. Inferior landmarks are the sternal notch and the spine or inferior angle of the scapula.

Materials

The L0170 is constructed of polymer with or without lining. Lining increases the bulk but may increase wearing comfort.

Philadelphia Collar (CO) (L0172)

Biomechanical Efficacy

The Philadelphia collar is a prefabricated orthosis that provides total contact in the cervical spine and provides a mild degree of motion control.

Indications

The Philadelphia collar is indicated for stable midcervical injuries, strain, sprain, and stable bony or ligamentous injury. It is frequently used when a patient is weaned from a more rigid cervical orthosis to limit sudden strain on the neck after weeks or months of immobilization. Similar yet more expensive orthoses that provide better control are the commercially available Newport, Miami, and Malibu collars.[19]

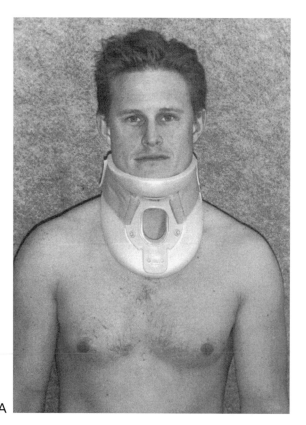

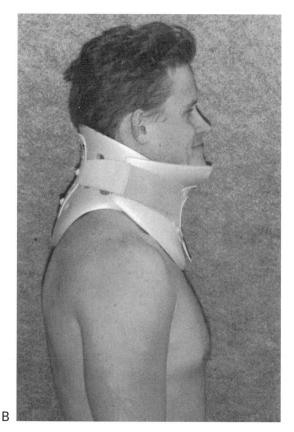

A   B

Fig. 4-3. **(A & B)** Philadelphia collar. A cervicothoracic style is available.

Contraindications

The Philadelphia collar is contraindicated for conditions in which the chin, occiput, sternum, or upper thorax cannot tolerate pressure. It is also contraindicated in the presence of cervical spine instability.

Fitting Parameters

The Philadelphia collar is available in several sizes according to circumference of the neck and the height from the chin to the sternal notch when the head is in neutral alignment.

Materials

This prefabricated orthosis is manufactured from plastizote foam and has rigid kydex (high-temperature) plastic reinforcements. It consists of anterior and posterior shells that are connected by Velcro, and a tracheotomy design is available.

Philadelphia Collar With a Thoracic Extension (CTO) (L0174) (Fig. 4-3)

Biomechanical Efficacy

Better leverage is gained with the thoracic extension on a Philadelphia-type orthosis. Because of the extension, this is classified as a CTO, and it affects motion control on the lower cervical spine as well as the mid cervical.[12]

Indications

This CTO is indicated for stable bony, ligamentous, or soft tissue injury to the mid and lower cervical spine.

Contraindications

This orthosis is contraindicated for any unstable injury of the spine, or if total contact cannot be tolerated on the occiput, mandible, sternum, or upper thoracic spine.

Fitting Parameters

The fitting parameters for this CTO are the same as for the Philadelphia collar. The thoracic extension is fitted to follow the sternum and ends at the xiphoid inferiorly. It is fixed with a strap around the torso at the xiphoid level.

Materials

The Philadelphia collar with a thoracic extension is commercially available and fabricated from plastizote foam with kydex (polymer) to lend rigidity.

Two or Four Poster (CO) (L0180) (Fig. 4-4)
Two or Four Poster With a Thoracic Extension (CTO) (L0200) (Fig. 4-5)

Biomechanical Efficacy

This orthosis provides end-point control through the chin and occipital components opposed by the chest

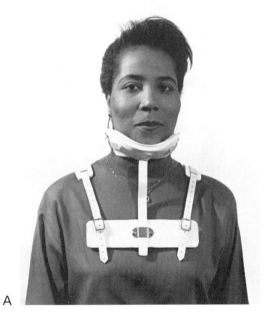
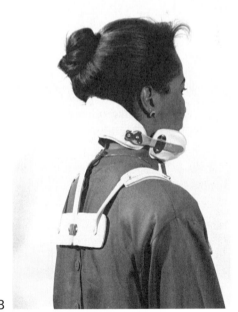

A   B

Fig. 4-4. **(A & B)** Cervical orthosis—two poster. (Courtesy of C.D. Denison Orthopaedic Appliance Corp.)

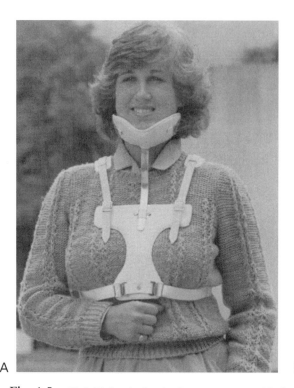 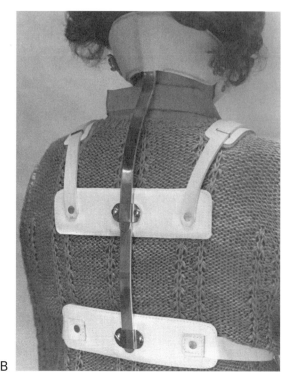

A   B

Fig. 4-5. **(A & B)** Cervical orthosis—two poster with thoracic extension. (Courtesy of C.D. Denison Orthopaedic Appliance Corp.)

pieces. Cervical motion in the sagittal plane is held. Lateral flexion and rotation are not well controlled.[16] Adding a thoracic extension converts an L0180 to the L0200. This addition adds two three-point pressure systems to treat the lower cervical spine.

Indications

This orthosis is indicated for mid or low (with extension) stable cervical fractures and arthritis.

Contraindications

Contraindications are unstable cervical fractures or conditions of the head and neck in which pressure from the orthosis cannot be tolerated.

Fitting Parameters

This orthosis is fitted from a small number of prefabricated sizes based on chin to sternal notch distances.

Materials

Padded metal components include sternal and posterior upper thorax sections connected by one or two vertical bars to occipital and mandibular pieces.

The total number of vertical bars give this orthosis its name.

SOMI (Sternal Occipital Mandibular Immobilizer) (CTO) (L0190) (Fig. 4-6)

Biomechanical Efficacy

The SOMI provides end-point control, and it stops sagittal plane flexion. It provides poor extension control secondary to weak aluminum components and a rotating occipital pad.

Indications[12,16]

The SOMI is indicated for cervical arthritis, postsurgical fusions, and stable cervical fractures. It is frequently used as the orthosis used on removal of a halo.

Contraindications

The SOMI is contraindicated for unstable injuries, especially those unstable in extension.

Fitting Parameters

This prefabricated orthosis is recommended for its relative ease of fitting because it can be fitted without moving

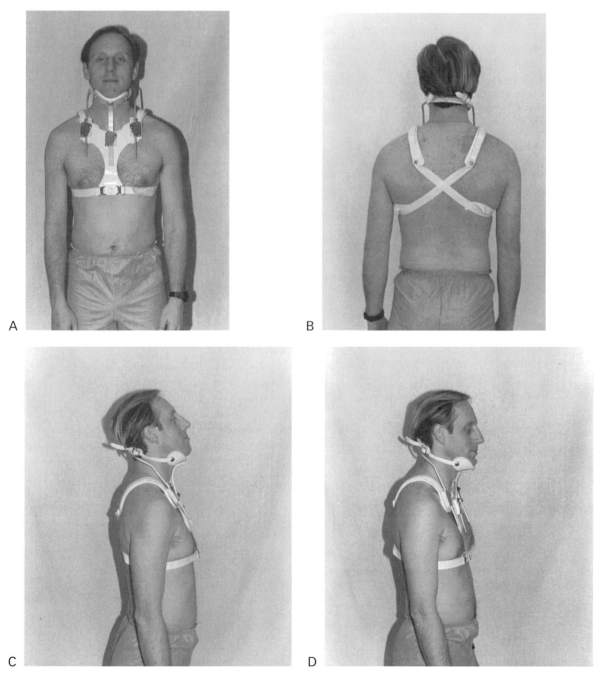

Fig. 4-6.   SOMI cervicothoracic orthosis (sternal occipital mandibular immobilizer). **(A & B)** Anterior and posterior views. **(C & D)** Side views. Note that the neck extension is allowed through a rotating occipital pad.

a supine patient. It is readily adjustable, is radiolucent, and unfortunately, is readily removable.

Materials

The SOMI is constructed of aluminum and plastic with foam padding. It has a chest piece with a detachable chin and occipital pieces. The chest piece has adjustable shoulder components. It is available in two sizes to fit most adults. The commercially available SOMI Jr. resembles an aggressive Philadelphia collar more than a less aggressive SOMI.

SOFT SPINAL ORTHOSES

Thoracic Rib Belt—Prefabricated (L0210)
Thoracic Rib Belt—Custom (L0220)
Biomechanical Efficacy

The thoracic rib belt applies circumferential pressure to the thorax to prevent maximum rib expansion and thus prevent discomfort associated with rib fractures or dislocations. The orthosis is worn as tight as possible to effect this goal.

Indications

This orthosis is indicated for rib fractures or dislocations.

Contraindications

The thoracic rib belt is contraindicated for multiple rib fractures when mechanical stability of the thorax is compromised.

Fitting Parameters

For males, the orthosis wraps around all the ribs, axilla to xiphoid. For females, to avoid the breast tissue, the orthosis passes from the inferior breast margin to waist.

Materials

The orthosis is usually made from either elastic or canvas. Elastic is more expandable and possibly more comfortable. Canvas provides better limitation of terminal expansion of the ribs.

Flexible Sacroiliac—Prefabricated (SIO) (L0600)
Sacroiliac—Custom (L0610)
Semirigid Sacroiliac—Custom (L0620)
Biomechanical Efficacy

These orthoses provide total contact and circumferential pressure about the pelvis. They also provide external reinforcement to the sacroiliac joints.

Indications

These orthoses are used for sacroiliac strain. SIOs are widely used by construction workers, weight lifters, or others at risk for spinal strain. They have little advantage over corsets with molded posterior plastic supports but may appeal to men more than corsets.

Fitting Parameters

These orthoses wrap around the pelvis, from the pubis to the iliac crests. Various styles and designs are available.

Materials

Most are elastic, although some styles are fabricated from canvas. They may use a simple Velcro closure or corset-type adjustments on the lateral aspects.

LSO Corset—Prefabricated (L0500) (Fig. 4-7)
LSO Corset—Custom (L0510)
LSO Elastic—Prefabricated Warm and Form (L0515)
Biomechanical Efficacy

These orthoses provide variable hold in the sagittal and coronal plane for the lumbar spine only. Total contact and circumferential pressure contribute to an increase in the intracavitary pressure of the abdomen.[2,13,20] This increase is thought to limit motion and redistribute load from the intervertebral discs to the surrounding soft tissue of the abdomen.

Indications

Low back pain or muscle strain. Abdominal ptosis may be supported through the use of a specially designed corset (L0500, L0510). Designs are also available for patients with pendulous abdomens (L0520, L0530). These corsets are longer anteriorly to serve several objectives. The added length contains the pendulous abdomen, increasing intracavitary pressure, which improves comfort as the orthosis is worn. It moves the patient's center of gravity posteriorly to a more normal position and hence reduces lumbar strain. Maternity-style elastic corsets are used to reduce lordosis and support the abdomen to decrease the low back pain commonly experienced in pregnancy.[21,22]

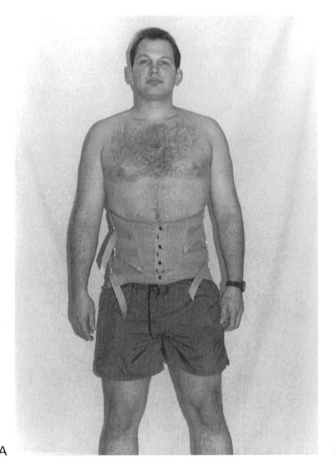 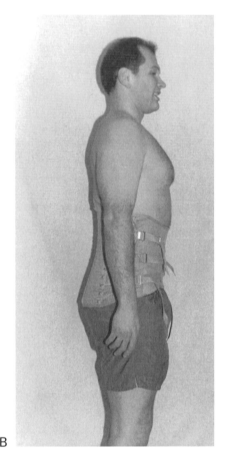

A   B

Fig. 4-7.   **(A & B)** Corset—LSO type.

Contraindications

These orthoses are contraindicated for severe respiratory distress.

Fitting Parameters

Prefabricated corsets are sized based on circumferential measurements at the waist and hips. Custom-fabricated orthoses are fabricated using patterns. The patterns are developed from multiple measurements including lengths, diameters, and circumferences of the torso. For unusual body shape or asymmetry, a custom-fabricated corset can be designed. Custom corsets are mostly used on adult scoliosis patients to limit pain by reduction in axial load on the spine through increased intracavitary pressure.

Materials

Corsets as a rule can be fabricated from elastic, mesh, canvas, or synthetic fabrics. The elastic is the most expandable material and creates the most flexible garment. The canvas and synthetic styles are the least expandable fabrics and provide the most restriction. Increased rigidity can be afforded through the use of corset stays, thin spring steel bars added longitudinally to the orthosis. Stays provide structural integrity to the fabric and prevent the fabric edges from rolling when the corset is worn. Instead of stays, a low-temperature thermoplastic material can be heated, molded to the spine, and placed in a sleeve on some prefabricated styles (L0515). This technique also lends structural rigidity and improves total contact on the spine.

TLSO Corset (L0300) (Fig. 4-8)
TLSO Corset Custom (L0310)
Elastic TLSO Corset Warm and Form (L0315)
TLSO Corset Warm and Form (L0317)

Biomechanical Efficacy

These orthoses provide variable hold in the sagittal and coronal plane for thoracic and thoracolumbar spine. This orthosis provides total contact around the torso and circumferential pressure, which increases intracavitary pressure. Further, the orthoses extend with straps, which wrap around the shoulders to limit motion in the thoracic spine.

Indications

These orthoses are indicated for soft tissue injuries to the thoracic and lumbar spine. They are frequently used for kyphosis secondary to osteoporosis.

Contraindications

These TLSOs are contraindicated for severe respiratory compromise and asymmetry of the spine. Although asymmetry is not necessarily a contraindication for fitting the lumbosacral corset, the length of thoracolumbosacral corsets make prefabricated corsets difficult to allow fitting for a scoliotic deformity. Custom-fabricated thoracolumbar corsets have been used on scoliosis in adults who present with pain but no progression.

Fitting Parameters

Circumferential and height measurements allow selection of the best prefabricated style.

Materials

Corsets as a rule can be fabricated from elastic, mesh, canvas, or synthetic fabrics. Elastic is the most expandable material. The canvas and synthetic are the least expandable. Increased rigidity can be obtained through the

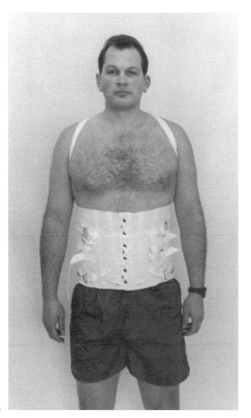
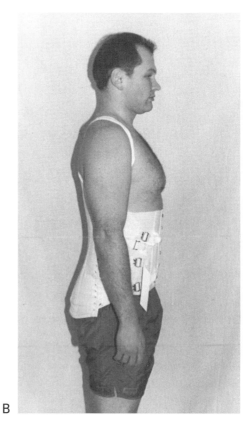

A   B

Fig. 4-8. **(A & B)** Corset—TLSO type.

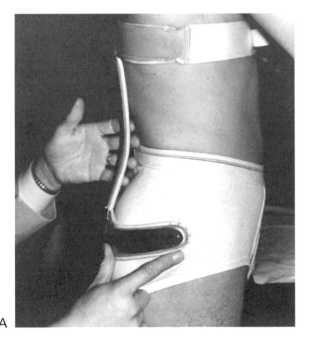 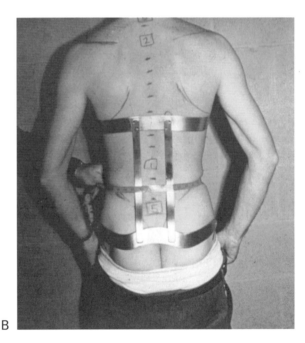

Fig. 4-9. **(A & B)** Chairback-style LSO. The thoracic band, pelvic band, and paraspinal bars provide sagittal movement control.

use of corset stays, thin spring steel bars added longitudinally to the orthosis in channels. Stays provide structural integrity to the fabric and prevent the edges from rolling as it is worn. Instead of stays, a low-temperature thermoplastic can be heated and placed in a sleeve on some prefabricated styles (L0317), as previously mentioned for the lumbosacral corsets.

TRADITIONAL METAL ORTHOSES

LSO Anteroposterior Chairback (MacAusland)—Custom: Sagittal Control (L0530) (Fig. 4-9)

This orthosis has been described by MacAusland[22] and consists of a thoracic band, a pelvic band, and paraspinal bars.

Biomechanical Efficacy

This orthosis provides, as most orthoses do, a three-point force system that affects motion control. The thoracic and pelvic bands provide two anteriorly directed forces, and the midpoint of the corset provides a third posteriorly directed force. These three forces are in equilib-

rium and serve to stop extension of the lumbar spine. Similarly, three points of force can be described that stop flexion, and thus the orthosis holds motion in the sagittal plane. Further, the corset increases intracavitary pressure to unload the intervertebral discs and transmit that load to the surrounding soft tissue.

Indications and Contraindications

This orthosis is sometimes recommended for low back pain and disc herniation. It may be used for stable fracture management, but its use for fractures is extremely limited. It provides inadequate superior leverage to control motion of thoracolumbar fractures and provides inadequate inferior leverage to control motion of most lumbosacral fractures. Thus, the only fracture levels potentially managed with this orthosis are stable midlumbar noncompression fractures.[23] For pain control, it is mostly a kinesthetic reminder to limit motion.

Fitting Parameters

This LSO is fabricated from measurements of circumference and heights in the torso. The superior border of the thoracic band is inferior to the scapula, and the inferior border of the pelvic band is the sacrococcygeal junction.

The pelvic band should contain the gluteal mass lateral to the midline to afford the best pelvic control. The pelvic band location is necessary for adequate leverage of the system, and the thoracic band location allows for containment of the ribs throughout inspiration. The thoracic band should also allow for full motion of the scapulae without impingement. The paraspinal bars follow the paraspinal musculature and connect the thoracic band to the pelvic band.

Materials
These components are fabricated from aluminum, and the orthosis is generally worn with a cloth corset.

LSO Anteroposterior/Lateral Knight—Custom: Sagittal Coronal Control (L0520) (Fig. 4-10)
Biomechanical Efficacy
This LSO provides a three-point force system and a circumferential corset to increase intracavitary pressure. This orthosis is similar to the sagittal-style LSO with the addition of lateral bars so that three-point force systems can be described in the sagittal and coronal planes.

Indications and Contraindications
James Knight invented this orthosis for use in tuberculosis.[24] It is presently recommended for low back pain and disc herniation. For fracture management, it has limited application because of its short leverage. The only fractures well managed are midlumbar, stable, noncompression-type fractures. Thoracolumbar injuries that require immobilization of the involved area necessitate the use of a TLSO.[25] Lumbosacral injuries that require complete immobilization necessitate the addition of a thigh interface and hip joint to control pelvic motion.[3,19,23,26]

Fitting Parameters
The Knight-style LSO is identical to the chairback with the addition of lateral bars, which afford lateral control and permit an anterior corset panel to be used instead of a full corset. (See Fig. 4-10.) The coronal plane control may be indicated in some situations, such as a transverse process fracture.

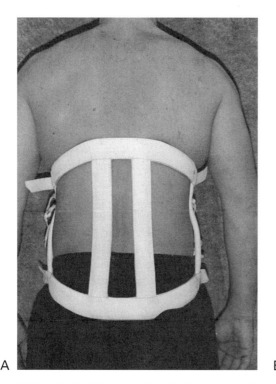
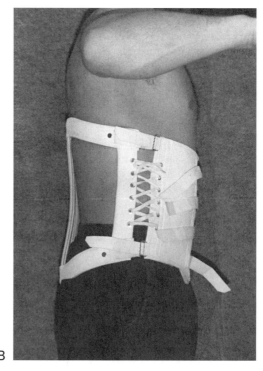

Fig. 4-10. **(A & B)** Knight-style LSO. Note the similarity to the chairback style but with the addition of lateral bars for coronal movement control.

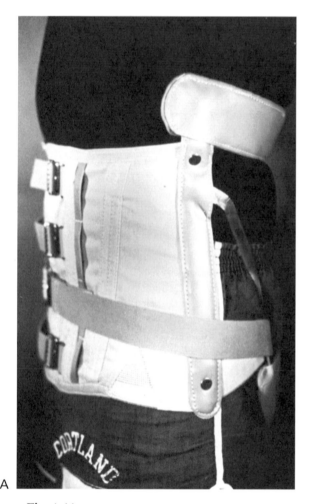

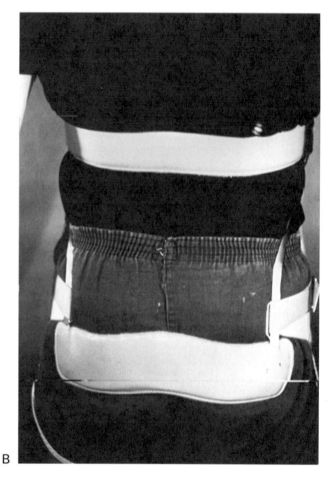

A   B

Fig. 4-11. **(A & B)** Williams-style LSO. This LSO stops coronal motion and extension but articulates in the sagittal plane to allow flexion.

Materials
The Knight LSO is constructed of an aluminum pelvic band, a thoracic band, lateral bars, paraspinal bars, and an anterior corset panel or, if desired, a full corset.

LSO Williams Flexion Type—Custom: Extension Coronal Control (L0540) (Fig. 4-11)
Paul Williams invented this orthosis in 1937.[27]

Biomechanical Efficacy
This unique orthosis is dynamic. Its component attachments and straps allow for free flexion yet stop extension in the lumbar spine. Coronal plane motion control is "hold" as per the technical analysis form. Lumbosacral flexion is thought to be maintained throughout its use as the patient stands, walks, and sits. For spondylolisthesis, maintenance of lumbar flexion is meant to reduce the shear placed on the fracture site, maintaining the fracture segments together and thus it prevents progressive lumbar slip.[28–31]

Indications
Williams described the orthosis as disease specific for spondylolysis and spondylolisthesis.

Contraindications

The Williams orthosis is contraindicated for any pathology for which flexion should not be allowed, as in traumatic compression fractures.

Fitting Parameters

The oblique bar of this orthosis makes fabrication and fitting of a custom-fabricated system more difficult than in the previous orthoses. The same circumferences and heights would be used for fabrication.

Materials

This orthosis is constructed of an aluminum thoracic band, a pelvic band, lateral bars, oblique bars, and an anterior panel. The anterior panel is elastic to allow full flexion. Lateral bars articulate with a thoracic band and are not attached inferiorly to the pelvic band. This articulation, combined with a nonelastic inferior pelvic strap contribute to the flexion allowance and restriction of extension provided by this orthosis.

Taylor—Custom (L0320)

This TLSO sagittal control orthosis was invented in 1863 by Charles Fayette Taylor,[32] an orthopedist in New York.

Biomechanical Efficacy

This orthosis provides two three-point forces systems in the sagittal plane to hold motion. The leverage provided by the system is good for motion control within the confines of the orthosis; however, motion may be increased at the end points of the orthosis, that is the cervical spine and the lumbosacral spine.[33]

Indications

This orthosis was originally designed to be used for Potts disease or tuberculosis of the spine. The Spinal Assistant, as originally described by Taylor, held the spine in extension to prevent gibbous deformity during recovery. Today, the orthosis is primarily used for kyphosis secondary to osteoporosis, although compliance with elderly patients can be difficult to achieve.

Contraindications

Because pelvic fixation is not a component of this orthosis, its use should not be recommended for adolescent thoracic kyphosis as in Scheuermann's disease.

Fitting Parameters

The motion control provided by the orthosis is provided through the paraspinal bars, interscapular band, and pelvic band, but also the addition of a corset for increased intracavitary pressure. The interscapular band is fitted to rest on the scapulae and provide an anteriorly directed force to decrease thoracic kyphosis. Prefabricated styles frequently possess an interscapular band that is short, resting between the scapulae, which diminishes the anteriorly directed force for maintenance of thoracic extension.

Knight Taylor—Custom: TLSO, Sagittal Coronal Control (L0330) (Fig. 4-12)

Biomechanical Efficacy

This orthosis is a combination of the Knight and Taylor orthoses, previously described, and thus provides control of the thoracic and lumbar spine in the sagittal and coronal planes. The orthosis consists of a Taylor-style TLSO with a thoracic band and lateral bars. These components provide lateral and sagittal three-point force systems as well as circumferential pressure and increased intracavitary pressure from a corset addition.

Indications

This orthosis could be used for postsurgical or nonsurgical stable fracture management of the thoracic and lumbar spine. Pain that is due to severe muscle strain can also be managed by a spinal orthosis such as this one.

Contraindications

Unstable fractures are contraindications for the Knight Taylor orthosis.

Fitting Parameters

The Knight Taylor-style TLSO[34] is made from circumferential and height measurements of a patient's torso and delineations of their spine. The thoracic band is fitted just inferior to the inferior angle of the scapula, and the pelvic band is fitted at the sacrococcygeal junction inferiorly. The lateral bars follow the lateral midline of the patient's body, and the paraspinal bars follow the apices of the paraspinal muscles, starting at the pelvic band, and ending at the spine of the scapula. These fitting parameters ensure the appropriate control without impingement on bony landmarks of the spine and torso.

Materials

Aluminum is almost exclusively used for all of the components of this orthosis. The orthosis is either encircled by a corset, or an anterior corset panel is worn. Either way, the corset maintains the orthosis on the patient while increasing intracavitary pressure.

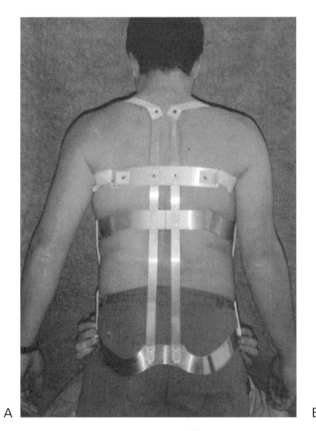
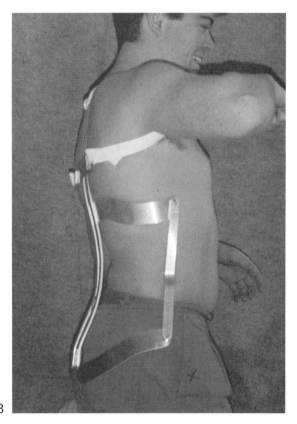

Fig. 4-12.   **(A & B)** Knight Taylor-style TLSO.

Cowhorn, Arnold, Magnusen, Steindler—Custom[22] (L0340)
TLSO, Triplane, Sternal Extension—Custom (L0380)

These orthoses all represent triplanar control TLSOs (Fig. 4-13)

Biomechanical Efficacy

Sagittal and coronal control of the thoracic and thoracolumbar spine is as described previously with three-point pressure systems. Control in the transverse plane comes from pelvic stabilization in conjunction with counterpressures from the superior subclavicular projections that arise from the thoracic band. These orthoses provide motion hold in all three planes for the thoracic and lumbar spine.

Indications

These traditional styles represent the metal alternative to a plastic TLSO body jacket. They are indicated for fracture management of the thoracic and lumbar spine.

Contraindications

These orthoses are contraindicated for high thoracic injuries. Orthotic recommendation for high thoracic fractures are discussed in the plastic body jacket section.

Fitting Parameters

These orthoses are difficult to fit, because the subclavicular projections must be custom made. They are difficult to don, because the patient must slide into the orthosis from the side. They provide good motion control of the involved area when plastic is not an option but must be carefully fitted and monitored.

Materials

These orthoses are constructed of an aluminum pelvic band, a thoracic band, subclavicular extensions, paraspinal bars, and lateral bars. They are worn with a corset.

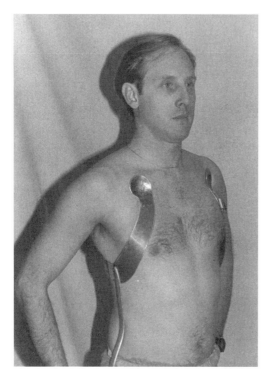

Fig. 4-13. Triplanar control TLSO. Subclavicular extensions help control rotation, giving it the name Cowhorn brace.

TLSO Flexion Control—CASH (Fig. 4–14), or Jewett[6] Type Prefabricated (L0370) (Fig. 4-15)

These are two different prefabricated orthoses that provide identical biomechanical control. CASH is an acronym for cruciform anterior spinal hyperextension, and Jewett is named for its inventor, a Florida surgeon.

Biomechanical Efficacy

These orthoses are classic examples of the three-point force system of orthotic management. Two posteriorly directed forces and one anteriorly directed force maintain spinal extension. These orthoses allow free extension but stop flexion.

Indications

Designed originally to replace plaster casts for spinal fractures, the Jewett brace or alternate styles are commonly and effectively[25] used for traumatic compression fractures of the thoracolumbar spine. Sometimes they are used for thoracolumbar Scheuermann's disease. They are used, although not effectively, for thoracic osteoporotic

kyphosis. They are not extremely effective in this instance, because the apex of curvature is frequently in the mid thoracic spine. The anteriorly directed force of this orthosis is located on the thoracolumbar junction, and the posteriorly directed force is inferior to the sternum or approximately the T5 level. This provides inadequate leverage to control the midthoracic spine. A more effective orthosis for holding osteoporotic deformities is the TLSO that provides sagittal control. However, effectiveness does not always meet compliance, and the TLSO with flexion control is sometimes better tolerated by osteoporotic patients.

Contraindications

Because these orthoses do not control trunk rotation, they are contraindicated in any unstable fracture or any pathology that requires limitation of spinal extension such as spondylolisthesis.

Fitting Parameters

These orthoses are fitted to lie between the sternal notch and the symphysis pubis anteriorly, and they produce two posteriorly directed forces. Posteriorly, the thoracolumbar pad acts as the anteriorly directed force. Anterolateral or lateral pads stabilize the orthosis.

Materials

These orthoses are prefabricated and are generally aluminum with plastic pads. The CASH style is cross shaped with sternal, pubic, posterior, and anterolateral pads. The Jewett style has sternal, pubic, and lateral pads connected by oblique bars counteracted by a posterior pad as well.

Body Jackets (Fig. 4-16)

CTLSO	Minerva type—custom (L0700)	
CTLSO	Minerva type with lining—custom (L0710)	
TLSO	body jacket—custom (L0390)	
TLSO	body jacket—custom with lining (L0400)	
TLSO	bivalve body jacket—custom (L0410)	
TLSO	bivalve body jacket with lining (L0420)	
TLSO	body jacket with lining—prefabricated (L0430)	
LSO	body jacket—custom (L0550)	
LSO	body jacket—custom with lining (L0560)	
LSO	body jacket—prefabricated (L0565)	

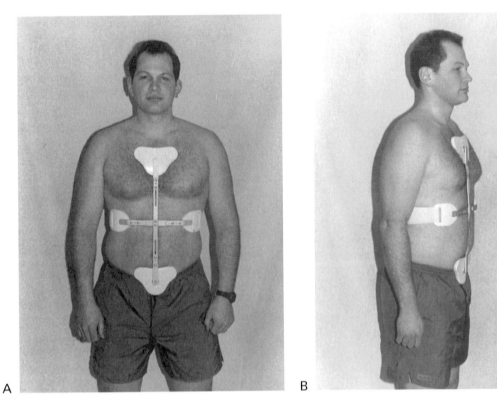

A   B

Fig. 4-14. **(A & B)** CASH (cruciform anterior spinal hyperextension orthosis) TLSO. Note the adjustable length bars. This orthosis primarily controls flexion.

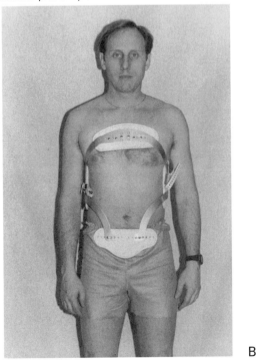
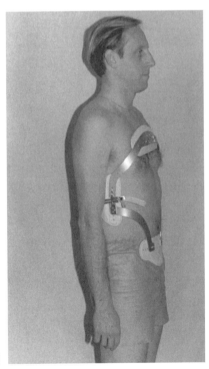

A   B

Fig. 4-15. **(A & B)** Jewett TLSO. Note the adjustable features at sides and at either end. This orthosis primarily controls flexion.

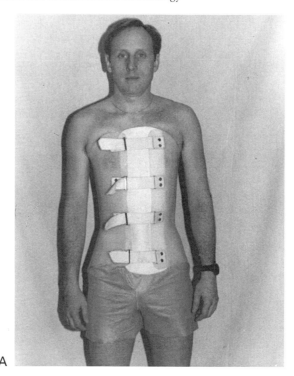

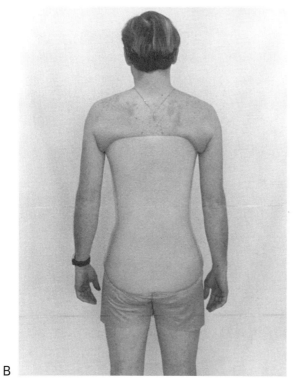

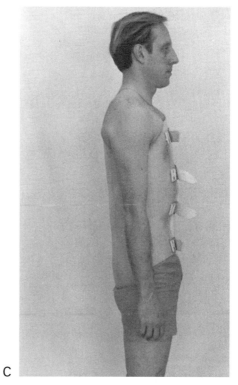

Fig. 4-16.   Plastic body jackets—custom-molded TLSOs. **(A–C)** One piece with anterior opening.

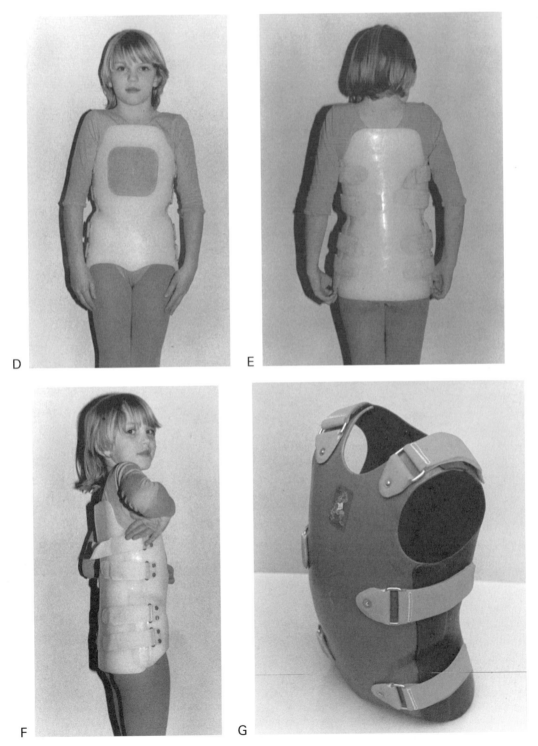

Fig. 4-16. *(Figure continued.)* **(D–F)** Bivalve design with lateral closure. **(G)** Bivalve design with shoulder extensions.

Biomechanical Efficacy

Body jackets are total contact systems that use all of the biomechanical principles previously described. The basic objective of these orthoses is to maintain spinal alignment through total contact. Motion is controlled, and the CTLSO and TLSO styles provide triplanar hold. The LSO does not provide counterpressure to provide transverse plane motion control and therefore would be classified having only sagittal and coronal plane control.

Indications

These body jackets are indicated for traumatic or postsurgical fracture management. Low back pain, disc herniation, disc surgery, and postsurgical fusions are also indications.

Contraindications

Body jackets are contraindicated when skin sensitivity or heat sensitivity would make total contact plastic inappropriate.

Fitting Parameters

A wide variety of styles of plastic body jackets are available. The choice of CTLSO, TLSO, or LSO depends on the level and number of fractures. TLSO designs have simple trimlines for fractures from midthoracic to midlumbar levels or can encompass subclavicular extensions as in the metal style for better immobilization of the midthoracic spine. TLSO designs can incorporate shoulder flanges. Shoulder flanges are used to reduce the flexion moment occurring in the thoracic spine when patients use their upper limbs in activities of daily living. In the presence of midthoracic level fractures, that flexion moment may interfere with fracture healing by compressing the fracture site.

High thoracic fractures should be managed with CTLSO or CTO depending on severity and multiple trauma. A CTO may be adequate for stable cervithoracic fractures,[16] however, with multiple injuries including lower thoracic or lumbar fractures, a CTLSO is indicated. A CTLSO is also recommended if posture is a contributing factor as in extreme thoracic kyphosis combined with the cervicothoracic level fracture.

The LSO body jackets provide inadequate superior leverage to control any fracture level other than midlumbar. Even then, the control provided in the orthosis may be questioned as producing nothing more than increased intracavitary pressure and postural alignment. For lumbosacral immobilization, the body jacket must

have a hip component added to it. During hip extension, lumbar and lumbosacral extension also occur (Fig. 4-17 and 4-18. If hip extension is not controlled, the simultaneous motion at the fracture site may contribute to poor healing.[3] The orthotic hip component consists of a molded thigh interface with a static or dynamic hip joint that stops or holds hip extension to a position of slight hip flexion.

The landmarks for fitting a TLSO body jacket are sternal notch to pubis anteriorly and spine or inferior angle of the scapula to sacrococcygeal junction posteriorly. The gluteal mass should be contained for most effective motion control. Laterally, the axilla and trochanter are allowed clearance. Total contact is effected in body jackets through compression of soft tissue and

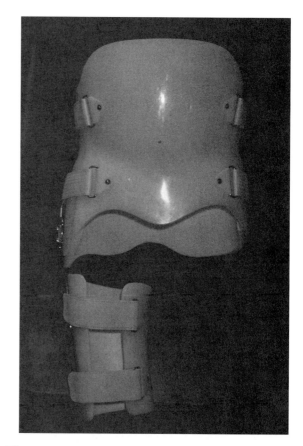

Fig. 4-17. Plastic body jacket modifications—custommolded LSO. Note that the hip joint and thigh piece are needed to control gross motion of the lumbosacral spine. (Courtesy of Ballert Orthopaedic of Chicago.)

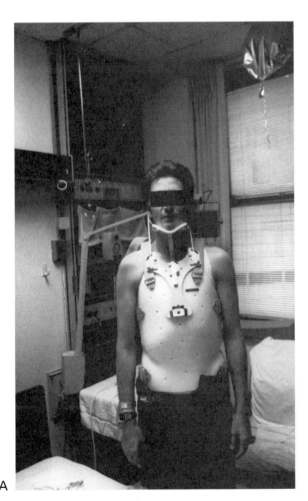

A

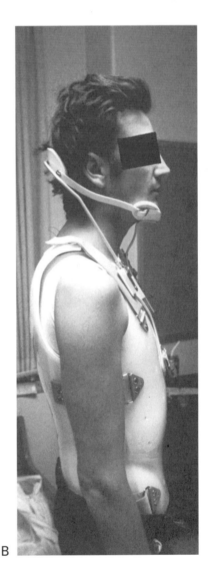

B

Fig. 4-18.   **(A & B)** Traumatic body jacket with SOMI-type cervical extension. Functionally, this is a CTLSO. (Courtesy of Lakeshore Prosthetics and Orthotics, Chicago, IL.)

relief of bony prominences. Body jackets are typically custom fabricated from an impression and measurements of the patient's torso. The impression is poured in plaster to create a positive casting. The casting is then modified to provide pressure in the abdomen and relief for the iliac crests and other bony prominences. Plastic is then vacuum formed over the casting to create the total-contact interface. The orthosis is cut off the casting, the edges are smoothed, and straps are applied to hold the orthosis together as it is worn.

Materials
Body jackets are typically fabricated from polymers such as polyethylene or a copolymer of polyethylene and polypropylene. Cervical extensions may be total contact and continuous with the plastic body jacket or may consist of occipital and mandibular pads connected to the rest of the body jacket by vertical metal bars. Body jackets may be lined for comfort, but linings increase the bulk.

If a hip component is added, it might be total-contact plastic that crosses the hip and contains the thigh or may consist of a thigh interface attached to the orthosis by a metal hip joint.

TLSO Flexion Jacket—Prefabricated (L0350)
TLSO Flexion Jacket—Custom (L0360)
This orthosis is the plastic equivalent for the Williams-style metal LSO. This is the Raney-type orthosis (Fig.4-19) described in the *Atlas of Orthotics*[34]; the orthosis purports to flex the lumbar spine and maintain flexion throughout activities, as in the control provided by the Williams orthosis.

Biomechanical Efficacy
This orthosis does provide additional control compared to the LSO extension/coronal control. Because of its cir-

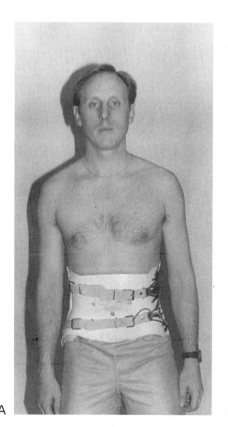
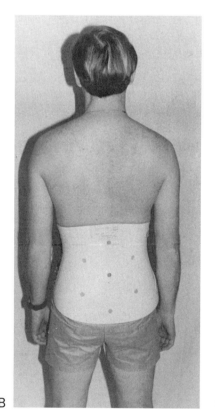
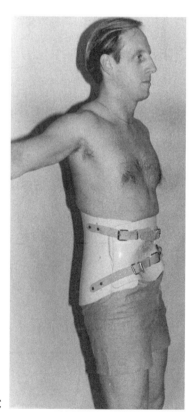

A   B   C

Fig. 4-19.   (A–C) Rainey-type LSO. Note the built-in abdominal compression to provide flexion control, which is its primary purpose.

cumferential design, and total-contact polymer, this orthosis is not dynamic as in the Williams, but rather static; it holds motion in the sagittal and coronal planes for the lumbar spine only.

Indications

This orthosis is indicated for spondylolysis spondylolysthesis.

Contraindications

Any pathology for which lumbar flexion or abdominal pressure cannot be tolerated is a contraindication for this orthosis. Recently, it has been shown that patients with disc herniation experience increased comfort with lordosis of the lumbar spine.[35] Thus, this orthosis, and all orthoses of this type, would be contraindicated.

Fitting Parameters

The fitting parameters for this orthosis are the same as those for all body jackets.

Materials

This orthosis is constructed of thermoplastic with a two-piece design and side closures.

Boston Overlap Brace (BOB) (L0440)

The BOB orthosis is commercially available, is made to measurements or impression, and is a thermoplastic lumbosacral orthosis. The orthosis can be fabricated in three different lumbar postures, 0, 15, and 30 degrees of lordosis or custom fabricated from an impression in any lumbar position. Patients who are to be fitted with the BOB should be evaluated for the most comfortable and stable posture of the lumbar spine before ordering the orthosis.

Biomechanical Efficacy

This orthosis holds motion in the sagittal and coronal plane for the lumbar spine only.

Indications

The BOB orthosis is indicated for stable noncompression fractures of the lumbar vertebra and for spondylolysis and spondylolisthesis.[28,31]

Contraindications

This orthosis is contraindicated for fractures outside the area treated by the orthosis, that is, any fracture more superior than the midlumbar region.

Fitting Parameters

The BOB orthosis is fitted snugly around the torso from the xiphoid to the pubis anteriorly and from the inferior angle of the scapulae to the sacrococcygeal junction pos-

teriorly. Functionally, the orthosis should allow free motion of the scapulae without impinging, and the orthosis should encompass the gluteal mass inferiorly.

Materials

This orthosis is constructed of thermoplastic that overlaps itself, and it has a nonelastic Velcro strap closure.

Halo[36] (L0810) (Fig. 4-20)
Halo and Plaster Body Cast (L0820)
Halo and Milwaukee (L0830)
MRI Compatibility (L0860)

Biomechanical Efficacy

These orthoses provide the best immobilization of the cervical spine of all the cervical orthoses. Immobilization in this orthosis is a result of long leverage for a three-point force system control and end-point fixation to the

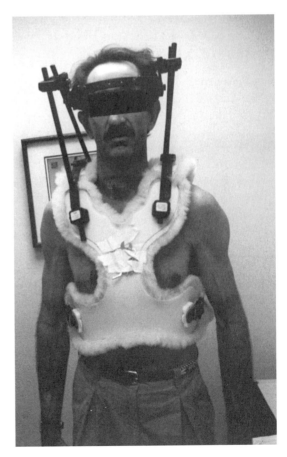

Fig. 4-20. Halo CTO. (Courtesy of Lakeshore Prosthetics and Orthotics, Chicago, IL.)

skull. Distraction may be used to reduce load on the spine, however, minimally to avoid separating fracture sites. These orthoses may allow small amounts of intersegmental motion, or snaking of adjacent vertebrae, and there are questions regarding whether intersegmental snaking is enough to warrant concern. Snaking that occurs actually does not risk stability and may assist healing by stimulating blood to flow to the involved area.[16–18,37,38]

Indications

These orthoses are indicated for unstable fractures of the cervical spine. A plaster body cast or Milwaukee-type interface may be added to the orthosis for multiple-level fractures or if the orthosis is to be worn after scoliosis surgery.

Contraindications

These orthoses are contraindicated for cranial fractures, because the halo ring requires pin fixation to the skull of the patient.

Fitting Parameters

The halo ring is fitted to be approximately 10 mm wider than the diameter of the skull at the equator of the skull. Pins are at least four in number and serve to tighten the halo ring to the patient's skull. Pins are located 10 mm superior to the lateral third of the eyebrow and two opposing posterior pins. The halo ring is attached to a superstructure which extends inferiorly to the halo vest system. The vest, which can be removed in emergencies, is a plastic two-piece shell, which serves as inferior fixation of the orthosis. The orthosis is applied with the patient supine and can be almost completely applied without moving the patient. Moving the skeletally unstable patient requires a well-trained careful team of professionals. Distraction is adjusted after application with the patient supine.

Materials

These orthoses are constructed of a thermoplastic vest with an aluminum, steel, or titanium superstructure, and a halo ring. The halo superstructure may be used attached to a plaster cast (L0820) or plastic body jacket to increase the area of control. Attaching the halo superstructure to a Milwaukee-type pelvic interface (L0830) was a historical alternative to bed traction before scoliosis surgery.

SCOLIOSIS

A definitive discussion of scoliosis management is not within the scope of this chapter. Entire books have been dedicated to scoliosis management. The reader is encourage to locate the referenced texts as excellent resources for decision making in scoliosis. The following is a brief discussion of two basic orthoses that are commonly used.

CTLSO Milwaukee-Style (L1000) (Fig. 4-21)

The Milwaukee CTLSO is a composite orthosis custom manufactured from a polymer pelvic interface and an aluminum and steel superstructure with a cervical ring. These components serve as the basic system to which pads are attached for correction of scoliotic or kyphotic curves of the spine.

Biomechanical Efficacy

The Milwaukee-type CTLSO[1] provides end-point control, three-point pressure systems, and counterpressures to gain correction of the triplanar deformities of scoliosis.[39] The Milwaukee-type CTLSO is recommended for flexible curves not caused by abnormal vertebral development or known neuromuscular disease and is used when growth remains. The objective of the orthosis is to maintain symmetry while the spine grows to encourage symmetric growth. Some consider the orthosis a training orthosis because the patient, wearing the orthosis up to 23 hours per day, must constantly maintain good posture. Slouching in the orthosis produces discomfort that encourages the patient to straighten again.

Indications

Scoliotic curves of 25 to 40 degrees have traditionally been treated with this orthosis if the curve apex is located superior to T8, shows signs of progression, and growth remains. The orthosis is indicated for idiopathic or flexible congenital scoliosis.[40–42] Thoracic Scheuermann kyphosis is a second indication for the orthosis.[39,42]

Contraindications

Typically, Milwaukee-style CTLSOs are contraindicated for neuromuscular scoliosis. Paralysis renders the patient unable to withdraw from the pads, and total contact in the thorax is then indicated. A *modified* Milwaukee-type orthoses has been used in neuromuscular scoliosis.[43] The objectives in neuromuscular scoliosis management are maintenance of trunk, neck, and head stability.

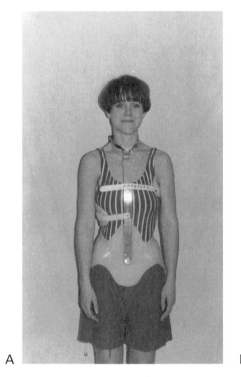 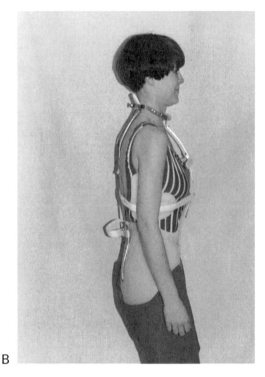

Fig. 4-21. **(A & B)** Milwaukee-style CTLSO.

Fitting Parameters

The pelvic interface is posterior opening and is fitted snugly with trim lines from the gluteal fold to the inferior costal margin posteriorly, and from the xiphoid process to the pubic symphysis anteriorly. The superstructure comprises two posterior paraspinal bars, which follow the paraspinal musculature and end at the cervical ring. One broad aluminum anterior bar follows the midline of the body and ends at the cervical ring. The cervical ring is circumferential with a posterior screw closure and anterior hinge to allow donning. It has occipital and mandibular pads, which should rest 20 to 30 mm inferior to occiput and mandible. These act as the superior end point of the orthosis and definite kinesthetic reminder to remain erect. This framework serves as end-point control, but within the framework are pads that apply a transverse load to the ribs and spine to correct scoliotic curvatures. Thoracic pads are attached with straps to the vertical bars. A thoracic pad applies a transverse load to the apex of the curve transmitted through the ribs. Many additional components can be added for increased curve correction or correction of decompensation as the ortho-

sis is worn. These components include lumbar, trochanteric, and derotation pads; axillary slings; and shoulder caps. The patient is evaluated in three planes as the orthosis is worn because scoliosis presents not only as lateral curvature but also concomitant rotation and reduced thoracic kyphosis.

Materials

As discussed, the Milwaukee CTLSO is a composite orthosis. The anterior aluminum bar is radiolucent, and the posterior steel bars span the vertebrae following the paraspinal musculature. These components allow for radiographs while the patient wears the orthosis, which gives the physician confirmation of correction achieved. The pelvic interface is fabricated from polymer and is held together with nonelastic straps to maintain a snug fit.

Custom Body Jacket for Scoliosis (L1300) (Fig. 4-22)

This orthosis is a custom-fabricated TLSO or LSO that effects control of scoliotic curve between 25 and 40 de-

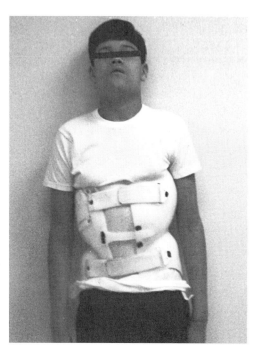

Fig. 4-22. Plastic body jacket. A custom-made TLSO for scoliosis specially modified to create snug interfaces to apply corrective forces to the scoliotic curves. (Courtesy of Bio-Concepts Laboratory, Burr Ridge, IL.)

grees and that has that apical vertebra at T8 and inferior. Many varieties of scoliosis body jackets are currently in use. Among these are the Boston, Miami, Wilmington, Charleston, and Lyon, named for the cities where they were invented. Also, the Rosenberger,[44] named for its inventor, is currently used in some settings. All of the orthoses use the same biomechanical principles to correct flexible scoliotic curves. Each orthotic design does have certain characteristics that make that system unique. The Boston system is described for the purposes of this discussion as a representative of TLSO management of scoliosis.

Biomechanical Efficacy

The orthosis provides three-point pressure systems, counterpressure systems, and torso shift to maintain symmetry or overcorrection during growth. The Milwaukee CTLSO and the TLSO for scoliosis share the same objectives; however, only the Milwaukee has effective leverage for curves superior to T8.

Indications

These orthosis are indicated for flexible scoliotic curves in growing spines between 25 and 40 degrees in magnitude. Scoliosis orthoses are indicated when scoliotic curves show evidence of progression.[42,45,46]

Contraindications

Nonprogressive, paralytic curves, curves above T8, and adult curves are contraindications for these orthoses.

Fitting Parameters

The orthosis should be fitted to provide pressure at the apex of curvature. For thoracic curves, pressure is applied through ribs to the apex. Additional points of pressure can be identified at the end points of curves. The inferior trim lines of the orthosis contain the gluteal mass and end at the pubic symphysis. Laterally, the trochanter may be contained for increased coronal control. The superior trim lines vary based on the apex of curvature.

Materials

These orthoses are fabricated from thermoplastic with or without lining. Closure is with nonelastic straps. Foam pads are used for curve correction.

CONCLUSION

When prescribing a cervical orthosis, the physician needs to keep certain objectives in mind. If the purpose is to provide motion control, as in most fractures, the orthotic criteria must be maximal restraint of motion and static posture. The two orthoses that provide the greatest limitation of motion are the Minerva-style CTO and the halo CTO. If, on the other hand, the purpose is to relieve pain, and the spine is stable, the criterion must be to give enough restraint to promote healing and reduce pain yet still act as a tolerable kinesthetic reminder to keep the neck and head immobilized.

In theory, spinal orthoses if properly applied should increase spinal stability by applying external forces to substitute for defective muscle action and, therefore, reduce pain. This may be true for neck pain, but in most cases of lumbar back pain of a chronic nature, the cause of pain is unknown. Whether increasing spinal stability by an external appliance is the reason why many patients find them helpful is debatable. Furthermore, the spine is very difficult to immobilize. The interposition of muscle and other soft tissue prevents an orthosis from gripping the bony segments. The long leverage of the trunk and its weight create very large moments needing control. Spinal shape varies from standing to sitting. Therefore, spinal orthoses that are fitted for standing may migrate superiorly when the patient is seated if improperly fitted. This migration is not only irritating but can minimize the control the orthosis provides.

Regardless of the cause of spinal pain and instability, it is impossible to restrict only one segment with an orthosis. All orthoses must achieve fixation somewhere—the skull, rib cage, or pelvis. The orthosis must encircle more than one segment; the greater the restriction needed, the wider the area that needs to be covered.

For the best use of spinal orthoses, physicians and other health professionals should understand what the supports can and cannot do. Compliance in wearing spinal orthoses is often a problem. The prescribing physician may have to judge whether or not the patient will wear an orthosis before causing undue expense by prescribing one. In comparison with other treatment issues in regard to back pain, scientific studies on the effects of orthoses on back pain are sparse.

With few exceptions, the use of restrictive spinal supports in treating neck or back disorders should be a temporary measure. Whenever possible, the aim should be to restore physiologic forces that support the spine through the action of muscles rather than through an external device. Another alternative is to advise patients how to avoid undue stress on the spine by correcting postural habits or by using some of the ergonomic furniture and automobile seats that prevent stress on the spine.

To manage spinal pathologies effectively, one must first consider the mechanics of the pathology and the level of injury. It is imperative that the orthosis achieve the mechanical goals for each. The recommendation of spinal orthoses is not easy; many variables need to be addressed for each orthotic recommendation. The patient's size, activity level, pain level, and severity of injury are only a few of the variables that affect orthotic recommendation. If one simplifies the patient's pathology to a pathomechanical condition, and if spinal orthoses are remembered generically, then orthotic recommendation will be simplified and individualized.

REFERENCES

1. Blount W, Moe J: The Milwaukee Brace. Williams & Wilkins, Baltimore, 1973

2. Keagy R: Biomechanics of the spine and orthoses. In: Spinal Disorders: Diagnosis and Treatment. Lea & Febiger, Philadelphia, 1977

3. White MM, Panjabi AA: Spinal braces: Functional analysis and clinical Applications. In: Clinical Biomechanics of the Spine. 2nd Ed. JB Lippincott, Philadelphia, 1990

4. Health Care Financing Administration (HCFA): Common Procedures Coding System, a combined effort of the American Orthotic Prosthetic Association (AOPA), HCFA and the Blue Cross and Blue Shield Association (BCBSA). AOPA, Alexandria VA

5. McCullough NC, III: Biomechanical analysis systems for orthotic prescription. In: Atlas of Orthotics. CV Mosby, St. Louis, 1975

6. Jewett EL: A three point hypextension back brace. J Bone Joint Surg 19:1128, 1937

7. Axelsson R: Influence of a lumbar orthosis on intervertebral mobility. A roentgen stereophotogrammetric analysis. Spine, 17:678, 1992

8. Habal M: Repair of nonossifying defects in the skull. J Craniofac Surg 4: 1993

9. Hyman SL, Fisher W, Mercugliano M, Cataldo MF: Children with self injurious behavior. Pediatrics 85:437, 1990

10. Vinson R: Head banging in young children, AFP 43:1991

11. Clarren SK: Plagiocephaly and torticollis: etiology, natural history and helmet treatment. J Pediatr 98:92, 1981

12. Johnson RM, Owen JR, Hart DL et al: Cervical orthoses: a guide to their selection and use. Clin Orthop Rel Res 154: 34, 1981

13. Keagy R: The spine. In: Principles of Orthotic Treatment. CV Mosby, St. Louis, 1976

14. Fischer SV, Bowar JF, Essam AA, Gullikson G: Cervical orthoses effect on cervical spine motion: roentgenographic and goniometric method of study. Arch Phys Med Rehabil 58: 109, 1977

15. Hartman JT, Palumbo F, Hill BJ: Cineradiography of the braced normal cervical spine. A comparative study of five commonly used cervical orthoses. Clin Orthop Rel Res 109: 97, 1975

16. Johnson RM, Hart DL, Simmons EF et al: Cervical orthoses: a study comparing the effectiveness in restricting cervical motion in normal subjects. J Bone Joint Surg [Am] 59:1977

17. Maiman D et al: The effect of the thermoplastic Minerva body jacket on cervical spine motion. Neurosurgery 25: 1989

18. Millington PJ, Ellingsen JM, Hauswirth BE et al: Theromoplastic Minerva body jacket, a practical alternative to current methods of cervical spine stabilization. A clinical report. Phys Ther 67:223, 1987

19. Lunsford T, Davidson M, Lunsford B: The effectiveness of four contemporary cervical orthoses in restricting cervical motion. J Prosthet Orthot 6: 1994

20. Grew ND, Deane G: The physical effect of lumbar spinal supports. Prosthet Orthot Int 6:79, 1982

21. Lucas D: Spinal orthotics for pain and instability. In: Orthotics Etcetera. Williams & Wilkins, Baltimore, 1986

22. Thomas A: Orthopaedic Appliances Atlas. Vol. 1. Appliances for the Spine and Trunk. American Academy of Orthopaedic Surgeons, Edwards Brothers, Ann Arbor, MI, 1952

23. Nachemson AL: Orthotic treatment for injuries and diseases of the spinal column. Phys Med Rehabil 1:11, 1987

24. Knight J: Orthopaedia (or a Practical Treatise on the Aberrations of the Human Form). JH Vail, New York, 1884

25. Patwardhan AG, Gavin TM, et al: Orthotic stabilization of thoracolumber injuries—a biomechanical analysis of the Jewett hyperextension orthosis. Spine 15:654, 1990

26. Fidler MW, Plasmans CMT: The effect of four types of support on the segmental mobility of the lumbosacral spine. J Bone Joint Surg 65:9434, 1983

27. Williams PC: Lesions of the lumbosacral spine-lordosis brace. J Bone Joint Surg 19:690, 1937

28. Burkus JK, Lonstein JE, Winter RB, Denis F: Long term evaluation of adolescents treated operatively for spondylolisthesis. A comparison of in situ arthrodesis only with in situ arthrodesis and reduction followed by immobilization in a cast. J Bone Joint Surg 74:693, 1992

29. Gramse RR, Sinaki M, Ilstrep DM: Lumbar spondylolisthesis a rational approach to conservative treatment. Mayo Clin Proc 55:681, 1980

30. Kim S: Factors affecting the fusion rate in adult spondylolisthesis. Spine 15: 1990

31. Steiner M, Micheli J: Treatment of symptomatic spondylolysis and spondylolisthesis with the modified boston brace. Spine 10: 1985

32. Taylor CF: On the mechanical treatment of Pott's disease of the spine—the spinal assistant. Treatise New York State Med Soc 6:67, 1863

33. Lumsden RM, Morris JM: An in vivo study of axial rotation and immobilization at the lumbosacral joint. J Bone Joint Surg [Am] 50:1591, 1968

34. Fishman S: Spinal orthoses. In: Atlas of Orthotics, AAOS. CV Mosby, St. Louis, 1985

35. Willner SW: Effect of a rigid brace on back pain. Acta Orthop Scand 56:40, 1985

36. Thompson H: The halo traction apparatus—a method of external splinting of the cervical spine after injury. J Bone Joint Surg [Br] 44:655, 1962

37. Benzel E, Hadden T, Saulsbery C: A comparison of the Minerva and halo jackets for stabilization of the cervical spine. J Neurosurg 70:411, 1989

38. Koch RA, Nickel VL: The halo vest; an evaluation of motion and forces across the neck. Spine 3:103, 1978

39. Bradford D: Vertebral osteochondrosis (Scheuermann's disease). Clin Orthop 158:83, 1981

40. Bunch WH: Scoliosis: Making Clinical Decisions. CV Mosby, St. Louis, 1989

41. Carr WA, Moe JH, Winter RB, Lonstein JE: Treatment of idiopathic scoliosis in the Milwaukee brace. J Bone Joint Surg [Am] 62:595, 1980

42. Lonstein J: Orthotic treatment of spinal deformities: scoliosis and kyphosis. In: Atlas of Orthotics, AAOS. CV Mosby, St. Louis, 1985

43. Mital MA, Belkin SC, Sullivan MA: An approach to head, neck and trunk stabilization and control in cerebral palsy by use of the Milwaukee Brace. Dev Med Child Neurol 18:198, 1976

44. Gavin T, Bunch W, Dvonch V: The Rosenberger scoliosis orthosis. J Assoc Child Prosthet Orthot Clin 21: 1986

45. Emans J, Kaelin A, Bancel P et al: The Boston bracing system for idiopathic scoliosis: follow up results in 295 patients. Spine 11: 1986

46. Hall J, Cassella M: Current treatment approaches in the non-operative and operative management of adolescent idiopathic scoliosis. Phys Ther 71: 1991

SUGGESTED READINGS

Asher: Orthotics for Spinal Deformity. Orthotics Etcetera, Williams & Wilkins, Baltimore, 1986

Axelsson P, Johnsson R, Stromqvist B: Lumbar orthosis with unilateral hip immobilization. Effect on intervertebral mobility determined by roentgen stereophotogrammetric analysis. Spine 18:876, 1993

Colachis SC, Jr, Strohm BR, Ganter EL et al: Cervical spine motion in normal women. Radiographic study of effect of cervical collars. Arch Phys Med Rehabil 54:161, 1973

Edmonson A: Spinal orthotics. Orthot Prosthet 31:31, 1977

Harris J: Cervical orthoses. In: Orthotics Etcetera. Williams & Wilkins, Baltimore, 1986

Johnnson R: Influence of spinal immobilization on consolidation of posterolateral lumbosacral fusion. Spine 17:1992

Lantz S: Lumbar spine orthosis wearing. I. Restriction of gross body motions. Spine 11:1986

Letts M, Rathbone D, Yamashita T et al: Soft Boston orthosis in management of neuromuscular scoliosis: a preliminary report. J Pediatr Orthop 12:470, 1992

Lusskin R: Pain pattern in spondylolisthesis. Clin Orthop 40:125, 1965

Marsolais E, Byron: Spinal pain. In: Atlas of Orthotics, AAOS. CV Mosby, St. Louis, 1985

McGill SM, Norman RW, Sharratt MT: The effect of abdominal belt on trunk muscle activity and intra-abdominal pressure during squat lifts. Ergonomic 33:147, 1990

Montgomery SP, Erwin WE: Scheuermann's kyphosis, long term results of Milwaukee brace treatment. Spine 6:5, 1981

Nagel DA, Koogle TA, Pizialli RL, Perkash I: Stability of the upper spine following progressive disruptions and applications of individual internal and external fixation devises. J Bone Joint [Am] Surg 63:62, 1981

Norton PL, Brown T: The immobilizing efficacy of back braces: their effect on the posture and motion of the lumbosacral spine. J Bone Joint Surg [Am] 39:1958

Walpin L: The role of orthotic devices for managing neck disorders. Phys Med Rehabil: State Art Rev 1: 1987

Waters RL, Morris JM: Effect of spinal supports on the electrical activity of muscles of the trunk. J Bone Joint Surg [Am] 52: 51, 1970

Upper Limb Orthoses

Linda J. Miner
Virginia S. Nelson

This chapter presents an introduction to the most common upper limb (UL) orthoses. Functions and indications (appropriate conditions/diagnoses) are delineated for each orthosis. Information is provided regarding proper placement, biomechanical efficacy, materials, and contraindications. Orthotic devices used strictly to enhance activities of daily living are not included. These are considered adaptive equipment and are discussed in Chapters 9 and 10.

GENERAL CONSIDERATIONS

Upper limb orthoses may be used in a number of different circumstances, including congenital disorders, trauma, degenerative conditions, and after surgery to (1) immobilize a body part to promote tissue healing; (2) prevent contractures; (3) increase range of motion (ROM); (4) correct deformities; (5) strengthen muscles; (6) reduce tone; (7) reduce pain; or (8) restrict motion to prevent harmful postures.

Before the prescription of an orthosis, an analysis of the anatomy, function, and deficits must be performed by the physician and/or therapist. With this information, realistic goals may be determined and an appropriate or-

thosis prescribed, specifying type of orthosis, materials, and wearing schedule. Unlike lower limb orthoses, most UL orthoses are designed for temporary rather than long-term use. Whenever possible, the patient should be included in the decision-making process to increase patient acceptance. Patient compliance is also increased with thorough patient/family education and orthotic design that successfully achieves its goal.

Orthoses may be fabricated from rigid or flexible materials. Flexible splints, which allow limited midrange motion, are often used with nonacute cumulative trauma disorders. Whenever possible, off-the-shelf or prefabricated orthoses should be used to decrease cost and delivery time, with modifications made for the individual patient as needed. Custom upper extremity orthoses may be fabricated by occupational, physical, and hand therapists, or orthotists.

CLASSIFICATION AND NOMENCLATURE

Upper limb orthotic terminology can be very confusing. Historically, many different orthotic classification systems have been described in the literature. Orthoses are often grouped by design, purpose, location, materials, and/or source of power. Each system has its advantages and disadvantages. In this chapter, orthoses will be grouped generically by anatomic location, purpose, and/or design. Common names, acronyms, and eponyms are listed under the generic name to assist the reader and provide further clarity.

The terms *orthosis* and *splint* are used interchangeably. Traditionally, these devices have also been described as *static* or *dynamic*. Static orthoses hold a body part in a fixed position, whereas dynamic orthoses allow or create movement. Unfortunately, these terms are potentially confusing because static splints are often used to create movement. This is the case when a splint or cast is used to hold soft tissue on low-load stretch for long periods. Tissue is elongated after cell mitosis occurs, and the end result is increased range of motion. Additionally, dynamic splints can also include components that restrict arc of movement or statically hold one joint while allowing or creating movement at another.[1] Therefore, in this chapter, the terminology recommended by the American Society of Hand Therapists Splint/Orthotic Classification System[2] is used because it further clarifies the purpose of an orthosis as immobilizing, mobilizing, restricting, or a combination of these. A humeral fracture brace is a static orthosis used to immobilize or stabilize a humeral fracture. A resting hand splint may be used to either mobilize or immobilize joints of the wrist and/or hand. A dynamic elbow extension splint is used to mobilize or increase elbow extension. A balanced forearm orthosis is a combination of all three, designed to mobilize some joints, immobilize other joints, and restrict motion in still other joints.

Mobilizing orthoses may be (1) body-powered/internally powered (e.g., hinged elbow orthosis); (2) externally powered (e.g., dynamic extension outrigger splint); or (3) a combination of both (e.g., tenodesis splint). The simplest form of external power is provided by elastic materials, coils, or springs used to create movement through traction. Unfortunately, these forms of external power do not provide much force. Electric motors and the McKibben muscle with carbon dioxide actuators have been historically poorly accepted by patients. Upper limb orthoses may be externally powered with the same myoelectric or switch-controlled electronic components used in UL prostheses. These potentially can provide more power but may be cumbersome as well.

Digits and metacarpals are identified numerically as follows:

1. Thumb
2. Index finger
3. Middle finger
4. Ring finger
5. Small finger

Seddon's numeric system is used to describe muscle strength[1]:

0	No contraction
1	Palpable contraction without movement
2−	Less than full ROM, gravity eliminated
2	Full ROM, gravity eliminated
2+	Full ROM, gravity eliminated, minimal resistance
3−	Less than full ROM against gravity
3	Full ROM against gravity
3+	Full ROM against gravity with minimal resistance
4−	Full ROM against gravity with less than moderate resistance
4	Full ROM against gravity with moderate resistance
4+	Full ROM against gravity with full resistance/but breaks with resistance
5	Normal

The following medical acronyms are used in the text of this chapter:

AAROM	Active assistive range of motion
AC	Acromioclavicular joint
ADL	Activities of daily living
ALS	Amyotrophic lateral sclerosis
AROM	Active range of motion
BFO	Balanced forearm orthosis
BPL	Brachial plexus lesion
CMC	Carpometacarpal joint of the thumb
CP	Cerebral palsy
CPM	Continuous passive motion
CTD	Cumulative trauma disorders (also known as repetitive stress syndrome—RSS)

CTS	Carpal tunnel syndrome
CVA	Cerebrovascular accident
DBS	Dorsal blocking splint
DIP	Distal interphalangeal joint
EO	Elbow orthosis
EWHO	Elbow–wrist–hand orthosis
FO	Finger orthosis
GBS	Guillain-Barré syndrome
GH	Glenohumeral joint
IP	Interphalangeal joint (both PIP and DIP)
LMN	Lower motor neuron
MC	Metacarpal bone
MCP or MP	Metacarpophalangeal joint
MD	Muscular dystrophy
MS	Multiple sclerosis
ORIF	Open reduction internal fixation
PIP	Proximal interphalangeal joint
PO	Postoperative
PROM	Passive range of motion
RA	Rheumatoid arthritis
ROM	Range of motion
RSD	Reflex sympathetic dystrophy
SCI	Spinal cord injury
SEO	Shoulder–elbow orthosis
SEWHO	Shoulder–elbow–wrist–hand orthosis
SLE	Systemic lupus erythematosus
SO	Shoulder orthosis
TBI	Traumatic brain injury
TOS	Thoracic outlet syndrome
UL	Upper limb
UMN	Upper motor neuron
WHFO	Wrist–hand–finger orthosis
WHO	Wrist–hand orthosis

TYPES OF ORTHOSES

Groups of generic orthoses are presented below by their location on the UL from proximal to distal. Common names are listed under each generic heading. Note that L codes, when known, are given with the names of the orthoses. Standardized names (e.g., WHO, SO) are given after the common names.

Clavicular orthoses
Arm slings (Figs. 5-1, 5-2)

Arm abduction orthoses (Fig. 5-3)
Functional arm orthoses (Fig. 5-4)
Arm suspension slings (Fig. 5-5)
Balanced forearm orthoses (Fig. 5-6)
Arm supports
Nonarticular fracture orthoses
Elbow orthoses
Elbow–forearm–wrist orthoses (Fig. 5-7)
Elbow or wrist mobilization orthoses (Fig. 5-8)
Articulated orthoses
Epicondylar straps (Fig. 5-10)
Forearm mobilization orthoses (Fig. 5-9)
Forearm–wrist orthoses (Fig. 5-10)
Forearm–wrist–thumb orthoses (Fig. 5-11)
Forearm–wrist–MP orthoses (Fig. 5-12)
MP mobilization orthoses (Fig. 5-13)
Forearm–wrist–finger(s) orthoses (Fig. 5-14)
Digit flexion mobilization orthoses
Tenodesis orthoses (Figs. 5-15, 5-16)
Forearm–wrist–hand orthoses (Fig. 5-17)
Tone reduction orthoses (Figs. 5-18, 5-19)
Flexor tendon repair orthoses (Fig. 5-20)
Thumb orthoses (Fig. 5-21)
MP-restriction orthoses (Figs. 5-22, 5-23)
Partial hand opposition orthoses (Fig. 5-24)
Finger orthoses (Fig. 5-25)
Ring orthoses (Fig. 5-26)
IP mobilization orthoses (Figs. 5-27, 5-28)
DIP orthoses (Fig. 5-29)
Web orthoses (Fig. 5-30)
Gloves
Continuous passive motion orthoses

CLAVICULAR ORTHOSES[3,4] (L3650)
Figure-of-Eight Harness, Clavicular Brace/Harness, SO

Functions	Indications
Restrict motion to promote tissue healing	Clavicular fractures
Improve posture	Forward shoulder posture TOS
Reduce scapular myofascial pain	CTD
Increase/maintain PROM	Pectoral contractures

Placement
Material goes over clavicles, under arms, and crosses over high thoracic spinous processes.

Biomechanical Efficacy
These orthoses restrict movement of the clavicle and to some extent inhibit scapular protraction while allowing free movement at the GH joint.

Materials
Webbing straps, padding, and Velcro. Prefabricated orthoses are often used.

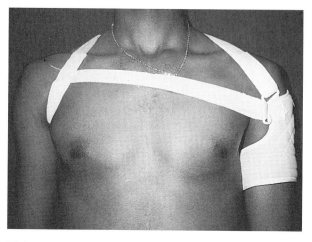

Fig. 5-2. Rolyan Hemi Arm Sling. (Courtesy of Smith & Nephew Rolyan Inc., Germantown, WI.)

ARM SLINGS[5–7] (L3660)
Figure-of-Eight Sling (Fig. 5-1), Universal Sling, Nothern Ring Sling, Cuff Sling, Hemi Sling, Orthopedic Sling, Flail Arm Sling, Homemade Bandanna-Type Sling, Glenohumeral Support, Hook Hemiharness, Rolyan Hemi Arm Sling (Vertical Arm Sling) (Fig. 5-2), SO

Functions	Indications
Immobilize to promote tissue healing	AC joint injury Scapular, humeral fractures PO shoulder repair/ arthroplasty PO tendon, artery, or nerve repairs Rotator cuff injury Bicipital tendinitis
Prevent overstretching of GH musculature/ ligaments	BPL
Decrease shoulder pain related to arm distraction and shoulder–hand syndrome	UMN lesions: hemiparesis with subluxation
Keep hand and forearm elevated to reduce edema	

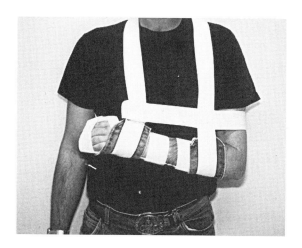

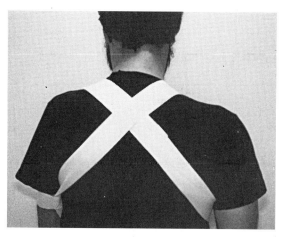

Fig. 5-1.   Figure-of-eight sling.

Placement
Most slings support the forearm with the elbow flexed, shoulder internally rotated, and arm adducted. The Ro-

lyan hemi arm sling supports the humerus and allows the elbow and forearm to be free by using a humeral cuff with figure-of-eight suspension. The Hook Hemiharness has two humeral cuffs connected by a posterior yoke and abducts each arm slightly while allowing the elbow and forearm to be free.

Biomechanical Efficacy
Slings may be static or dynamic. Dynamic slings use elastic straps and are designed to allow some motion of the forearm while supporting the arm. The wrist should be supported by the sling to prevent wrist drop if there is distal weakness. Hand should be higher than the elbow to decrease edema. Care must be taken to mobilize the

shoulder as soon as possible to prevent adhesive capsulitis.

Materials
Cloth, webbing, elastics, metal rings or fasteners, and Velcro. Prefabricated slings are often used.

Contraindications
Slings have fallen out of favor with a neurodevelopmental treatment approach to UMN lesions because they are thought to encourage flexion synergy, increase flexor tone, and promote contractures. The Rolyan hemi arm sling or the Hook Hemiharness may not approximate the GH joint in large patients.

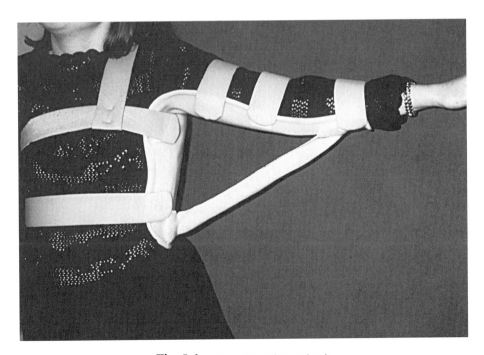

Fig. 5-3. Arm abduction orthosis.

ARM ABDUCTION ORTHOSES[2,4,5] (L3960)
(Fig. 5-3); Airplane Splint, SEWHO

Functions	Indications
Immobilize to promote tissue healing	Axillary burns PO shoulder fusion PO axillary scar release Shoulder dislocation
Increase PROM by soft tissue elongation via low-load, prolonged stretch (serial static splinting)	Burns Contractures

Placement
Medial arm and lateral trunk, with weight of arm borne primarily on the iliac crest or lateral trunk.

May be one piece or separate waist piece with arm attachment.

Biomechanical Efficacy
The shoulder should be positioned in abduction, with the degree determined by the pathology. Care should be taken not to overstretch skin, nerves, or vascular structures.

Materials
Casting, thermoplastics, metal, pillow, padding, strapping, and Velcro.

Contraindications
In persons with TOS, the arm should be in less than 90 degrees of abduction.

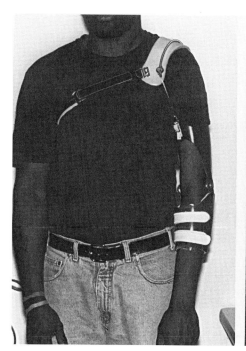
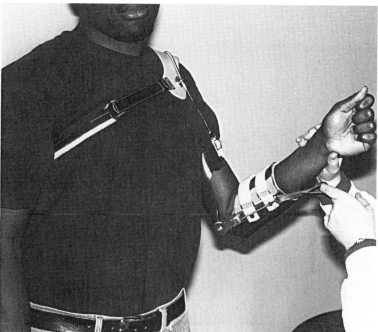

Fig. 5-4. Functional arm orthosis with external locking elbow hinge (humeral and forearm cuffs suspended from Bowden cable on shoulder saddle).

FUNCTIONAL ARM ORTHOSES[4,5,8] (L3999)

(Fig. 5-4); Functional Arm Brace (L3963), Flail Arm Splint, SEWHO

Functions	Indications
Substitute for weak/absent shoulder and elbow muscles	BPL LMN lesion with proximal weakness
Enhance ADL	

Placement

The circumferential proximal forearm cuff (and humeral cuff if the elbow is externally hinged) is suspended from a shoulder saddle by straps and/or a Bowden cable. Orthosis is suspended from a chest strap.

Biomechanical Efficacy

The GH joint should be approximated to minimize subluxation. This is best achieved by compression through the elbow joint (from the forearm or humeral cuff) to the shoulder saddle. Prosthetic components are often used. Suspension from a Bowden cable allows free arm swing while maintaining GH joint approximation and minimizing migration of the shoulder saddle. Suspension solely from a humeral cuff is usually ineffective. The external elbow hinge should have a manual lock in several ratcheted positions if the orthosis is substituting for weak or absent elbow flexion. Dynamic (elastic) assists may be added to assist weak elbow flexors. A removable palmar strut may be added to the forearm piece, or a forearm–wrist orthosis may be worn when wrist extension is weak.

This orthosis may be used temporarily while muscle reinnervation occurs and is most useful in treating those lesions severely affecting proximal function (shoulder, elbow) while sparing hand and wrist muscles.

The flail arm splint[8] differs from the orthosis mentioned above. It is a UL prosthetic shell that fits on a flail arm. This orthosis combines all of the prosthetic components noted above with the addition of a split hook protruding from a volar hand support. This functional hook is activated by a single control cable running up the flail arm, around the back, to the sound shoulder. Scapular protraction of the normal shoulder will open the hook. The hook will automatically close by rubber bands when the shoulder is relaxed.

Materials

Thermoplastics, metal, laminates, padding, cables, Neoprene, elastics, strapping, and Velcro.

Contraindications

Functional arm orthoses are not recommended when pathology indicates that the shoulder must be immobilized.

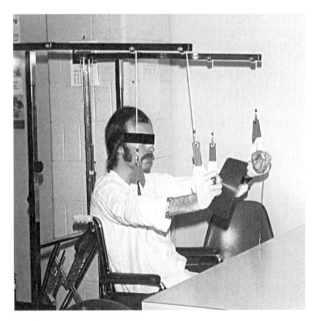

Fig. 5-5.   Deltoid aid.

ARM SUSPENSION SLINGS[4,5]

Deltoid Aid (L3969) (Fig. 5-5), Swedish Slings, Overhead Slings, Counterbalance Arm Slings, SEWHO

Functions	Indications
Position arm to allow hand use when shoulder/arm muscles are less than antigravity in strength	UMN lesions: CVA, TBI Myopathy with proximal weakness GBS
Exercise arm muscles in gravity eliminated position	SCI MD Arthrogryposis

Placement

Elbow and wrist straps are suspended from an overhead support that is freestanding or attached to table/wheelchair.

Biomechanical Efficacy

The forearm swings like a pendulum from elastic or static straps attached to the overhead support. With the deltoid aid, the weight of an arm can be counterbalanced to assist weak humeral flexors or abductors. Suspension slings can also be used to reduce or prevent CTD in factory workers assembling small parts.

Materials

Wheelchair/table mounting unit, overhead suspension bar, freestanding metal frame, leather or elastic straps, cloth sling(s).

Contraindications

The bulk of the overhead suspension assembly may prevent use outside of an institutional setting.

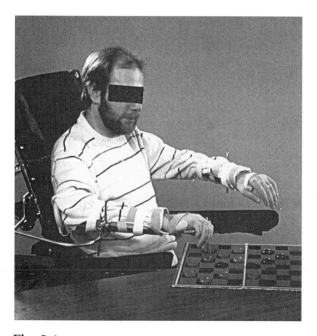

Fig. 5-6. Bilateral balanced forearm orthoses with forearm–wrist orthoses.

BALANCED FOREARM ORTHOSES[4,5,9] (L3964, L3965)

BFO (Fig. 5-6), Mobile Arm Support, Ball-Bearing Forearm Orthosis/Feeder, Friction Feeder (L3968), Body-Based BFO, "Gun Slinger," SEWHO

Functions	Indications
Support/position arm and assist weak proximal muscles to strengthen muscles and perform ADL	Severe proximal weakness BPL SCI Polio GBS MD
Allow patients with high tone to self-feed (dampen/control tone via friction feeder)	UMN lesions with high tone

Placement

BFOs may be clamped to a table, mounted on a wheelchair upright (Fig. 5-6) or attached to a body jacket worn on an ambulatory patient's trunk, resting on the iliac crests.

Biomechanical Efficacy

The patient must have 2+ or better strength in either neck, trunk, shoulder, *or* elbow muscles to successfully depress the elbow, thus elevating the hand. Orthosis setup is very complicated and usually accomplished by an occupational therapist or orthotist who has received extensive training. Successful "balanced" setup depends on the therapist's/orthotist's skill as well as the patient's sitting tolerance and motivation. Patients may be able to achieve tabletop activities (page turning, writing, keyboarding) even if self-feeding is not possible. A forearm–wrist orthosis may be required for distal support.

BFO Components (Proximal to Distal)

Bracket Ball-Bearing Housing (L3966)

The ball-bearing housing allows or can be tilted to assist horizontal arm adduction/abduction (a reclining bracket is available although mechanical leverage is compromised).

Proximal Arm

1. Standard (used in absence of deltoid function): The patient uses scapular elevation/retraction/relaxation to achieve internal rotation/elbow extension or external rotation/elbow flexion.

2. Elevating (L3970) (for deltoids graded 2 or 3): Assists humeral flexion/abduction in addition to the above.

Proximal Ball-Bearing Housing
Anterior or posterior tilt facilitates elbow extension or flexion.

Distal Arm
A bowed lateral bar is positioned from elbow to forearm trough.

Distal Ball-bearing Housing
1. Standard rocker arm assembly: allows internal/external rotation.
2. Offset swivel (L3972): dampens extreme ranges of internal/external rotation.
3. Supinator assist (L3974): allows supination with elbow flexion/external rotation and pronation with elbow extension/internal rotation.
4. Vertical trough stop: dampens extremes of motion with either standard or supinator assist rocker arm.
5. Risers: elevate trough 1.5 inches to reach the mouth.

Forearm Trough With Elbow Dial
This component supports the weight of the arm.

Materials
Metal, ball-bearing assembly.

Contraindications
Lack of sitting tolerance, low motivation, extreme spasticity, contractures.

ARM SUPPORTS (L3999)
Wheelchair Arm Trough, Forearm Elevators, Wrist Rests, Wheelchair Lapboard, Pillows

Functions	Indications
Reduce GH subluxation Prevent overstretching of muscles	Arm paresis due to UMN lesions: CVA, TBI
Elevate hand and forearm to prevent/reduce edema	Hand/forearm injury After hand surgery
Prevent/reduce pain/ inflammation (wrist rests)	CTD

Placement
The trough is attached to the armrest of the wheelchair. Forearm elevators may be placed on any surface. Wrist rests support distal volar forearm and are useful for keyboarding.

Biomechanical Efficacy
The arm is positioned so the shoulder is neutral and the hand and forearm are supported. The height of the trough is adjusted so the shoulder joint is approximated without undue compression. Forearm elevators position the hand higher than the elbow at the midchest level or higher.

Materials
Thermoplastics, high-density closed cell foam for troughs, metal, fabric, wood, and pillow. Prefabrications are most often used.

NONARTICULAR FRACTURE ORTHOSES[2,10]
Humeral Fracture Splint/Brace (L3980), Forearm Fracture Splint/Brace (L3982), Clamshell Brace, Isoulnar Splint, Galveston Splint[11]

Functions	Indications
Immobilize to promote tissue healing	Nondisplaced fracture of humerus, ulna or 2–5 MCs.
Protect bones	Osteogenesis imperfecta

Placement
Circumferential, covering the entire length of bony segment.

Biomechanical Efficacy
Brace immobilizes bony segment yet permits proximal and distal joint AROM. The Galveston brace works on a three-point fixation system to stabilize MCs 2, 3, 4, or 5 without immobilizing MPs or wrist.

Materials
Thermoplastics, padding, strapping, Velcro. Prefabrications are available.

Contraindications
Young or unreliable patients, severe edema or obesity.

ELBOW ORTHOSES[2,5] (L3999)
Posterior Elbow Splint, Elbow Cast, Air Splint, EO

Functions	Indications
Immobilize or restrict elbow motion to promote tissue healing	Medial/lateral epicondylitis Cubital tunnel syndrome PO tendon, artery, nerve repair Olecranon fracture Burns
Increase elbow PROM via low-load, prolonged stretch (serial static splinting)	Burns Elbow contractures

Placement
The splint is positioned circumferentially or on the posterior side of the distal two-thirds of the humerus and proximal two-thirds of the forearm. The angle of the elbow is dictated by pathology.

Biomechanical Efficacy
Posterior splints may be clam-shelled.

Serial casts may be used to provide low-load, prolonged stretch to promote soft tissue elongation and to increase PROM. Simultaneously, they provide neutral warmth, which tends to decrease/inhibit tone. Casts are changed every 3 to 4 days.

Wedge casts, a variation of serial casts, are used to increase elbow extension. After 2 to 4 days, the original cast is grooved anteriorly with a cast saw from the medial to the lateral epicondyle (the posterior portion is left intact). The elbow is stretched into greater extension, and a wooden wedge is inserted into the groove to maintain the stretch. New casting material is applied over the groove and wedge. After 2 to 4 additional days, the entire cast is removed, and the procedure is repeated until full extension is achieved.[12]

An airsplint (circumferential inflatable arm sleeve) or posterior elbow splint may also be used to maintain elbow extension for the purpose of weight bearing or to increase or maintain elbow extension.

Materials
Thermoplastics, casting, padding, strapping, and Velcro.

Contraindications
Serial casting is not recommended if the arm has open wounds, bony deformity, or recent fracture. Airsplint is contraindicated in patients intolerant of heat on extremity or allergic to this plastic material.

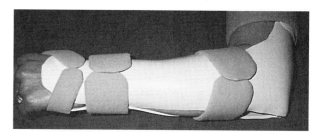

Fig. 5-7.   Sugar-tong elbow–forearm–wrist splint.

ELBOW–FOREARM–WRIST ORTHOSES (L3999)
Sugar-Tong Splint (Fig. 5-7), EWHO

Functions	Indications
Immobilize elbow/forearm/wrist to promote tissue healing	CTD Forearm fractures PO elbow arthroplasty PO ulnar nerve transposition

Placement
Circumferential with elbow in 90 degrees of flexion and forearm/wrist in neutral.

Biomechanical Efficacy
Orthosis should totally restrict elbow, wrist, and forearm AROM yet should allow full active use of all digits.

Materials
Thermoplastics, strapping, and Velcro.

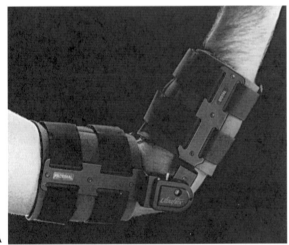

A

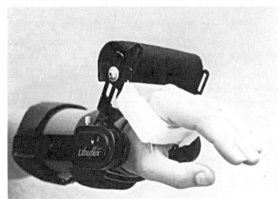

B

Fig. 5-8. **(A)** Empi Ultraflex dynamic elbow flexion orthosis and **(B)** dynamic wrist extension orthosis. (Courtesy of Ultraflex Systems Inc., Malvern, PA.)

ELBOW OR WRIST MOBILIZATION ORTHOSES[1,5,13,14]

Dynamic Elbow (L3730) (Fig. 5-8A), or Wrist Flexion/Extension Splint (Fig. 5-8B), Dynasplint, Ultraflex Splint, Static Progressive Splint (L3999), Phoenix Wrist Hinge, Turnbuckle Splint, EO or WO

Functions	Indications
Increase PROM by soft tissue elongation via low-load, prolonged stretch	Contractures PO scar release Burns Fracture (late phase)
Replace or assist weak wrist extensors to enhance ADL	Radial nerve lesion SCI BPL Polio

Placement

Dorsal (posterior), volar (anterior), or circumferential.

Biomechanical Efficacy

Two distinct methods can be used to stretch soft tissue, thereby encouraging tissue elongation and increased PROM. With either method, submaximal load for long periods of time achieves the best results:

1. Serial splinting with low-temperature thermoplastics (progressive static splinting) or serial casting. *Advantage:* Good conformity, little shifting. *Disadvantage:* Potential skin breakdown.
2. Traction (via elastics, coils, or springs) is applied across the joint (often a hinged joint) *Advantage:* Amount of load can be adjusted. *Disadvantage:* Forces can cause shifting of orthosis. Such splints are more difficult to fabricate unless prefabrications are used. Noncompliant patients can remove the orthosis.

Materials

Casting, thermoplastics, elastics, Neoprene, metal, strapping, Velcro, and springs.

Contraindications

Dynamic traction put on muscles with high tone may increase tone.

ARTICULATED ORTHOSES[1] (L3999)

Elbow (EO), Wrist (WO), PIP Hinged Splints (FO)

Functions	Indications
Provide mediolateral stability/support and in some cases limit AROM Control AROM in one plane	Joint instability PIP strains/sprains PIP volar plate injury (hinged with extension block) PO PIP surgery: partial ligament tear repair Total elbow resection PO wrist arthroplasty

Placement

Splint is applied circumferentially with the splint joint adjacent to anatomic joint.

Biomechanical Efficacy

The splint limits mediolateral motions (including forearm supination/pronation and wrist ulnar/radial deviation). Stops may be added to limit extension/flexion.

Materials

Thermoplastics, metal or plastic joints, strapping, and Velcro.

EPICONDYLAR STRAPS[2,15,16] (L3999)

Tennis/Golfer's Elbow Strap, Proximal Forearm Orthoses, Counterforce Brace, Forearm Band (see Fig. 5-10)

Functions	Indications
Reduce pain during activity Promote tissue healing at tendinous origins (theory)	Medial/lateral epicondylitis

Placement

Epicondylar straps are applied circumferentially to forearm distal to epicondyles without impeding elbow AROM. (Sleeve can extend above elbow.)

Biomechanical Efficacy

Compression over the tendon/muscle (counterforce) is hypothesized to reduce the muscular forces at the osteotendinous junction (origin on lateral or medial epicondyles) by redirecting the line of pull. This is felt to reduce inflammation and promote tissue healing without elbow or wrist immobilization.

Materials

Thermoplastics, elastics, Neoprene, Velcro, and D-rings.

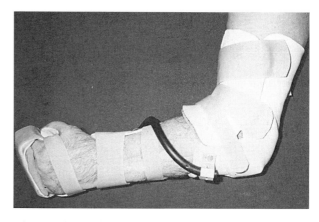

Fig. 5-9. Forearm supination mobilization orthosis using Rolyan Dynamic Pronation/Supination Kit. (Courtesy of Smith & Nephew Rolyan Inc., Germantown, WI.)

FOREARM MOBILIZATION ORTHOSES[1,2,14,17,18] (L3999)

Dynamic Supination/Pronation Splints, EWHO (Fig. 5-9)

Functions	Indications
Increase supination or pronation Increase PROM or AAROM	Forearm rotational contracture Upper trunk BPL (Erb's palsy) SCI

Placement

These orthoses are often composed of two pieces: (1) posterior elbow orthosis (2) forearm–wrist (see p. 115) or forearm–wrist–hand orthosis (Fig. 5-9). These are connected by a piece of rubber tubing. Circumferential serial casting may also be used.

Biomechanical Efficacy

The elbow splint is applied first. Distal splint is twisted three or four times then applied to the wrist and/or hand. The splint applies low-load, prolonged stretch to increase supination or pronation (depending on the direction the tube is twisted).

Increased passive pronation or supination can also be achieved with another two-piece orthosis, which seems to exert more even, direct rotational traction but is more difficult to fabricate. The proximal piece anchors on the humerus and immobilizes the elbow in 90 degrees of flexion. Two lateral bars protrude from the distal humerus and run parallel to the forearm (without touching it). The distal piece is a forearm–wrist orthosis, which has four to five loops in the low-temperature thermoplastic material on both the radial and ulnar borders of the splint. These loops are spaced evenly from the distal palmar crease to the proximal brim of the splint. Elastic traction is applied from the loops to the lateral bars.

Materials
Casting, thermoplastics, padding, tubing or pretightened coiled spring, metal hardware to attach tubing, strapping, Velcro. For children, the entire splint may be made of low-temperature thermoplastics.

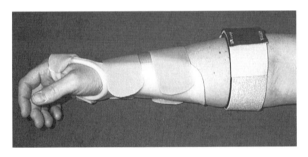

Fig. 5-10. Forearm–wrist orthosis with Rolyan epicondylar strap. (Courtesy of Smith & Nephew Rolyan Inc., Germantown, WI.)

FOREARM–WRIST ORTHOSES[1,13,15]
Wrist–Hand Orthosis, Thumb Hole Wrist Cock-up (L3906), Wrist Extension Splint, Static Wrist Splint, Bunnell Dorsal Wrist Splint, Bunnell Spring Cock-up Splint, Serpentine Splint, Futuro, Neoprene or Leather Prefabricated Wrist Extension Splints (L3908), Gutter Splint, WHO

Functions	Indications
Immobilize to promote tissue healing	CTD
	CTS
	Flexor/extensor tendinitis
	Lateral/medial epicondylitis
	Wrist sprain/contusion
	Arthritis
	Forearm/wrist fractures
	PO wrist extensor tendon repair
	PO wrist fusion
	PO skin grafting
Substitute for weak wrist extension	SCI
	BPL

Continues

Functions	Indications
Prevent overstetching of wrist extensors	ALS
	Radial nerve lesion
Stabilize the wrist for maximal grasp and pinch prehension/strength	Polio
	GBS
	Arthrogryposis
	UMN lesions: CVA, TBI, CP, MS
Immobilize wrist/forearm to maintain PROM	Burns
	PO scar release
Restrict motion to prevent harmful wrist postures during activity	CTD
	Arthritis
	Athletes or performing artists
Elongate soft tissue via low-load, prolonged stretch (serial static splinting)	Burns
	Wrist contractures

Placement
These orthoses are volar, dorsal, circumferential, or gutter based, extending from the proximal MP to two-thirds of the distal forearm. (If volar-based, palmar material should end $\frac{1}{4}$ inch proximal to the distal palmar crease to allow unrestricted MP flexion.)

Biomechanical Efficacy
The wrist can be positioned in flexion or extension, but for optimal hand function, the wrist should be in 15 to 30 degrees of dorsiflexion. (For carpal tunnel syndrome, the wrist should be neutral to maximize carpal tunnel lumen and to minimize median nerve compression.)

Base for Attachments
Outriggers, utensil holders.

Materials

Rigid: Metal, thermoplastics, casting, strapping, Velcro

Flexible: Neoprene, leather, elastics, fabric, strapping, Velcro

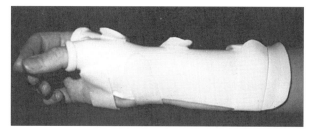

Fig. 5-11.   Forearm–wrist–thumb orthosis (long opponens splint).

FOREARM–WRIST–THUMB ORTHOSES[15] (L3907)

Long Opponens Splint (Fig. 5-11), Thumb Spica, WHFO

Functions	Indications
Immobilize thumb/wrist to promote tissue healing	CMC/MP synovitis/arthritis
	CTD
	de Quervain's tenosynovitis
	Thenar tendinitis
	Thumb sprain
	CMC/MP collateral ligament injury (gamekeeper's thumb)
	Scaphoid/thumb fracture
	PO thumb
	ORIF
	Surgical CMC/MP fusion
	Arthroplasty/reconstruction
	Tendon transfer
	Tendon/ligament repair
	Nerve repair
	PO trapeziumectomy

Continues

Functions	Indications
Substitute for weak thumb muscles; stabilize thumb in opposition for three jaw chuck pinch	Median/ulnar nerve lesion
	UMN lesions: CVA, TBI, CP
Maintain thumb PROM	Burns
Restrict motion to prevent harmful thumb positions during activity	CTD
	Arthritis
	Athletes or performing artists
Elongate soft tissues via low-load, prolonged stretch (serial static splinting)	Burns
	Thumb contractures

Placement

The orthotic material usually covers two-thirds of the distal radial forearm and surrounds the thumb to the IP (but can extend to tip).

Biomechanical Efficacy

In most cases, the thumb should be positioned in palmar abduction so that three jaw chuck prehension is easily achieved, unless pathology dictates otherwise. Material should not restrict motion of digits 2 to 5.

Materials

Rigid: Thermoplastics, metal, strapping, Velcro, casting, padding

Flexible: Neoprene, elastics, fabric, leather, strapping, Velcro.

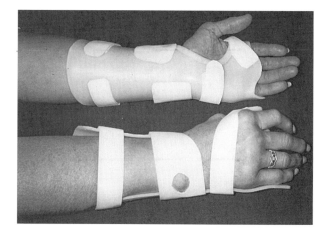

Fig. 5-12.   Forearm–wrist–MP orthosis.

FOREARM–WRIST–MP ORTHOSES[1,5]

(Fig. 5-12); MCP/Wrist Cock-up Splint, Molded Gauntlet (L3906), WHFO

Functions	Indications
Immobilize wrist/MPs to promote tissue healing	RA SLE PO intrinsic release
Protect wrist and MPs from internal/ external stresses during activity	RA SLE
Restrict ulnar deviation of digits 2–5 MPs	

Placement

The volar base spans the distal two-thirds of the forearm with material extending ¼ inch proximal to the PIP crease and a lateral ulnar stop extending to the middle of the small finger middle phalanx.

Biomechanical Efficacy

The wrist should be placed in neutral or 15–30 degrees of dorsiflexion. The MP ulnar deviation should be corrected to neutral. Thumb and digits 2 to 5 IP joints should have unrestricted motion to allow pinch and gross grasp during activity.

Materials

Thermoplastics, metal, strapping, and Velcro.

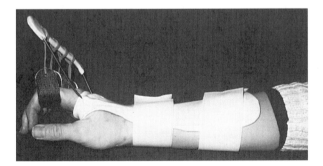

Fig. 5-13. MP extension mobilization orthosis.

MP MOBILIZATION ORTHOSES[1,5,14,19]

(Fig. 5-13); Dynamic MP Flexion/Extension Splint (L3916), Radial Nerve Splint (L3916), MP Arthroplasty Splint (L3916), MCP Extension or Flexion Assist, Dynamic Outrigger (L3916), Elephant Splint, Spider Splint, Swanson Splint (L3910), Bunnell Knuckle Bender (L3918), WHFO or FO

Functions	Indications
Improve hand function by substituting for lost or weak finger extension or thumb abduction	Radial nerve lesion BPL (dorsal outrigger)
Protect reconstruction while allowing active MP flexion, maintaining proper alignment, and restricting deviation during functional activities	PO MP arthroplasty PO extensor tendon repair (dorsal outrigger)
Increase passive thumb abduction/MP extension via low-load, prolonged stretch	Burns Contractures PO MC fracture ORIF (radial outrigger)
Increase passive MP flexion via low-load, prolonged stretch (volar outrigger)	Burns MP collateral ligament contractures Extensor tendon shortening Median/ulnar nerve lesion Claw hand PO MP capsulotomy PO MC fracture ORIF

Placement

Volar, dorsal, or circumferential (usually forearm-based) placement is used.

Biomechanical Efficacy

This splint is essentially a forearm–wrist orthosis (see p. 115) with high- or low-profile volar, dorsal, or radial outriggers for fingers and/or thumb. (The thumb will need a separate outrigger.) Best results are achieved when a submaximal load is exerted at a 90-degree angle from the proximal phalanx. The splint may be hand based to stretch MP collateral ligament contractures or to assist weak extensor digitorum when the wrist extension is muscle grade 4 or better.

Materials

Base: Metal, thermoplastics, casting, strapping, Velcro
Traction: Elastics, springs, coils, monofilament lines
Finger slings: Back-to-back moleskin, fabric, suede

Contraindications
Dynamic traction put on muscles with high tone may increase tone.

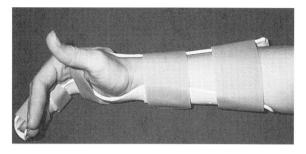

Fig. 5-14. Ulnar gutter splint (digits 4 and 5 with intrinsic plus positioning).

FOREARM–WRIST–FINGER(S) ORTHOSES[1] (L3906)
Radial/Ulnar Gutter Splint (Fig. 5-14), Forearm-Based Finger Splint, Long Finger Immoblization Splint, WHFO

Functions	Indications
Immobilize to promote tissue healing	2–5 MC fractures PO MC fracture ORIF PO ulnar/digital nerve repair Trigger finger Dupuytren's contracture
Maintain PROM/neutral positioning	Radial/ulnar ray congenital deficiency

Placement
Placement is radial/ulnar gutter or volar based extending from the tip of the fingers to two-thirds of the distal forearm.

Biomechanical Efficacy
The wrist is usually positioned in neutral to slight dorsiflexion with the digits in an intrinsic plus position unless pathology dictates positioning otherwise (e.g., for Dupuytren's contracture, MPs are positioned in maximal extension to maintain stretch on palmar soft tissue). "Intrinsic plus position" is a term used to describe positioning of digits 2 to 5 with MPs flexed at 70 to 90 degrees

and IPs in full extension (Figs. 5-14 and 5-17). Immobilization in this position is preferred because the MP and IP collateral ligaments are kept on stretch, minimizing future joint capsule contractures.[1]

> *Radial gutter:* Unrestricted thumb, ring and small fingers
>
> *Ulnar gutter:* Unrestricted thumb, index and middle fingers

Materials
Casting, thermoplastics, metal, strapping, Velcro.

DIGIT FLEXION MOBILIZATION ORTHOSES[1]
Dynamic Finger/Thumb Flexion Splint (L3912), Finger Flexion Glove/Mitt, WHFO

Functions	Indications
Increase passive composite digit flexion (MP/PIP > DIP)	Extrinsic extensor tendon shortening MP collateral ligaments Contractures of digits 2–5
Elongate extensor extrinsics via low-load, prolonged stretch	Claw hand/intrinsic tightness Extensor tendon repair (late) Burns Stiff hand
Substitute for lost/weak grasp (cylindric objects are held in palm by mitt or glove)	SCI Polio GBS ALS
Enhance ADL	MS BPL Median/ulnar nerve lesion UMN lesions: CVA, TBI, CP

Placement
Volar or circumferential.

Biomechanical Efficacy
To increase PROM, forearm/wrist orthosis (see p. 115) with volar outriggers (good for extrinsic stretch) or a hand-based flexion glove/mitt (good for MP more than PIP capsule stretch) is used. Note: without a pulley in

the palm (located at the distal palmar crease), little DIP flexion can be expected.

Materials

Thermoplastics, elastics, fabrics, leather, vinyl, metal, strapping, and Velcro.

Contraindications

A flexion mitt with static traction (Velcro strap) is favored over a flexion glove with rubber-band traction for UMN lesions, because dynamic traction put on muscles with high tone may increase tone.

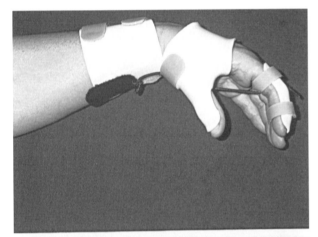

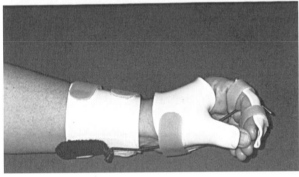

Fig. 5-15. Rehabilitation Institute of Chicago (RIC) tenodesis splint.

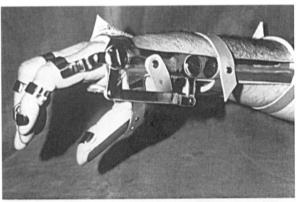

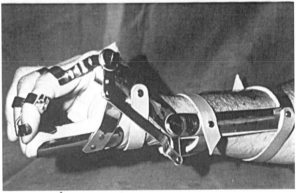

Fig. 5-16. Wrist-driven flexor hinge splint.

TENODESIS ORTHOSES[4,5,9]

(Figs. 5-15, 5-16); RIC Tenodesis Splint (L3999), Wrist-Driven Flexor Hinge Splint (L3900), Dynamic Cable-Driven Flexor Hinge (L3901), WHFO

Functions	Indications
Facilitate three jaw chuck pinch prehension via natural tenodesis	SCI Polio GBS
Augment strengthening via functional activities	

Placement

See Figures 5-15 and 5-16.

Biomechanical Efficacy

As wrist is extended, thumb is pulled into opposition with the index and middle fingers. For orthoses using natural tenodesis, wrist extensors should be 3 + or better muscle strength. The maximum pinch force that can be achieved is approximately 1 to 2 pounds. Some degree of shortening in extrinsic finger flexors is beneficial, so care should be taken during PROM and transfers to avoid overstretching. Externally powered orthoses often use proximal muscles and do not require distal muscle strength.

Rehabilitation Institute of Chicago (RIC) Tenodesis Splint (Fig. 5-15)

This orthosis is usually made of low-temperature thermoplastics in two or three separate pieces (wristlet, short opponens, dorsal plate over index and middle finger).

> *Advantages:* Lightweight, easily and quickly fabricated, good for temporary situations
> *Disadvantage:* Splint migration

Wrist-Driven Flexor Hinge Splint (Fig. 5-16)

This orthosis is usually made of metal, fabricated by a certified orthotist, and considered a definitive orthosis. Some designs include adjustable ratchets. The MP spring-activated ratchet lock facilitates sustained pinch after the wrist relaxes. The wrist ratchet accommodates various wrist positions and pinching of different-sized objects. All ratchets are disengaged passively, by the other extremity, or by pushing against chest or chin.

> *Advantages:* Stronger pinch force may be achieved, with less splint migration. Components are more adjustable.
> *Disadvantages:* Lengthy fabrication time. Heavier materials require stronger wrist extension (4−) and better endurance.

Externally Powered Tenodesis Orthoses (L3902)

Powered by an electric motor or the McKibben muscle (CO_2 actuators), these orthoses have been poorly accepted by patients. However, external power is possible with more recent technology that is used in upper extremity prostheses (myoelectric or switch control).

Functional Electrical Stimulation (FES) (L3904)

Some facilities use implanted or surface electrodes located in a dorsal forearm cuff to recruit stronger wrist extension and natural tenodesis prehension.

Materials

Base: Thermoplastics, padded metal, laminates, strapping, Velcro
Traction: Elastics, springs, coils, cord

Contraindications

Insufficient range of motion.

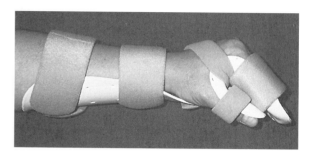

Fig. 5-17. Resting hand splint (digits with intrinsic plus position).

FOREARM–WRIST–HAND ORTHOSES (L3907)

(Fig. 5-17); Resting Hand/Pan Splint, Static Hand Splint, Functional Resting Splint, Burn Splint, Weight Bearing Splint, WHO, or WHFO

Functions	Indications
Immobilize to promote tissue healing	Open wounds, cellulitis
	Arthritis
	CTD
	Extensor digitorum tendinitis
	Extrinsic flexor tendinitis
	Lateral/medial epicondylitis
	PO forearm–wrist–hand
	ORIF
	Tendon/nerve/artery repair
	Skin graft
	Dupuytren's release
Maintain PROM wrist and hand (often used at night)	UMN lesions: CVA, TBI, MS
Maintain stretch on MP/IP collateral ligaments	ALS
	SCI
	Polio
	Burns
	BPL
	GBS
Position wrist/digits in extension for crawling (weightbearing)	Pediatric UMN lesions
	Pediatric BPL
Elongate soft tissue via low-load, prolonged stretch (serial splinting)	Burns
	Contractures

Placement

Placement of these orthoses is circumferential, dorsal, or volar based, extending from the tips of the fingers and/or thumb to two-thirds of the distal forearm. (Sometimes the thumb is left free.) These orthoses may extend above the elbow for a pediatric weightbearing splint.

Biomechanical Efficacy

The wrist is usually positioned in neutral to slight dorsiflexion with the digits in an intrinsic plus position unless pathology dictates positioning otherwise (e.g., after an extensor tendon repair, MPs should be positioned in full extension to minimize tension on the suture site while healing occurs). Note: "Intrinsic plus position" is a term used to describe positioning of the fingers with the MPs flexed at 70 to 90 degrees, the IPs in full extension, the thumb with CMC in palmar abduction, and the MP/IP in full extension (Fig. 5-17). Immobilization in this position is preferred because MP and IP collateral ligaments are kept stretched, minimizing future joint capsule contractures. In addition, the thumb is maintained in a functional position for opposition/three jaw chuck pinch prehension.[1]

Materials

Casting, thermoplastics, metal, strapping, and Velcro.

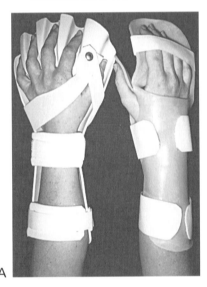

Fig. 5-18. **(A)** Rolyan Preformed Anti-Spasticity "Ball" Splint and **(B)** Snook Splint. (Courtesy of Smith & Nephew Rolyan Inc., Germantown, WI.)

TONE-REDUCTION ORTHOSES[20]

(Fig. 5-18, 5-19); Antispasticity Ball Splint (L3907), Snook Splint (L3908),[21,22] Cone Splint, Bobath Splint, Becker Splint,[22,23] Finger Abduction Splint, WHFO

Functions	Indications
Flexor tone reduction	UMN lesions: CVA, TBI,
Prevent maceration of palm by fingernails	MS, CP
Increase PROM via low-load, prolonged stretch (serial static splinting)	

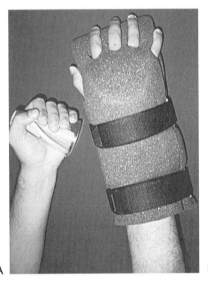

Fig. 5-19. **(A)** Rolyan Clear Hand Cone and **(B)** MIT Dynafoam Wrist–Hand Orthosis. (Courtesy of Smith & Nephew Rolyan Inc., Germantown, WI.)

Placement

Tone-reduction orthoses can be hand based (volar or circumferential) or forearm based (volar, dorsal, or circumferential).

Biomechanical Efficacy

UL high tone can be reduced throughout the limb with reflex-inhibiting positioning (digit extension combined with abduction, a neurodevelopmental treatment [NDT] technique) or firm pressure into the palm (a Rood technique). Hand-based splints, such as a rigid cone strapped firmly into the palm (Rood), shown in Figure 5-19, or foam finger extension abduction splints (Rood) may reduce mildly increased flexor tone.[24] Forearm-based splints are generally more effective because of the extension positioning of the extrinsic finger flexors.

The rationale for the dorsal-based Snook splint is different.[20,21] Broad contact over a body surface tends to facilitate contraction of underlying muscles. Therefore, it is theorized, stimulation to the extensor surface might balance muscle tone and/or avoid increasing flexor tone.

A typical wearing schedule for a tone reduction splint is 2 hours on and 2 hours off throughout the day.

Some therapists feel that an airsplint is helpful in reducing flexor tone by providing neutral warmth and breaking up synergy patterns. The circumferential inflatable sleeve of clear plastic extends from fingertips to axilla. Before inflation, the arm is positioned in slight external rotation/adduction with the digits abducted, the wrist neutral, the forearm supinated 45 degrees, and the elbow extended. The length of application is usually 20 minutes. Clothing or a stockinette sleeve under the splint may increase wearing tolerance.[25]

Materials

Thermoplastics, foam, strapping, Velcro, and clear plastic.

Contraindications

Open skin lesions, fractures. Air splints are contraindicated with plastic allergies or skin lesions exacerbated by sweating.

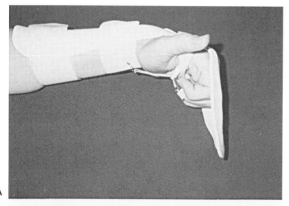

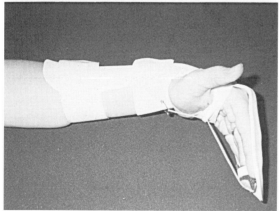

Fig. 5-20. Dorsal blocking splint (DBS) with finger flexion mobilization (early controlled motion Washington protocol). **(A)** Relaxed position. **(B)** Active finger extension against resistance.

FLEXOR TENDON REPAIR ORTHOSES[1]
(L3999)

DBS (Fig. 5-20), Kleinert splint, Early Controlled Motion Splint, Strickland Splint, WHFO

Functions	Indications
Protect flexor tendon reconstruction/promote tissue healing	PO flexor tendon repair in zones 2–5 (between DIP and distal volar forearm)
Allow tendon gliding to decrease adhesions (early controlled motion protocols)	

Placement

Flexor tendon repair orthoses are placed on the dorsal forearm, wrist, and/or hand (Fig. 5-20).

Biomechanical Efficacy

The DBS is positioned with the wrist in 20 to 45 degrees of flexion, the MPs in 40 to 70 degrees of flexion, and the IPs in full extension. (Protocols vary slightly for wrist and MP positioning.)

Duran Protocol[26]

The DBS is used without mobilizing components. The patient is instructed to remove the straps, holding the digits in place to perform PROM exercises every waking hour.

Early Controlled Motion Protocols
Kleinert[27]

The DBS is combined with elastic traction, pulling digits into flexion. Traction is applied from the volar wrist to a distal fingertip hook, which is either sewn on by the surgeon, glued to the nail, or taped in place. The patient is told to actively extend the digit(s) against the resistance of the elastic traction to the limits of DBS and then to allow the elastic traction to pull the digit(s) back into flexion without contracting the repaired flexor tendon(s). This exercise is performed 5 to 10 times during each waking hour. Traction is removed at night, and the digit(s) are immobilized in the DBS by straps or elastic bandage.

Washington[28]

The Washington protocol is similar to the Kleinert protocol with the addition of a pulley at the distal palmar crease to increase passive DIP flexion (Fig. 5-20).

Strickland[29]

A specific surgical suture technique is required. The patient is started with a modified Duran protocol, but within the first 4 weeks PO, an additional mobilizing splint is provided. This splint is a DBS with digits positioned similarly, but the wrist hinged with a stop to permit full wrist flexion and up to 30 degrees of dorsiflexion. The patient continues to wear the immobilizing DBS most of the time but is instructed to change to the hinged wrist DBS every waking hour for a brief period of AAROM exercises.

Materials

Base: Thermoplastics, strapping, Velcro
Traction: Elastics, springs, monofilament line, hooks, safety pin pulleys, tape

Contraindications

Early controlled motion is contraindicated with coinciding nerve repairs and in very young or noncompliant patients.

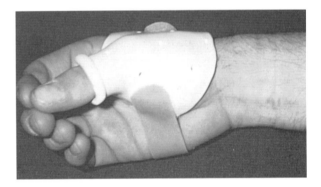

Fig. 5-21. Hand-based thumb or opponens splint.

THUMB ORTHOSES[1,5,19]

Cone Splint, Hand-Based Opponens Splint (Fig. 5-21), Short Opponens Splint (L3800), Static Thumb Splint, C-Bar (L3810), FO

Functions	Indications
Immobilize thumb to promote tissue healing	CMC/MP arthritis CMC/MP fracture (late phase) CMC/MP dislocation/ subluxation CMC/MP collateral ligament injury (gamekeeper's or skier's thumb) CTD PO MP fusion PO collateral ligament repair
Protect thumb CMC/MP from internal/external stresses during activity	Arthritis CTD Athletes or performing artists
Improve hand function by facilitating three jaw chuck pinch	Ulnar/median nerve lesion SCI GBS

Placement

Thumb orthoses are placed circumferentially from just proximal to the IP to the base of the thumb, clearing the thenar crease in the palm.

Biomechanical Efficacy

Motion in the thumb CMC and MP is restricted, and the IP is usually left free to facilitate pinch prehension. In most cases, the thumb should be positioned in palmar abduction so that three jaw chuck prehension is easily achieved, unless the patient's condition dictates otherwise. In children, the thumb can be abducted and brought into opposition using a Neoprene strap.

Materials

Rigid: Thermoplastics, casting, strapping, Velcro
Flexible: Neoprene, fabric, elastics, strapping, Velcro

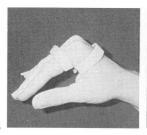 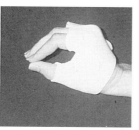

Fig. 5-22. **(A)** MP-blocking figure-eight splint and **(B)** hand-based intrinsic plus splint.

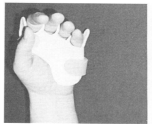 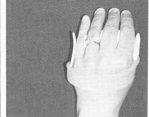

Fig. 5-23. Hand-based ulnar deviation correction splint.

MP RESTRICTION ORTHOSES[5,30,31] (L3999)

Anticlaw Splint, Hand-Based Intrinsic Plus Splint (Fig. 5-22B), Pretzel Splint, Figure-of-Eight Splint (Fig. 5-22A), Ulnar Palsy Splint, Lumbrical Bar, Clam Digger, Ulnar Deviation Splint (Fig. 5-23), FO

Functions	Indications
Block MP extension and permit full MP flexion	Median/ulnar nerve lesion
Allow active IP extension in intrinsic minus hand	UMN lesions: CVA, TBI BPL GBS
Protect 2–5 MPs from external stresses during activity by restricting MP ulnar deviation and maintaining proper alignment	RA SLE
Immobilize MP to promote tissue healing/reduce inflammation	Tenosynovitis (trigger finger)

Placement

Placement of MP joint-restriction orthoses is volar, dorsal, or circumferential hand based.

Biomechanical Efficacy

For the intrinsic minus hand, MPs are blocked in 70 to 90 degrees of flexion. Ulnar nerve lesions may require MP blocking on the ring and small fingers only. This splint should be worn throughout the day and night for two reasons: (1) It prevents contractures of the MP, PIP, and DIP collateral ligaments (claw hand deformity), and (2) it allows the patient to actively extend the PIPs and DIPs in the absence of intrinsic function, thereby increasing hand function while simultaneously maintaining strength in the extensor digitorum. The splint should be used until the neuropathy resolves or until tendon transfers are performed.

For arthritis, ulnar deviation should be corrected to neutral, and MP flexion/extension should be unrestricted if possible (depending on the amount of MP subluxation/deformity). Patients with early MP ulnar drift are encouraged to use this splint while performing ADL. Realignment enhances hand prehension and reduces the forces pushing the digit into ulnar deviation. Patients may find this orthosis cumbersome and may opt for MP arthroplasty.

For tenosynovitis, the MP is typically immobilized in full extension while allowing unrestricted motion in IPs.

Materials

Thermoplastics, metal, elastics, fabrics, strapping, and Velcro.

Contraindications

Psoriatic arthritis skin lesions that do not allow pressure from splint. An ulnar drift splint is generally ineffective with moderate-to-severe MP subluxation (arthritics).

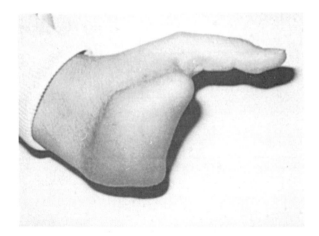

PARTIAL HAND OPPOSITION ORTHOSES[32] (L3999)

(Fig. 5-24); Opposition Post, Temporary "Prosthesis," Child Amputee Prosthetics Project (CAPP) Opposition Platform

Functions	Indications
Improve hand prehension—enable hand to pick up/hold objects	Congenital/traumatic partial hands Absent thumb Radial ray deficiency Transmetacarpal amputations

Placement

Placement is in opposition to the residual hand.

Biomechanical Efficacy

Opposition orthotic design may include a ratcheting device if multiple positions are desired. Opposition material must be placed carefully so active motion of the residual hand is unrestricted.

Materials

Metal, laminates, thermoplastics, strapping, Velcro, and leather.

Contraindications

Open wounds are contraindications.

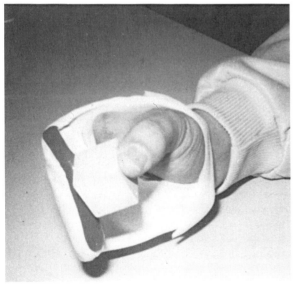

Fig. 5-24. Partial hand opposition splint.

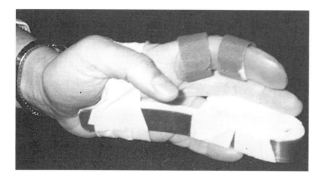

Fig. 5-25. Finger orthoses: finger gutter (index finger) and aluminum/foam hand-based digit immobilization splint (ring finger).

FINGER ORTHOSES[1,33] (L3999)

Gutter Splint (Fig. 5-25), Eggshell Finger Cast, Static Finger Splint, FO

Functions	Indications
Immobilize to promote tissue healing	Phalanx fracture PIP/DIP dislocation PIP/DIP collateral ligament injury PIP volar plate injury
Exercise extensor digitorum in the absence of intrinsic function	Ulnar nerve lesion
Elongate soft tissue via low-load, prolonged stretch (serial static splinting)	Burns Contractures

Placement

Placement of finger orthoses is circumferential, lateral, dorsal or volar based, usually restricting motion at the PIP and DIP only. These orthoses can also be hand based to include immobilization of MP.

Biomechanical Efficacy

In general, IPs are immobilized in full extension to keep collateral ligaments stretched and to prevent IP flexion contractures, unless the patient's condition dictates otherwise.

Materials

Padded metal, casting, thermoplastics, tongue depressor, strapping, and Velcro.

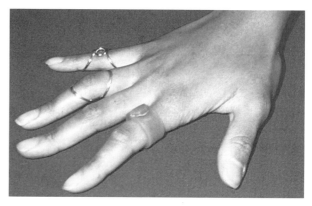

Fig. 5-26. Ring orthoses: A2 pulley ring (index finger), Siris swan neck splint (ring finger), Siris boutonniere splint (small finger). (Courtesy of Silver Ring Splint Co., Charlottesville, VA.)

RING ORTHOSES[5] (L3999)

(Fig. 5-26); Silver Ring Splints, Swan Neck Splint, Figure-Eight Splint, PIP Hyperextension Block Splint, Murphy Ring Splint, Boutonniere Splint, Pulley Ring, PIP Extension Stop, FO

Functions	Indications
Block PIP/DIP hyperextension but allow normal IP flexion/extension Prevent overstretching of PIP or DIP volar plate Prevent deformity	Arthritis Swan neck posture/deformity PIP/DIP volar plate injury
Immobilize PIP in extension (DIP free) Prevent deformity	Arthritis Boutonniere posture/deformity
Prevent bowstringing of flexor tendons	A2 pulley injury (annular pulley for flexor tendon located on volar surface of proximal phalanx)
Protect reconstruction/allow dynamic motion, without immobilizing finger	PO A2 pulley repair

Placement

Placement of the ring orthoses is shown in Figure 5-26.

Biomechanical Efficacy

Rings are custom fitted and worn at all times.

Swan neck ring: Prevents IP hyperextension via three points of pressure but allows full IP flexion. Lateral or distal supports may be added for stability.

Boutonniere ring: Immobilizes the IP in extension via three points of pressure. This splint needs to be removed several times daily for ROM.

A2 pulley ring: Fits firmly around the proximal phalanx from the PIP volar crease to the MP volar crease.

Materials

Metal, thermoplastics (temporary).

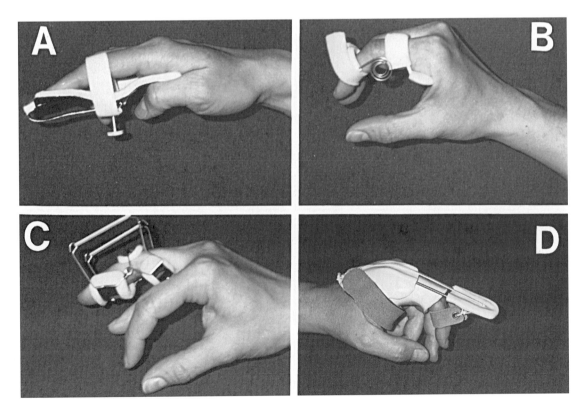

Fig. 5-27. Interphalangeal joint extension mobilization orthoses: **(A)** Rolyan Joint Jack splint. **(B)** Rolyan Spring Coil Finger Extension (Capener) Splint. **(C)** Rolyan Reverse Knuckle Bender Splint. **(D)** Hand-based PIP extension splint with low-profile outrigger (elephant splint). (Courtesty of Smith & Nephew Rolyan Inc., Germantown, WI.)

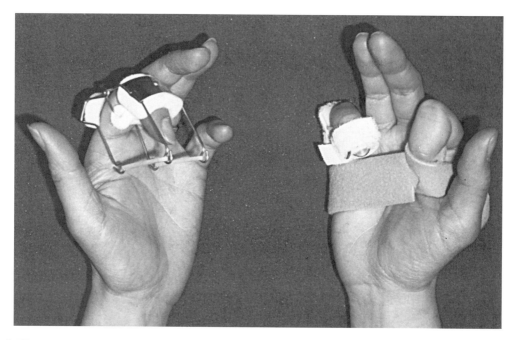

Fig. 5-28. Interphalangeal joint flexion mobilization orthoses: Rolyan Finger Knuckle Bender Splint (left index), Rolyan Dynamic Finger Flexion Loop (right small), flexion strap (right index). (Courtesy of Smith & Nephew Rolyan Inc., Germantown, WI.)

IP MOBILIZATION ORTHOSES[5,14,34–38]

(Figs. 5-27, 5-28); *Extension:* Dynamic IP Extension Splint (L3934), Reverse Knuckle Bender (L3942), Joint Jack, Neoprene "Banana" Splint, Safety-Pin Splint, IP Serial Casting, Spring-Coil Assist, Capener Splint, Elephant Splint (L3800, L3820), Dynamic Thumb IP Extension Splint (L3805, L3845), FO

Flexion: Dynamic IP Flexion Splint/Thumb Flexion Splint, Knuckle Bender (L3948), Buddy Strap/Tape/Trapper, Flexion Strap (L3999), Joint-Cinch, FO

Functions	Indications
Increase passive IP extension	IP flexion contracture (capsular tightness) Boutonniere deformity PO Dupuytren's release
Increase passive IP flexion	IP extension contracture (capsular tightness)

Placement

Placement of hand-based orthoses is circumferential. Forearm-based orthoses may be dorsal, volar, or circumferential (Figs. 5-27 and 5-28).

Biomechanical Efficacy

Two methods can be used to stretch soft tissue, thereby encouraging tissue elongation and increased PROM in the IPs. With either technique, submaximal load for long periods achieves the best results:

1. Holding the IP statically on low tension circumferentially (eggshell finger casts, flexion straps, Joint Jack, Neoprene "banana" splint, serial static splints)
2. Traction (via elastics, coils, or springs) applied across the joint from proximal to distal, equally balanced on both radial and ulnar sides of digit, and requiring three points of contact (knuckle benders, reverse knuckle benders, spring coil extension assist [Capener], safety-pin splint, outriggers with rubber band traction)

Buddy straps/tape/trappers use normal ROM in an adjacent digit to support and increase IP motion in the involved finger.

Materials

Base: Thermoplastics, metal, padding, casting, strapping, Velcro

Traction: Elastics, coils, springs, monofilament lines

Slings: Fabric, moleskin, suede

Contraindications

Dynamic traction on muscles with high tone (UMN lesions) may result in increased tone. Note: These orthoses are only effective in reducing capsular contractures (not contractures related to extrinsic tendon shortening).

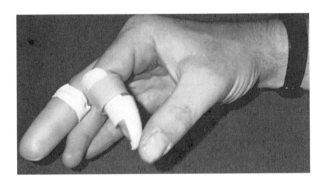

Fig. 5-29. Stax splint (index finger) and circumferential DIP immobilization splint (middle finger) (Courtesy of Smith & Nephew Rolyan Inc., Germantown, WI).

DIP ORTHOSES[1] (L3999)

(Fig. 5-29); Stax or Stack Splint, DIP Gutter Splint, Static DIP Splint, FO

Functions	Indications
Immobilize to promote tissue healing	DIP fracture Distal extensor tendon repairs

Placement

Placement of DIP orthoses is volar, dorsal, or circumferential from the tip of the finger to just distal to the PIP volar crease.

Biomechanical Efficacy

Motion at the PIP should be unrestricted. Extensor tendon repairs distal to the DIP should be immobilized in slight DIP hyperextension to take tension off repair.

Materials

Padded metal, casting, thermoplastics, tongue depressor, strapping, tape, and Velcro.

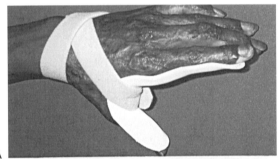

A

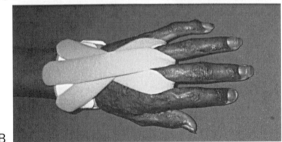

B

Fig. 5-30. **(A)** Thenar web spacer (C-Bar Split); **(B)** finger web spacers.

WEB ORTHOSES[19]

(Fig. 5-30); C-Bar Splint (L3800, L3810), Web Spacers, FO

Functions	Indications
Increase or maintain space between digits Prevent web space contractures	Burns PO syndactyly reconstruction PO scar revision Web space contractures

Placement
The orthotic material is held firmly in web space.

Biomechanical Efficacy
These orthoses are most effective if tension is applied over the web spacer. (This can be achieved with the use of a compression glove or straps applied perpendicular to the web space.)

Materials
Otoform, Elastomer, silicone-based, low-temperature thermoplastics, Neoprene, Strapping, and Velcro

Contraindications
Open wounds.

GLOVES[(L3999)]
Shock Absorbing Gloves, Isotoner/Tubigrip/Jobst Compression Gloves

Functions	Indications
Absorb shock/vibration entering palm or hand	CTD
	CTS
Prevent CTD (shock absorbing gloves)	Flexor tendinitis
	Wheelchair users
	Hypersensitive palmar skin/ scars
Reduce hand/wrist swelling via circumferential compression (compression gloves)	Traumatic hand injuries with edema
	Burns
	RSD
	CTD
	SCI
	UMN lesions: CVA, TBI
Reduce hypertrophic scarring (compression gloves)	Burns (maturation phase)
	Scars

Placement
Gloves are placed circumferentially on the hand and wrist. (Tips or whole fingers of the glove may be omitted if not needed.)

Biomechanical Efficacy
Shock absorption: The palmar aspect of the glove and volar wrist can be padded with various materials (e.g., silicone gel).[39]

Edema reduction: Low-to-moderate compression (10 to 15 mmHg[40] capillary pressure).

Scar reduction: Pressure garments with high compression (15 to 25 mmHg[40] capillary pressure).

Materials
Elastics, fabrics, leather, silicone, nylon, and spandex.

Contraindications
Open wounds. Compression with vascular occlusive conditions can further compromise blood flow and must be cautiously undertaken. Scars must be able to tolerate shear forces occurring during donning and doffing of gloves.

CONTINUOUS PASSIVE MOTION ORTHOSES[41]

Electrically powered continuous passive motion (CPM) orthoses are available for mobilizing joints. They are usually made of metal and plastic and provide continual, reciprocal passive joint range within a uniaxial plane. Adjustable controls program the arc of range, speed, and force of movement. Most of these devices are portable. They are usually rented to the client for use at home but can be purchased.

The rationale for use is to maintain or increase PROM, promote tissue healing, prevent complications by providing connective tissue homeostasis, facilitate neuromuscular reeducation, and control pain. CPM is particularly useful in the treatment of burns or in individuals experiencing stiffness.

A typical wearing schedule is several weeks with the patient encouraged to wear the orthoses as much as possible throughout the day.

CPM orthoses are an adjunct to ongoing therapy and should be closely monitored by the therapist. Patients should be educated that CPM is no substitute for AROM or AAROM and strengthening exercises.

ACKNOWLEDGMENTS

The authors thank the following members of the Department of Physical Medicine and Rehabilitation at the University of Michigan Medical Center for their invaluable assistance in the preparation of this chapter: Christine Hoban, OTR, CHT; Janette Baker, OTR, CHT; Brenda Myers, OTR; Ruth Lamphiear, OTR; Ann Morley, OTR; and James A. Leonard, MD. We are especially grateful to Alycia Sykora, BA, and Carol Gajar Pullen, BA, for their assistance in preparing this manuscript.

REFERENCES

1. Fess E, Phillips C: Hand Splinting Principles and Methods. 2nd Ed. CV Mosby, St. Louis, 1987

2. Bailey JM, Cannon NM, Casanova J et al: Splint classification system. American Society of Hand Therapists, Chicago, 1992

3. Thomas KA: Use of clavicle brace for upper extremity cumulative trauma. J Hand Ther 5:242, 1992

4. Long C: Upper limb orthotics. p. 190. In Redford JB (ed): Orthotics Et Ceters. 2nd Ed. Williams & Wilkins, Baltimore, 1980

5. Fishman S, Berger N, Edelstein J, Springer W: Upper limb orthoses. p. 163. In American Academy of Orthopaedic Surgeons (eds): Atlas of Orthotics. 2nd Ed. CV Mosby, St. Louis, 1985

6. Kenney DE, Klima RR: Modified arm sling for soft-tissue injuries of the shoulder and glenohumeral subluxation. J Hand Ther 6:215, 1993

7. Ryerson S, Levit K: The shoulder in hemiplegia. p. 117. In Donatelli RA (ed): Physical Therapy of the Shoulder. 2nd Ed. Churchill Livingstone, New York, 1991

8. Frampton FM: Management of brachial plexus lesions. J Hand Ther 1:115, 1988

9. Rehabilitation Institute of Chicago, Education and Training Center, Northwestern University Medical School, Chicago, 1988

10. King JW: Upper extremity fracture bracing. J Hand Ther 5:157, 1992

11. Sorensen JS, Freund KG, Kejla G: Functional fracture bracing in metacarpal fractures: the Galveston metacarpal brace versus a plaster-of-Paris bandage in a prospective study. J Hand Ther 6:263, 1993

12. Backer G, Mercer R, Dabrowski E, Nelson VS: Wedge casting for pediatric knee and elbow flexion contractures. Dev Med Child Neurol, suppl. 69:34, 1993

13. Schutt AH: Upper extremity and hand orthotics. Phys Med Rehabil Clin North Am 3:223, 1992

14. Flowers KR, Schultz-Johnson K: Static-progressive splints. J Hand Ther 5:36, 1992

15. Henshaw JL, Satren JW, Wrightsman JA: The semi-flexible support: an alternative for the hand-injured worker. J Hand Ther 2:35, 1989

16. Powell SG, Burke AL: Surgical and therapeutic management of tennis elbow: an update. J Hand Ther 4:64, 1991

17. Hokken W, Kalkman S, Blanken WC, VanAsbeck FW: A dynamic proration orthosis for the C6 tetraplegic arm. Arch Phys Med Rehabil 74:104, 1993

18. Colello-Abraham K: Dynamic pronation-supination splint. p. 1134. In Hunter J, Schneider L, Mackin E, Callahan A (eds): Rehabilitation of the Hand: Surgery and Therapy. 3rd Ed. CV Mosby, St. Louis, 1990

19. Colditz JC: Splinting for radial nerve palsy. J Hand Ther 1:18, 1987

20. McPherson JJ: Objective evaluation of a splint designed to reduce hypertonicity. Am J Occup Ther 35:189, 1981

21. Snook JH: Spasticity reduction splint. Am J Occup Ther 33:648, 1979

22. Feldman PA: Upper extremity casting and splinting. p. 149. In Glenn MB, Whyte J (eds): The Practical Management of Spasticity in Children and Adults. Lea & Febiger, Philadelphia, 1990

23. McPherson JJ, Becker AH, Franszczak N: Dynamic splint to reduce the passive component of hypertonicity. Arch Phys Med Rehabil 66:249, 1985

24. Mathiowetz V, Bolding DJ, Trombly CA: Immediate effects of positioning devices on the normal and spastic hand as measured by electromyography. Am J Occup Ther 37:247, 1983

25. Trombly CA: Neurophysiological and developmental treatment. p. 96. In Trombly CA, Scott AD (eds): Occupational Therapy for Physical Dysfunction. 3rd Ed. Williams & Wilkins, Baltimore, 1989

26. Duran RJ, Coleman CR, Nappi JF, Klerekoper LA: Management of flexor tendon lacerations in zone 2 using controlled passive motion postoperatively. p. 410. In Hunter J, Schneider L, Mackin E, Callahan A: Rehabilitation of the Hand: Surgery and Therapy. 3rd Ed. CV Mosby, St. Louis, 1990

27. van Strien G: Postoperative management of flexor tendon injuries. p. 390. In Hunter J, Schneider L, Mackin E, Callahan A: Rehabilitation of the Hand: Surgery and Therapy. 3rd Ed. CV Mosby, St. Louis, 1990

28. Dovelle S, Kulis HP: The Washington regimen: rehabilitation of the hand following flexor tendon injuries. Phys Ther 69:1034, 1989

29. Strickland JW (ed): Strickland protocol. The Indiana Hand Center Newsletter. Vol. 1. Foundation for Hand Research and Education, Indianapolis, 1993

30. Gilbert-Lenef L: Splinting the arthritic hand: soft ulnar deviation splint. J Hand Ther 7:29, 1994

31. Patel MR, Bassini L: Trigger fingers and thumb: when to splint, inject, operate. J Hand Surg 17A:110, 1992

32. Bunnell S: The management of the nonfunctional hand: reconstruction versus prosthesis. p. 997. In Hunter J, Schneider L, Mackin E, Callahan A: Rehabilitation of the Hand: Surgery and Therapy. 3rd Ed. CV Mosby, St. Louis, 1990

33. Laseter GF: Postoperative management of capsulectomies. p. 364. In Hunter J, Schneider L, Mackin E, Callahan A: Rehabilitation of the Hand: Surgery and Therapy. 3rd Ed. CV Mosby, St. Louis, 1990

34. Colditz JC: Anatomic considerations for splinting the thumb. p. 353. In Hunter J, Schneider L, Mackin E, Callahan A: Rehabilitation of the Hand: Surgery and Therapy. 3rd Ed. CV Mosby, St. Louis, 1990

35. Colditz JC: Spring wire splinting of the proximal interphalangeal joint. p. 1109. In Hunter J, Schneider L, Mackin E, Callahan A (eds): Rehabilitation of the Hand: Surgery and Therapy. 3rd Ed. CV Mosby, St. Louis, 1990

36. Lamey G: Buddy splint. J Hand Ther 7:30, 1994

37. Mignardi MM: Dynamic PIP stabilizing splint. J Hand Ther 7:31, 1994

38. Paynter P, Schinderler-Grasse P: Techniques for improving distal interphalangeal motion. J Hand Ther 6:216, 1993

39. Brown AP: The effects of anti-vibration gloves on vibration-induced disorders: a case study. J Hand Ther 3:94, 1990

40. Richard RL, Staley MJ: Burn Care and Rehabilitation Principles and Practice. FA Davis, Philadelphia, 1994

41. Dimick MP: Continuous passive motion for the upper extremity. p. 1140. In Hunter J, Schneider L, Mackin E, Callahan A (eds): Rehabilitation of the Hand: Surgery and Therapy. 3rd Ed. CV Mosby, St. Louis, 1990

SUGGESTED READINGS

1. Boozer J: Splinting the arthritic hand. J Hand Ther 6:46, 1993

2. Milford L: The Hand. 3rd Ed. CV Mosby, St. Louis, 1988

Appendix 5-1

International Classification of Disease Codes and Diagnoses[a]

ICD Code	Diagnosis	ICD Code	Diagnosis
840.00	Acromioclavicular joint injury, separation	834.02	DIP dislocation
886.00	Amputation, transmetacarpal	842.10	DIP sprain, volar plate injury
335.20	Amyotrophic lateral sclerosis	728.60	Dupuytren's contracture
842.10	Annular pulley injury	718.42	Elbow contracture
715.90	Arthritis, degenerative, osteoarthritis	812.41	Elbow fracture
714.00	Arthritis, rheumatoid	726.31	Epicondylitis, medial
728.30	Arthrogryposis	726.32	Epicondylitis, lateral
726.12	Bicipital tendinitis	767.60	Erb's palsy
736.21	Boutonniere posture/deformity	727.81	Extrinsic extensor/flexor tendon shortening
353.00	Brachial plexus lesion	958.60	Forearm contracture
949.00	Burns	813.80	Forearm fractures
943.04	Burns, axillary	357.00	Guillain-Barré syndrome
354.00	Carpal tunnel syndrome	344.40	Hemiparesis: arm, UMN lesion, CVA, TBI
681.00	Cellulitis, thumb or fingers		
682.40	Cellulitis, hand	342.00	Hemiparesis with subluxation, UMN lesion
343.10	Cerebral palsy		
436.00	Cerebrovascular accident	812.20	Humeral fracture
810.00	Clavicular fracture	718.80	Joint instability
736.06	Claw hand, acquired	354.90	LMN lesion with proximal weakness, arms
716.90	CMC arthritis	354.10	Median nerve lesion
842.10	CMC collateral ligament injury	815.00	Metacarpal fracture
833.04	CMC dislocation, subluxation	716.90	MP arthritis
728.89	Collateral ligament contracture	842.12	MP collateral ligament injury
354.20	Cubital tunnel syndrome	718.44	MP contracture
727.04	de Quervain's tenosynovitis	834.01	MP dislocation, subluxation
718.44	DIP contracture	815.00	MP fracture

Continues

133

Continues

ICD Code	Diagnosis	ICD Code	Diagnosis
340.00	Multiple sclerosis	718.41	Shoulder contracture
359.10	Muscular dystrophy	831.00	Shoulder dislocation
359.90	Myopathy with proximal weakness	709.20	Skin contractures
756.51	Osteogenesis imperfecta	344.00	Spinal cord injury (quadriparesis)
885.00	Partial hand, absent thumb	736.09	Swan neck posture/deformity
759.89	Partial hand, congenital	710.00	Systemic lupus erythematosus
886.00	Partial hand, traumatic (fingers missing)	727.05	Tendinitis, extensor digitorum, extrinsic flexors
885.00	Partial hand, traumatic (fingers and thumb missing)	727.00	Tenosynovitis
718.41	Pectoral contracture	726.90	Thenar tendinitis
816.00	Phalanx fracture	353.00	Thoracic outlet syndrome
718.44	PIP contracture	816.00	Thumb CMC fracture
834.02	PIP dislocation	718.44	Thumb contracture
842.10	PIP sprain, volar plate injury	842.10	Thumb sprain
138.00	Polio	854.00	Traumatic brain injury
955.30	Radial nerve lesion	727.03	Trigger finger, acquired
813.42	Radius (distal) fracture	813.22	Ulna fracture (shaft)
813.44	Radius/ulnar (distal) fractures	354.20	Ulnar nerve lesion
887.00	Radial ray deficiency	755.20	Ulnar ray congenital limb deficiency
337.21	Reflex sympathetic dystrophy, upper limb	718.43	Wrist contracture
959.20	Rotator cuff injury	814.00	Wrist fracture
811.00	Scapular fracture	842.00	Wrist sprain

a For expansions of acronyms, see pp. 104–5.

Appendix 5-2

International Classification of Disease Codes and Surgical Procedures[a]

ICD Code	Surgical Procedure	ICD Code	Surgical Procedure
39.59	Artery repair	86.84	Scar release, revision
80.40	Capsulotomy	81.83	Shoulder arthroplasty
82.35	Dupuytren's contracture	81.23	Shoulder arthrodesis (fusion)
	release	86.69	Skin graft, flap
81.85	Elbow arthroplasty	86.89	Syndactyly release
81.28	Finger arthrodesis (fusion)	83.88	Tendon repair
79.10	Fracture open reduction with	83.76	Tendon transfer
81.96	internal fixation	82.57	Tendon transfer, hand
	MP arthroplasty	81.26	Thumb CMC fusion
81.72	Ligament repair	81.27	Thumb MP fusion
80.40	MP capsulotomy	80.93	Trapeziumectomy
04.79	Nerve repair	04.60	Ulnar nerve transposition
83.63	Rotator cuff repair	81.26	Wrist fusion

[a] For expansions of acronyms, see pp. 104–5.

Orthotic Management of Children

Gabriella E. Molnar

6

PRINCIPLES

The principles of orthotics for children are the same as those for adults in terms of design and biomechanical characteristics. Only a few devices were designed specifically for children. As in adults, improvement of function and prevention of deformities constitute the two major reasons for using orthoses. From a clinical viewpoint, this conceptual distinction is often artificial, because both functional and preventive purposes may be achieved simultaneously. Prescription of an appropriate orthosis for children is based on the universally applicable principles of biomechanics and is determined by the extent of functional loss, kinesiologic abnormalities, and anticipated musculoskeletal complications.[1,2]

Clinical Applications and Goals

In the clinical application of orthotics, there are differences between children and adults. They stem from the fact that throughout childhood, growth and development act as dynamic forces. Although their influence is modified or curtailed by a disability of early onset, the element of change created by the pervasive effect of these processes is a distinctive feature in the rehabilitation of children. This chapter discusses orthotic management from the perspective of growth and development.

Rehabilitation goals and, within this framework, orthotic intervention are contingent on developmental expectations. They must be consistent with the child's current level of function and adjusted as maturation proceeds. The well-known standards of normal child development that relate accomplishment of certain milestones to chronological age are helpful only as a limited guide for handicapped children and need to be individually adapted in each case.

To define expectations, a number of factors are considered:

1. Anticipated deviations in motor development commensurate with the nature and extent of physical dysfunction
2. Personality development, because restricted mobility tends to perpetuate dependence and emotional immaturity
3. Mental age, in case of intellectual deficit, which affects learning ability and adaptive and cognitive functions
4. Possible medical complications associated with the motor disability that may influence the child's health and development

It should be apparent that a physical deficit is significant in the sense that it determines the pace and the highest attainable level of motor accomplishments. To what extent this potential is fulfilled will depend, however, on the interaction of some or all of the aforementioned factors. One should also be cognizant of the role of parents and family. Their contribution is crucial in fostering the child's development and independence toward realistic goals. Without their consistent participation, professional efforts are doomed to fail.

An important aim in the rehabilitation of children is to provide experiences that stimulate or approximate the usual developmental sequence. In this context, an orthosis is a functional device for sitting or standing in infancy and early childhood, as much as it is for walking at a later age. Bracing may be used to assist individuals with less advanced gross motor skills when the likelihood of achieving functional independence is slight or perhaps nonexistent.

An example is a standing brace for a child who is not expected to ambulate. Although it would be difficult to measure the effect of this intervention, the assumption seems reasonable that handicapped children in the sensorimotor stage of development also need to be exposed to a variety of new experiences, such as the sensation of being in the upright position and viewing the surrounding environment from a different perspective. Prevention of contractures and the physiologic effect of weight bearing on bone metabolism and on the formation of hip joints are additional benefits of this activity. A standing device may be particularly desirable and satisfying for a young child with normal intellectual endowment and severe physical impairment. Clinical experience indicates that eventually both parents and children are inclined to give up the use of an orthosis for such limited functional gain, usually by the end of the early school years.

Ambulation

For a bright, well-motivated young child, training in ambulation may be initiated in spite of the possible need for extensive orthotic application, bearing in mind that functional walking is not within the scope of long-range projection. A primary motivation for young children is to achieve physical mobility. The importance of this desire is well illustrated by youngsters with spinal cord injury, who often surpass adults with similar neurologic lesions in actual achievement and functional level of ambulation. Small stature, low center of gravity, and shorter leverage are mechanical factors in favor of greater mobility.

When walking efficiency and proficiency are marginal and require extensive bracing and other assistive devices, a regression tends to occur around adolescence. At this stage, intellectual, vocational, and other pursuits may take priority over ambulation. In the resulting emotional turmoil, the earlier interest in walking may well be lost. Also, the changing relationship between muscle strength and forces of gravity as a result of a sudden growth spurt and weight gain make the effort of ambulation more strenuous.[3] Progression of deformities that cannot be controlled successfully can be an additional adverse influence.

Contractures

That long-standing or permanent neuromuscular deficits, if untreated, lead to soft tissue contractures is well known. These complications are more prone to appear in a growing child and tend to progress rapidly when the rate of growth is physiologically accelerated. During adolescence, a combination of sudden increase in stature with functional decline enhances the threat of progressive deformities. The skeletal frame is molded by muscular and gravitational forces. In childhood, when bone tissue is more malleable and the epiphyseal plates are not ossified, bone and joint deformities can develop if these forces are unbalanced or abnormal. Protective orthotic stabilization of the lower limb may be needed to decrease skeletal changes resulting from neuromuscular dysfunction, defects or diseases of the joints, or their connective tissue support.

For the reasons previously stated, the preventive use of orthoses is given greater emphasis in children than in adults. The same considerations account for the tendency to apply more extensive bracing at an early age and to decrease it gradually as neuromuscular coordination and strength develop or as growth ceases.

Night splints and braces represent a form of preventive orthotic intervention used more often in children than in adults. The term "night brace" is actually a misnomer, because few children tolerate these devices through the night. Rather than deprive the whole family of peaceful sleep, it is more practical to incorporate the use of resting braces in the afternoon nap or evening play activities.

Deformities

A comment on the role of orthotics in correcting deformities seems appropriate, because it is sometimes mentioned as a feasible goal. Although braces are very useful for prolonged stretching of tight soft tissues, it is rarely, if ever, possible to expect correction of significant fixed contractures. Instead, the aim is to restrain further deterioration. An orthosis should accommodate deformities that cannot be corrected by passive manipulation; otherwise, children do not tolerate the device, and their tender skin can easily develop pressure ulcers. In properly selected cases, serial or progressive casting can be an effective method for reducing less fixed contractures, followed by orthotic fitting after a reasonable correction of the deformity has been achieved.

Appropriate Age

A question frequently raised is the appropriate age when an orthosis should be provided for a child with delayed development as a result of motor disability of early onset. Understandably, no hard rules can be applied to every case, because a great variability is seen in motor and associated deficits. When bracing is contemplated for functional purposes, one useful consideration is the level of gross motor accomplishments rather than chronological age.

If the child has attained at least fair or preferably good head control, an orthotic device may be indicated for sitting or standing. Active trunk control or an ability to maintain passive alignment of the torso above the weightbearing surface in the erect position is needed to plan functional ambulation with braces and crutches.

Aside from the physical attributes, a mental age of 2 to 3 years is usually required to learn the skill of crutch walking, although a few exceptional children in our clinical experience mastered it by 18 months of age. In children who have a relatively slight delay of motor development and a good outlook for unassisted walking, one can usually wait until they pull to stand and begin to cruise to decide whether an orthotic device is necessary. Nonhandicapped children sit, pull to stand, and walk approximately at 6, 10, and 12 months of age, respectively. Keeping the previously mentioned developmental and physical requirements in mind, the chronological age when orthotic assistance would be considered is around the third or fourth quarter of the first year for passive sitting and 12 to 18 months for passive standing. Walking requires active participation under any circumstance.

The timing of orthotic intervention solely for preventive purposes depends primarily on the changing status of the musculoskeletal system. Evidently, the more severe the motor deficit, the earlier and the faster will deformities occur. Splints made from low-temperature thermoplastic or other easily workable materials can be used in infancy or in older children as a substitute for a costly and cumbersome orthosis when functional gains are not feasible. It is beyond the scope of this chapter to dwell on the difficulties of early prognostication of function in physical disabilities of prenatal, perinatal, or early postnatal onset, or to discuss the uncertainties of predicting exact life expectancy in some progressive neurologic diseases of variable course. However, these considerations stress the importance of instituting proper and timely measures for averting or delaying deformities, regardless of the ultimate outcome.

Choice of Materials

When considering the choice of various materials for orthotic fabrication, light weight is a desirable feature at all ages. Synthetic materials offer an advantage over conventional braces made entirely of metal used in the past. Limited adjustability for growth is a disadvantage of plastic materials in childhood. Snugly fitted parts, such as the ankle–foot component, may require annual or even more frequent replacement during periods of rapid growth. A combination of extensible metal uprights with plastic cuffs provides room for growth and combines the advantage of lighter weight with adjustability in knee–ankle–foot–orthoses (KAFOs) or hip KAFOs (HKAFOs.) Prescription of extensible uprights is a standard procedure in pediatric orthotics. Occasionally, in a very active, ambulatory youngster, one may resort to a conventional AFO for durability. However, with the total contact plastic AFOs, soft tissue containment and control may be optimized. Such plastic AFOs can easily be combined with extensible uprights for higher level bracing.

Re-evaluation and Adjustment

All children who wear orthoses must be periodically re-evaluated. Progress in motor function may permit decrease or discontinuation of braces. In other cases, changing musculoskeletal findings warrant modifications.

During reviews of orthotic fitting, shoes should also be regularly examined since adjustment for growth is necessary. Generally, evaluation every 6 months is advisable, but the exact frequency depends on the rate of growth, which is fastest in the earliest years of childhood, and from about 10 years on through adolescence. However, some primary or secondary diseases of the skeletal system, neurologic deficits of cerebral origin, and especially lower motor neuron lesions are associated with decreased extremity growth. In the rapid phases of growth, adjustable metal uprights can usually accommodate increase in leg lengths for 2 to 3 years. Thigh cuffs and other plastic components may need more frequent adjustment or replacement for increasing size and girth.

Shoes

Similarly, in the fitting of shoes, growth should be taken into account. Correct shoe size should leave a 1/4- to 1/2-inch distance between the tip of the toes and the toe box. When the toes touch the end of the toe box, new shoes are needed. Width should be appropriate for both the hindfoot and the forefoot. Shoes should be fitted in the standing position, because foot configuration changes on weight bearing. The examiner should palpate the tip of the first and second toes for proper length and should feel the tension at the first and fifth metatarsal heads, over the instep and heel, to determine the correct width. During the fast-growing phase of early childhood, new shoes may be needed every 3 months. Some active youngsters with pathologic gait wear out their shoes in a matter of weeks and should be provided with two pairs. In young children, high-top shoes are used with orthoses. For older children or those with less extensive orthoses, Oxford shoes may be adequate. Many commercially available sport shoes provide adequate support when used with an orthosis. They are generally well accepted by children and parents. Split-size shoes are required if the difference between the two feet exceeds one shoe size. For further details of shoe types and modifications, see Chapter 3.

Counseling

The parents must be carefully instructed when the orthosis is first worn, and these recommendations are reinforced in physical therapy. It may require several weeks until children tolerate their first orthosis for the desired length of time. The brace should be applied for gradually increasing periods, the skin should be inspected for evidence of pressure marks, and these measures should be taken with special care when there is a sensory deficit. Repeated counseling is needed about the implications of absent sensation. Benefits expected from the use of orthoses should be clearly explained. In the case of limited goals, the parents must be advised in specific practical terms about how and when the orthosis can be best used. Parents should also be reminded that adjustments and changes that are due to growth must be initiated on time to avoid problems caused by ill-fitting orthoses and shoes during the waiting period.

CEREBRAL PALSY

Cerebral palsy is defined as a nonprogressive damage to the immature brain that can occur in the prenatal, perinatal, or postnatal period. The leading clinical sign is a neuromuscular dysfunction. Associated deficits may be present when cerebral structures other than those contributing to motor function are impaired.

Among these, mental retardation and seizure disorders are the most frequent. In some instances, impairment of vision and hearing may be present; the latter is most likely in the athetoid type following bilirubin encephalopathy. Cortical sensory deficit of the affected extremities, found in about half of the cases with hemiplegia, represents a limiting factor in functional use. It is often accompanied by a growth disturbance of central origin.

Clinical classification of cerebral palsy is based on neurologic signs and their topographic distribution.[4] Spastic clinical types have the highest incidence and include hemiplegia, diplegia, and quadriparesis. Dyskinetic clinical types are less frequent and encompass a range of athetoid-dystonic movement disorders. A mixture of spasticity and athetosis may occur. Ataxic and atonic clinical types are rare.

In spite of the static brain lesion, the natural history of cerebral palsy is characterized by changing clinical findings. In addition to delayed motor development, hypotonicity is a frequent early sign. Spastic hypertonicity usually makes its appearance in infants between 6 and 12 months of age, whereas definite dyskinetic movements may not become evident until 18 months or later. These changes are related to maturation of the defective central nervous system. Natural development leads to functional progress over the years; its pace and final out-come reflect the extent of cerebral damage. Musculoskel-etal sequelae of the neurologic dysfunction represent a simultaneous, potentially opposing influence.

Cerebral palsy is not a homogeneous disease entity regarding etiology, pathology, clinical manifestations, and course. From the viewpoint of ultimate prognosis, severity of motor deficit, intellectual function, and emo-tional adjustment were found to have the most signifi-cant influence.[4] As in all childhood disabilities with the potential for multiple handicaps, planning of overall management is based on all aspects of function.

The motor deficit in cerebral palsy is a disturbance of central movement control. Defective coordination of selective muscle action is compounded by tone abnor-malities, pathologic reflex activity, and persistent primi-tive infantile reflexes.[5] Undifferentiated synergistic movement patterns are more prevalent in the spastic clin-ical types. From an orthotic standpoint, the goal is to control abnormal and excessive muscle activity that can lead to deformities and causes biomechanical abnormali-ties of stance and gait. Surgical lengthening of spastic muscles and correction of deformities are effective meth-ods to improve postural deviations. Although this aspect of treatment is not discussed here, coordinated use of bracing and surgery is an essential part of management plans.

The greatest changes in the orthotic management of children have probably occurred in cerebral palsy. Long leg braces with a pelvic band,[6,7] often with a spinal at-tachment, have been replaced by less extensive and more selective action orthoses.[8,9]

Congenital and Acquired Hemiplegia

Children with congenital hemiplegia are generally 4 to 6 months behind in early motor achievements. Attain-ment of walking may be delayed somewhat longer, but the majority walk by 2 years, and virtually all walk by the age of 3.[4] Rare exceptions are youngsters with profound mental retardation who achieve these milestones much later or in some cases not at all.

A cortical sensory deficit in the leg tends to prolong the delay of walking and is often accompanied by under-development of the extremity. Size and length discrep-ancy usually become evident in infants between 12 and 18 months and continue to increase until 6 to 8 years of age. Length difference rarely exceeds 1 inch. A shoe lift is not necessary for this amount of discrepancy, be-cause the resulting functional lateral curvature of the spine is mild and nonprogressive. Moreover, in the pres-ence of plantar flexor hyperactivity, length difference makes toe clearance easier during the swing phase. How-ever, leg length must be measured regularly, and spinal alignment should be observed. Underdevelopment of the affected foot necessitates split-size shoes in some cases.

In general, an orthosis is not required until the child pulls to stand and begins to cruise holding on, because range of motion can be maintained by other means be-fore the stage of upright mobility. From this time on, a brace may be needed to correct ankle and foot abnormali-ties.

Gait deviations in children with hemiplegic cerebral palsy resemble the familiar kinesiologic features of exten-sor synergy.[10] Plantar flexor overactivity results in spastic equinus attitude of the ankle, which makes toe clearance difficult; weight is borne mostly or completely on the forefoot. Inadequate knee flexion, and consequently cir-cumduction, are particularly marked when walking is first started but decrease as coordination improves. Con-trary to the usual synergistic pattern of hip adduction and internal rotation, a more common postural attitude in the early stages of walking is abduction and external rotation at the hip. One might assume that this is an adaptation of the normal toddler's walk, superimposed on a pathologic gait. External rotation–abduction pos-turing needs no corrective bracing, such as a twister or other cumbersome device. It merely requires patience on the part of the examiner and reassurance of the parents that this is a temporary phenomenon.

Orthotic Management of Hemiplegic Cerebral Palsy

The most universal problem of orthotic concern is plan-tar flexor spasticity and, consequently, assistance for toe pickup.[11] Inversion or varus attitude results from spas-ticity of the tibialis posterior muscle and often accompa-nies the equinus foot posture.[12–15] A combination of pronation and plantar flexion is less common in hemiple-gia.[16] One might speculate that the duration of early walking patterns has some influence on subsequent foot deformity. When the limb is in abduction and external rotation, most of the weight is transmitted to the medial border of the foot, forcing pronation.

AFOs

An AFO adequately controls mild-to-moderate plantar flexor spasticity and provides toe clearance.[1,17] Both rigid and hinged ankle designs are available.[17] The hinged AFO offers the mechanical advantage of dorsiflexion during stance phase when the center of gravity passes anteriorly over the rotational axis of the ankle joint.[18] In more significant spastic hypertonicity, reinforcement of the plastic material extending from the heel to the posterior shaft provides a greater force for stretching and for assisting dorsiflexion.[17] A tone-reducing AFO (TRAFO) inhibits extensor synergy by maintaining the toes in dorsiflexion and should be considered particularly in those cases with persistent hyperactive plantar grasp reflex.[19]

In the majority of cases, a properly constructed AFO can control supination or pronation attitude.[17,20,21] To be effective, the foot and ankle must be encased with a high anterior trim extending over the instep and the forefoot. Anatomic alignment of the calcaneus is the essential feature for correcting any mediolateral instability of the foot and ankle.

Correction for lateral or medial tilt of the os calcis, talar displacement, and forefoot deviation must be incorporated during the process of casting for the orthosis. A soft lining or padding over the lateral malleolus, prominent part of the midfoot curve, and the medial forefoot is advisable to decrease excessive pressure and discomfort from corrective contact in varus attitude, especially when it is partly inflexible.

The less frequent valgus attitude is usually flexible and, therefore, less difficult to correct in young children with hemiplegia. Our experience has not been satisfactory with plastic molded shoe inserts attached to double metal bars, which have been recommended for foot and subtalar joint stabilization.[17,22] Because corrective forces are applied over a small area, stabilization is inadequate, and discomfort from pressure occurs.

In children with hemiplegia, a conventional AFO[17] is reserved for those instances when, for some reason, surgical correction of a fixed deformity is not possible. The aim is containment rather than correction. Spring-loaded or limited plantar flexion ankle joints are some options

for a fixed equinus deformity.[17] In case of equinovarus or equinovalgus deformity, a lateral or medial Y-strap and shoe modifications are added to a conventional double-bar AFO.[23]

KAFOs

Prescription of a KAFO for postural deviations of the knee is a rare exception in hemiplegia. Hyperextension of the knee is a compensation for triceps surae spasticity to achieve full plantar support in stance phase rather than resorting to the characteristic toe walking.[24] For the most part, genu recurvatum is correctable by plantar flexion control with an AFO, although gait readjustment may require several weeks or perhaps months. Correction from ankle realignment cannot be expected if there is an inflexible fixed gastrocnemius contracture. Otherwise, setting the ankle at 5 degrees of dorsiflexion or using a spring-loaded joint decreases genu recurvatum induced by plantar flexion.[25,26] Positioning the knee joint in slight flexion in a KAFO also encourages knee flexion. In small children, an adjustable elastic posterior strap that crosses the knee may be tried to assist flexion of this joint. A plastic supracondylar KAFO has been described as another method to control genu recurvatum.[27–29]

A knee hyperextension splint, which is less cumbersome than a KAFO, may be used for training purposes and will be discussed subsequently.[30]

An occasional but important application of KAFOs is for acquired hemiplegia in young children who have severe parietal lobe syndrome with profound cortical sensory deficit, apraxia, and disregard for the affected lower extremity, and who therefore will not bear weight on the hemiplegic leg. A KAFO is used for training purposes, which usually requires a long time. In the majority of cases, the KAFO can be decreased to an AFO when ambulation is accomplished.

Spastic Diplegia and Quadriparesis

Spastic diplegia and quadriparesis are clinical types of cerebral palsy that shows a wide range of neuromuscular dysfunction. The clinical course and orthotic management are less uniform than in hemiplegia. Approximately 85 percent of diplegic children walk independently or with assistive devices, the majority by 4 years of age.[4]

Two-thirds of those with quadriparesis become ambulatory with or without appliances, the majority after 4 years. Sitting at 2 years or earlier is a good indicator that the child will walk, whereas youngsters who do not sit by 4 years are not expected to ambulate.[4]

Posture

Postural deviations of diplegic stance and gait were originally observed by Little and studied more recently by others.[12,13,31,32] As a result of increased adductor tone, the legs are approximated. The supporting base is narrowed, and there is a scissoring gait. When this is severe, the feet cross, and it becomes difficult or impossible to take a forward step.

Gait

Often there is increased internal rotation at the hips because of spasticity and frequent underlying femoral anteversion.[12,33] This will cause the knees and feet to turn inward and adds to the difficulties of advancing the leg in swing phase. The relative weakness of hip abductors produces a gluteus medius lurch. Knee flexion in swing phase is usually inadequate, creating the impression of a stiff gait. Yet the child may stand and walk with flexed hips and knees. The feet are in equinus attitude, and toe clearance is impeded; weight is supported mostly or entirely on the forefoot.[13] Additional foot deformities, more frequently a valgus rather than varus attitude, can be observed.[14,15] Over the years, abnormal muscular and gravitational forces lead to progressive deformities with a predominance of different components of this basic pattern. The many complex postural deviations that can evolve cannot be elaborated here.[12,13,15] Only a brief description is given of those that are most commonly of orthotic concern.

Vase Stance

The so-called vase stance is initiated by excessive adductor spasticity, pulling the thighs so close that they are virtually propped against each other.[12,13] The associated, rather marked genu valgum allows the feet to be farther apart than the knees, hence the descriptive term. Internal hip rotation and equinovarus attitude of the feet may be present. A more common accompanying foot abnormality is equinovalgus as a result of medial displacement of the weightbearing line associated with genu valgum.[14]

In the supple foot of a child, a valgus deformity of the hindfoot can hide a plantar flexion contracture.[12] In stance, the foot appears plantigrade, and the heel may be in contact with the supporting surface. On observation, however, it becomes evident that there is a lateral angulation between the vertical axis of the calf and heel and that the plantigrade position is possible only because the contracted heel cord is displaced laterally. Persistent fetal configuration of the talar neck and spasticity of the peroneal muscles may also contribute to the development of pes planovalgus.[12]

Crouch Gait and Posture

Another frequent pattern, seen in spastic diplegia and quadriparesis the crouch gait, is an exaggeration of the abnormal hip and knee flexion.[34] In part, this may be a maturational phenomenon related to the cerebral dysfunction. Early predominance of extensor posturing and subsequent evolution of flexor pattern have been described as the natural course of spastic diplegia and quadriparesis.[35] Once this reversal occurs, biomechanical forces come into play, and the combined effects of relative weakness and contractures enhance the postural malalignment. Crouch posture and gait can either develop or become more severe after surgical overcorrection of heel cord contractures with resultant excessive ankle dorsiflexion.[12]

Last, it should be noted that in the presence of plantar flexion attitude or deformity, genu recurvatum is a compensatory mechanism more frequent in this group than in hemiplegic cerebral palsy.[12,13,15] The severity and extent of postural abnormalities depend on the degree of neuromuscular deficit. In mild cases, when spasticity around proximal joints is minimal, pathologic features may be confined only to the ankles.

Children with milder degrees of spasticity rarely require braces until they stand with support. Because they have active motor function and move about in a variety of ways, contractures are unlikely to develop in early years. Orthoses may be needed for correcting abnormalities of stance and gait and to prevent deformities that appear, sometimes insidiously, once the upright position is attained. Many less affected children gradually acquire better volitional control, and braces worn in early years can be discarded later as postural deviations ameliorate. In other cases, braces can be discarded after corrective surgical procedures.

Orthotic Management of Spastic Diplegia and Quadriparesis

Principles and Innovations

Improving postural control by distal stabilization and less extensive orthoses remain the current approach to orthotic management of cerebral palsy with bilateral spasticity. In the last several years, a spurt has occurred in the development of new plastic and thermoplastic designs for spastic foot deformities. This trend originated partly from incorporating the principles of inhibitive casting.[36–39] Another impetus was the relatively lower cost of ankle–foot splints (AFSs), which permits more experimentation.[30] Although inhibitive and serial progressive below- and above-knee casts are not orthotic devices, a discussion is included, because they are used as adjuncts for postural and gait deviations in ambulation training.[40] Two important rules should be remembered when assessing abnormalities of gait and posture and when selecting appropriate orthoses for this group of children: (1) Posture at any one joint will influence the alignment of all others, (2) Muscles crossing two joints further enhance this biomechanical interaction.

Foot Deformities

Foot deformities are the most frequent concern of orthotic treatment in bilateral spastic cerebral palsy.[11] In mild cases, especially in diplegia, foot correction may be all that is required. When more extensive correction of the foot and ankle is required, plastic AFO is preferred not only for its light weight and better cosmesis but also for more effective support from direct contact with the foot.[1,17,21] Considerations for those exceptional instances when a conventional metal AFO might be selected are described in the above section entitled "Congenital and Acquired Hemiplegia." Solid ankle[41] or hinged AFO is prescribed for equinus deformity without mediolateral ankle–foot malalignment[18] (Fig. 6-1). Because the hinged AFO seems to provide less distal and proximal stability than the rigid ankle design, it should be used

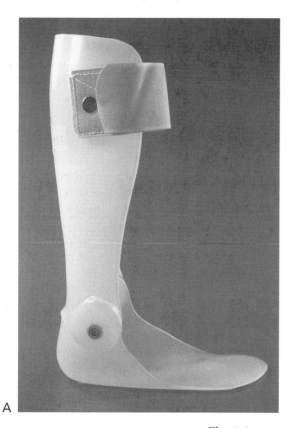

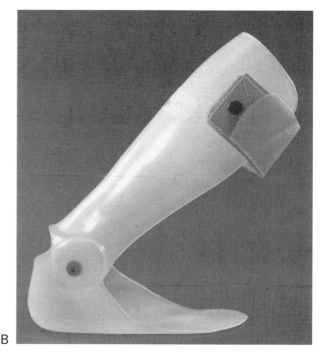

A   B

Fig. 6-1. **(A & B)** Hinged plastic AFO.

selectively.[18] Crouch posture and hamstring contracture are enhanced by ankle dorsiflexion and are contraindications for a hinged AFO. Persistent positive supporting reaction and hyperactive plantar grasp reflex enhance the equinus attitude caused by spasticity of the calf muscles.[42] These manifestations of neuromuscular dysfunction call for a TRAFO, which is fabricated from a preconstructed footplate to maintain the toes in extension.[19]

Mediolateral ankle–foot instability is a commonly associated component with spastic equinus.[16] In contrast to hemiplegia, pronation or equinovalgus deformity prevails in bilateral spastic cerebral palsy.[12,14] Meticulous fitting of an AFO is needed to maintain the calcaneus in anatomic position, to prevent medial displacement of the talus, and to support the unstable subtalar joint.

Supramalleolar orthoses (SMO) may achieve these goals in the presence of full passive range of dorsiflexion without tone increase at least to plantigrade and a supple pronation deformity (Fig. 6-2). Good postural control of proximal joints is an additional prerequisite.

The SMO is less effective in preventing plantar flexion than an AFO. Some degree of adaptation, however, is possible in this respect by using an open or reinforced posterior split and by changing the height of extension above the malleoli.

Hallux valgus develops as a result of a pronated foot, hyperactive plantar grasp reflex, or both. Addition of a toe loop to AFO or SMO is an attempt to prevent this progressive and often painful deformity. Orthotic management of the less frequent equinovarus deformity is as discussed under hemiplegic cerebral palsy. When the foot deviates medially from the line of progression, one must determine whether it represents a supination–adduction foot deformity or, as is more often the case, internal rotation at the hip. An AFO cannot correct the latter problem. At times, internal tibial torsion also may be present, most likely caused by the deforming force of the spastic tibialis posterior muscle.[43]

Knee Problems

As a rule, postural deviations of the knee are secondary to ankle and/or hip malalignment. Orthotic correction requires an analysis of their origin. The four characteristic patterns are genu recurvatum, flexion attitude of crouch posture, genu valgum associated with vase stance, and internally rotated, so-called "kissing" knees.[12,34]

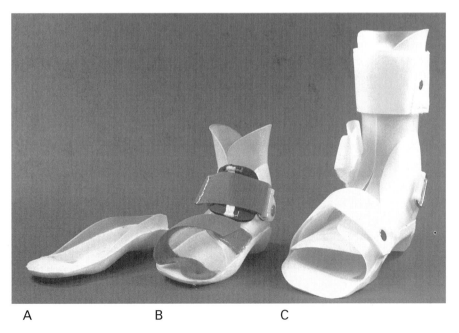

A   B   C

Fig. 6-2. **(A)** Shoe insert with reflex inhibitory features fabricated from a molded footplate. **(B)** SMO with high anterior trim, made from molded footplate for pes valgus with mild plantar flexor spasticity. **(C)** High SMO with high anterior trim and moderate plantar flexor spasticity.

Genu recurvatum is more frequent in diplegia and quadriparesis than in hemiplegia. It may be unilateral or more severe on one side since spasticity is rarely symmetric. Knee hyperextension is secondary to equinus position of the ankle.[24] Quadriceps spasticity indicated by a high riding patella alta may be a contributory factor. A rigid AFO in 5 to 10 degrees of dorsiflexion increases flexion moment at the knee and is effective for controlling, or at least improving, genu recurvatum.[44] Flexibility of the heel cord and knee stability both guide and limit the optimal or tolerable dorsiflexion angle. A thermoplastic knee hyperextension splint is recommended for the purpose of gait training and for determining the most appropriate dorsiflexion angle.[30] The splint consists of an anterior frame secured with Velcro straps and extends halfway along the thigh and calf. Because it is molded at 35 to 45 degrees of knee flexion and has a large anterior cutout, the splint permits knee flexion but limits extension.

Genu valgum of vase stance is a secondary deformity initiated by the spastic hip adductors.[12] Tight hamstrings and an equinovalgus foot alignment create additional deforming forces at the knee. Stretching and laxity of the medial collateral ligament lead to mediolateral knee instability. In severe long-standing cases, a bony deformity develops that is due to asymmetric growth of the open epiphyseal plates at the knee.[12,15]

Genu valgum is preventable in most cases if proper measures are taken in time to decrease hip adductor spasticity. Knee orthoses (KOs) of the cage type cannot provide the necessary knee stability when the hip is in adduction. Orthotic support for the abnormal hip and ankle alignment is a more reasonable approach, since it controls the primary origin of knee deformity.

The hip action orthosis provides mediolateral stabilization and effectively widens the supporting base[8,9] (Fig. 6-3). The orthosis consists of a pelvic band and wide thigh cuffs attached to it by lateral bars. The hip joint has selective action, permitting free flexion, extension, and abduction. The orthotic joint is adjustable so that it can be set at the desired angle of abduction, and adduction is not possible beyond that position. Reduction in the weight of the device compared to an HKAFO and unimpeded active knee movements, which also allow crawling, are definite advantages.

An extension of the hip action brace below the knee increases medial support when valgus attitude persists. A free motion ankle joint should be used for unrestricted knee flexion on walking. The child can also wear a separate unattached AFO with proper specification suitable to correct pes planovalgus.

A KAFO does not solve the problem of valgus knee as long as hip adductor spasticity is present. A standard KAFO with free motion knee joint or a supracondylar KAFO[27] may be necessary for persistent severe knee deformity or instability after adductor spasticity has been alleviated by surgery or phenol block.

Flexor Pattern

The flexor pattern of crouch gait is the most difficult problem to manage, and results are the least satisfactory with orthotic or any other means of treatment.[34,45,46] Hip flexion and excessive ankle dorsiflexion are part of this postural abnormality. Surgical release of fixed hamstring contractures improves but does not always correct a flexed knee posture.

Knee flexion attitude is sometimes caused or aggravated by surgical weakening of the triceps surae or overcorrection of a tendo Achilles contracture, particularly in combination with hamstring spasticity.[12,15,34] The simplest and preferred method for effective walkers is to control excessive dorsiflexion but allow plantar flexion to enhance knee extension moment.[44] A rigid ankle total-contact AFO with an anterior clamshell or a conventional AFO with a 90 degree anterior stop or adjustable plantar flexion spring assistance may be needed to achieve this purpose.[1,17,41]

Another device is the floor-reaction orthosis, which exerts knee extension force through a pretibial shell.[47,48] Problems with tolerating this orthosis tend to arise because pressure generated by the knee flexion tendency is distributed over a rather small area of the tibia. Construction of a separate, well-padded and molded pretibial shell may alleviate this difficulty, because extension force can be adjusted by graduated tighter application as tolerance improves.

The supracondylar KAFO with molded above-knee extension of the pretibial shell distributes pressure over a larger area and may be better tolerated. Neither the floor reaction orthosis[49] nor the supracondylar KAFO[27–29] are successful in the presence of fixed knee flexion contractures. At present, no articulated KAFO can offer adequate selective control of unwanted bent knee attitude throughout stance phase and yet allow flexion in the swing phase.

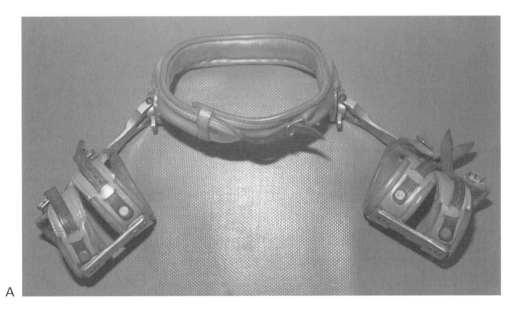

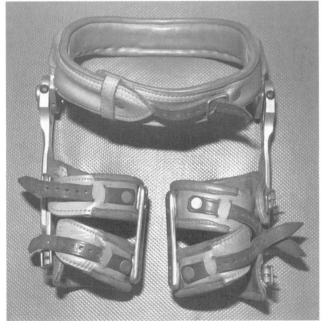

Fig. 6-3. **(A)** Hip action orthosis allowing free abduction and **(B)** limited adduction.

The eccentric free knee joint, spring-loaded knee joint, and other types of special knee joints generally require full-joint extension before their mechanical assistance has an effect, and they are not useful for spastic crouch posture. To place these children in KAFOs with the notion of improving their gait is a desperate measure that serves no useful purpose, because only with locked knee joints can the unwanted knee flexion be completely eliminated. When faced with the dilemma of an orthotic device for crouch gait in a functional ambulator, less is usually better than more, a decision that probably requires greater experience than prescribing extensive orthoses.

Hip and Pelvis

Excessive internal rotation of the hip causes a very unsightly gait because of the resultant in-toeing.[33,43] Although it very rarely occurs as a single deformity, the problem often draws special attention on account of cosmesis. To control abnormal rotational attitude of the leg arising from the hip joint, derotational moment must be applied around the longitudinal axis of the limb. To be effective, corrective forces must act at least along the length of the femur and must be transmitted to the foot.

Moreover, the derotational moment must be counteracted by balanced forces on the opposite side of the body. Otherwise, compensatory realignment of the pelvis and contralateral limb or rotation of the device occurs and makes corrective attempts ineffectual. HKAFO with a pelvic band can achieve this requirement, but again, it would be too extensive and unjustified for children who are active functional walkers.[6,7]

Twister Orthoses

For these situations, twister orthoses are available. The initial version of these devices was the wraparound twister, which consisted of a webbing strap.[1] To effect external rotation, the strap is attached to the lateral border of a pelvic band and winds anteromedially around the thigh. For the second loop of the twist, it courses in a posterolateral direction, and its distal end is attached anterolaterally to the dorsum of the shoe or calf cuff of an AFO. A more sophisticated construction is the cable twister.[8,9] Steel cables tightly coiled in a helical pattern are enclosed in a rubber housing. As they uncoil, an external rotation moment is generated. The twister extends over the lateral side between the pelvic band and shoe caliper or the calf portion of an AFO. The webbing straps hold them against the limb to keep them from flopping about in the swing phase. The rotational force can be adjusted with a key that winds or unwinds the cables at their proximal end.

Easy breakage may be a problem when the twister spans the entire limb length but is uncommon if it is attached to an AFO. In the rare event that a twister is used only for one leg, the pelvic band should be firmly anchored by a thigh corset on the contralateral limb to prevent derotation.

The cable twister is helpful in producing cosmetic gait improvement in young children, but its effectiveness decreases as they grow. Generally, after the patient reaches 10 years of age, no significant change can be achieved by the cable twister.

Cautions

When twisters are used, possible sites of rotation other than the hip should be observed regularly, specifically, the knee joints and tibial alignment. More often than not, internal hip rotation is caused by femoral anteversion rather than by muscle imbalance alone, although the latter usually contributes as an initiating factor. Rotational laxity of the knee joints and external tibial torsion can develop, particularly in the presence of an underlying bony hip deformity. These considerations have significantly decreased the initial enthusiasm for using twisters in children. Despite some claims, the hip action orthosis is not suitable to control rotational deformities at the hip, because it provides no derotational torque.

HKAFOs

In children who are already or expected to become functional ambulators, either independently or with crutches, the use of an HKAFO is hardly ever warranted, even if there is evidence of some adductor spasticity. These cumbersome and heavy braces do not promote earlier achievement of walking, and for children who already walk, they are a hindrance rather than a help in mobility.[50] Severe overactivity of the adductors causing actual crossing of the legs does not occur in this group. Milder degrees of adducted gait will either be overcome by maturation or may eventually require other means of correction. In rare cases with limited ambulatory potential and persistent adductor spasticity an HKAFO may assist in walking for exercise at a high energy cost which, by itself, will exclude functional ambulation.[3,7,51]

Positioning and Training Devices

When spasticity is severe and ambulation is not a realistic expectation, orthoses can serve as assistive or training devices in limited functional activities. For lack of head control, a cervical brace with or without a halo-type overhead suspension may be considered. The Milwaukee brace was also recommended for this purpose.[52] In children, however, mandibular deformity and dental malocclusion can occur from any device with head support anchored on the jaw. With an overhead suspension, pressure on the forehead can exceed skin tolerance, particularly when total passive support is needed for hours on end. Cosmetic appearance of an elaborate overhead suspension device is poorly accepted in everyday situations.

Orthotic devices have also been tried for trunk support in spastic quadriparesis. With severe extensor thrust, the pelvis and hips tend to slide out from the seated position. On the other hand, hypotonicity of the trunk leads to forward slumping of the torso.

The Milwaukee brace[52] or a thoracic suspension lumbosacralorthosis (TLSO) attached to the back panel of a wheelchair has been recommended for trunk stabilization in these cases.[53] A spinal orthosis with pelvic band, bilateral thigh cuffs, and hip joints that can be locked in flexion, while serving the same purpose, can also control hip adduction attitude.

Newer Approaches

Adapted seating and molded wheelchair inserts with neck and head stabilizers have largely replaced orthotic devices for head and trunk control in cerebral palsy. Similarly, the emphasis for passive standing has shifted from orthosis to other types of adaptive devices, such as a prone stander or a standing table. These devices have adjustable features to alleviate the various postural and tone abnormalities seen in cerebral palsy and are used during play and therapy activities. When upright position is elected for passive standing, the preferred orthosis is a parapodium, which has a simpler design and is easier to don and doff than an HKAFO with a spinal attachment.

Temporary Devices

Training braces, thermoplastic splints, inhibitory casts, and serial or progressive casting are temporary devices that use the same principles of support and correction as orthoses.[30,54–56] These temporary measures gained increasing popularity, mostly in physical therapy and in training.[30,57,58] The intent is to stretch predominantly spastic tight muscles and to overcome, at least temporarily, abnormal patterns of spasticity with the hope that eventually improved postural control will be facilitated.

Inhibitory casting was developed as an alternative to orthoses for spastic foot abnormalities.[59,60] The essential component is a molded prefabricated footplate which is then incorporated in a below-knee cast. The footplate is made of wood or layers of plaster of Paris from a tracing of the contour of the child's foot. Location of the meta-

tarsal heads is marked on the tracing and transferred to the plate. Fabrication of the molded footplate takes place with the child in sitting, lower extremity joints aligned at 90 degrees. The footplate has reamed out areas under the heel and under the second and third metatarsal heads. The forepart underlying the digits is raised to keep the toes in extension. While the calcaneus is stabilized in anatomic position and the anteromedial subluxation of the talus is passively reduced, a support is built in for the medial longitudinal arch (Fig. 6-2).

With the footplate in place, the above-ankle or below-knee cast is wrapped around the extremity. Inhibitive casts are made of plaster of Paris or various types of fast-setting synthetic cast materials with cotton stockinette padding adjacent to the skin. The cast may be left in place for several weeks, or it may be bivalved for application during the day.

Clinical studies report improved posture and gait with the inhibitory casts. The rationale and suggested mechanism of action include (1) reduction of abnormal tone by firm fixation of the ankle and by provision of a stable supporting base; (2) inhibition of hyperactive plantar grasp reflex; (3) decreased positive supporting reaction and extensor thrust by maintaining the toes in extension and the foot in plantigrade position; and (4) alleviation of spasticity by diminishing the stretch reflex response, while muscles of the ankle and the foot are placed and sustained in elongation.[42,55,57,58,61–63]

Another choice for spastic foot deformities is the ankle–foot splint (AFS) made of low-temperature thermoplastic material.[30] An AFS can be more easily adjusted than a plastic AFO. It serves as a substitute until the desired correction is achieved and a permanent orthosis is prescribed.

Training devices for improving knee control include the previously described knee hyperextension splint.[30] In crouch posture, a long leg cage with anterior support worn on alternating legs has been recommended.[9] Long leg, bivalved, or cylinder casts are suggested to decrease knee flexion attitude or contracture with progressive adjustment of corrective position.[30] A hip abduction splint maintains mediolateral alignment while crawling is practiced.[64] The device consists of two thigh cuffs and an adjustable spreader bar. It permits hip flexion and extension while adduction and abduction are controlled.

Resting Splints and Orthoses

The role of resting splints or braces in delaying contractures or in preventing their recurrence after surgical procedures is most important when spasticity is moderate to severe. A hip abduction brace maintains prolonged stretching of tight adductors and may contribute to a more satisfactory development of the hip joints.[65] Subluxation or dislocation of the hip is a serious threat in cerebral palsy and is most frequent in severely affected, nonambulatory children. It is caused by hip flexor and adductor overactivity that leads to coxa valga and femoral anteversion with a shallow, sloping acetabulum.[12,15,66]

Several types of abduction orthoses are available. In selecting the most suitable type, a number of biomechanical considerations must be weighed. Pelvifemoral symmetry should be ensured by maintaining both hip joints in the same degree of abduction, instead of separating the legs relative to each other (Fig. 6-4). Abduction of the hips should not create undue mediolateral stress at the knee joints, because it may lead to or enhance already existing genu valgum.

The previously described crawling brace can be used as an abduction orthosis.[64] Another simple method is a spreader bar attached to the soles of the shoes.[1,14] In this device, hip rotation and mediolateral ankle foot alignment can be also varied by setting the wing nut and serrated bolt at different angles. It is also used for torsional rotational deformities of the tibia. The device does not affect pelvifemoral alignment or mediolateral forces at the knee. It cannot prevent hip and knee flexion, a position that some children tend to assume while wearing an abduction orthosis.

A more elaborate abduction orthosis is the so-called A-frame, which consists of three bars arranged in a triangle shape. It is fastened to the legs by thigh and calf cuffs and holds the knees in extension. The A-frame provides medial counterpressure at the knees and maintains the legs in extension. It does not eliminate pelvifemoral asymmetry because it has no pelvic band. For equalization of abduction at both hips relative to the pelvis, an orthosis must extend above the hip. A pelvic band, or in severe asymmetry, a spinal extension must be attached. Addition of an orthotic hip joint that can be locked in flexion or extension permits both sitting and standing with the orthosis (Fig. 6-4).

Night splints or braces are used for stretching of the tight heel cords. Footplates with rigid ankles can be attached to an abduction orthosis when the aim is to control the position of both hips and ankles.

Dyskinetic Cerebral Palsy

The role of orthoses is relatively insignificant in dyskinetic cerebral palsy. Involuntary movements, most often athetosis or dystonia, accompanied by fluctuating tone, seem to prevent the appearance of fixed contractures. Tightness of soft tissues sometimes occurs by adolescence when the predominant feature is dystonia, and fixed contractures may develop by adulthood. Control of involuntary movements is the usually stated reason for an orthosis.[7] More precisely defined, orthoses provide joint stabilization rather than actual movement control. As in the bilateral spastic types, the severity of neuromuscular impairment varies a great deal. Approximately three-fourths of these children achieve independent ambulation, the majority by 3 years of age.[4]

Unlike spasticity, dyskinesias do not present typical gait patterns with predominant specific postural abnormalities. Each child develops his own way of walking that may look awkward and requires high energy consumption but is effective from a functional standpoint. Some severely affected youngsters use alternative means of locomotion in their home or in other familiar situations, such as positions resembling crawling or knee walking.

Prevention of deformities is not an important consideration. On occasion, braces may be helpful when the child has achieved the erect position and incipient stages of assisted walking. The usual problem that needs to be and can be successfully controlled is mediolateral ankle instability, often combined with plantar flexion attitude of the foot. Biomechanically, an AFO is appropriate. Sometimes, however, a conventional double-upright AFO is necessary to contain the strong dyskinetic movements. Little, if anything, is gained from more extensive orthoses. Involuntary movements may appear to be restrained, but there is no functional benefit, and in fact, the child usually finds it more difficult to move about. Orthoses cannot make the more severely affected children ambulate, particularly because upper extremity impairment generally precludes crutch walking.

A combination of spasticity and dyskinesia increases the chances of contractures, although contractures tend to appear later than in the purely spastic types. In these cases, orthotic management is similar to that discussed in conjunction with diplegia and quadriparesis.

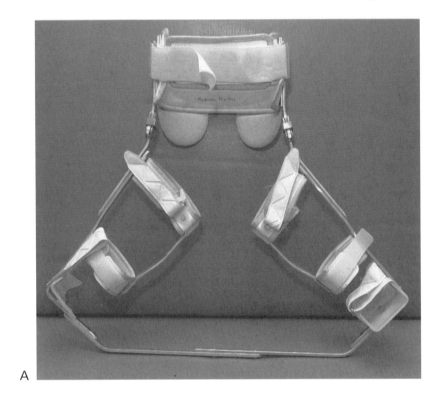

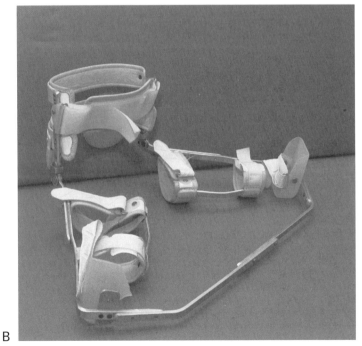

Fig. 6-4. Hip abduction positioning orthosis with pelvic band, double bars, and footplates. **(A)** Hip joint locked in extension for standing or supine positioning. **(B)** Hip joint in flexion for sitting.

Other Clinical Types

In the rare, true atonic type of cerebral palsy, prognosis for motor function is generally very poor. These children, however, can develop contractures much like those with extensive flaccid paralysis. Most frequent are foot deformities and contractures around the hips and knees, consistent with the so-called frog position in which they usually lie. Anterior hip dislocation can be an eventual consequence of this posture. Preventive positioning combined with splinting is needed before deformities occur. If the child has at least some head control, a parapodium can be used as a standing orthosis[67] (Fig. 6-5).

SPINA BIFIDA WITH MYELODYSPLASIA

Spina bifida represents a congenital dysrhaphism of the vertebral canal with or without an underlying malformation of the spinal cord.[15,68–70] The most common site of defect is the lumbosacral area. Thoracic and cervical segments are less frequently affected.

The spectrum of clinical manifestations includes spina bifida occulta and aperta. The occult type is generally symptomless. Only in rare instances is it accompanied by a partial dysplastic defect of the spinal cord. These are usually located in the lumbosacral segments and cause only mild gait abnormalities.

Spina bifida aperta is associated with malformation of the spinal cord. An exception is the very rare simple meningocele. The symptoms of myelodysplasia, determined by its location and extent are, motor paralysis; partial or complete absence of sensation, which predisposes to decubitus ulcers; and neurogenic impairment of bowel and bladder control which results in recurrent or chronic urinary tract infections. Characteristically, muscle weakness is of the lower motor neuron type. Less frequently, one may find a combination of upper and lower motor neuron signs as a consequence of other neurologic complications or malformations, particularly in myelodysplasia at higher thoracic levels.[71]

Additional neurectodermal defects that may accompany the spinal cord abnormality include Arnold-Chiari deformity and aqueductal stenosis leading to hydrocephalus, dilatation of the lateral and third ventricles, and abnormal cerebral gyri and sulci.[68] Among the associated mesodermal malformations, skeletal and urinary tract malformations are the most common.[68] Particularly significant are vertebral anomalies, congenital kyphosis, and hemivertebrae with relentless progression of scoliosis.

Hypoplasia, agenesis, horseshoe configuration of the kidneys, and ureteral abnormalities may contribute to deterioration of neurogenic bladder dysfunction and renal status. An intellectual deficit may occur, especially in the presence of hydrocephalus.[68]

The extent of paralysis is an important prognostic factor in that it curtails the upper limit of physical accomplishments, but by no means does it ensure their achievement.[72,73] Recurrent problems related to hydrocephalus, the urinary system, and decubiti can interrupt a child's development and functional training. Intellectual endowment, emotional adjustment, and home environment were also found to be of significance with respect to ultimate prognosis. Obesity is frequent among all the inactive children and compounds other complications.[72,74]

The management of children with myelodysplasia is a complex undertaking.[70] Bracing is an important aspect of this process and must be integrated with other therapeutic considerations.

Principles of Orthotic Prescription

The aim of orthoses is to provide mechanical substitution for weak or paralyzed muscles and to restrain the forces of those with unbalanced, unopposed action.[69,75,76] Orthotic prescription is based on an accurate assessment of neurologic deficit, which enables the examiner to project expected function and to anticipate musculoskeletal complications.

Different mechanisms contribute to the development of deformities in patients with spina bifida with myelodysplasia:

1. Selective paralysis and significant muscle imbalance at certain joints as a result of specific segmental neurologic lesions
2. Combined effect of gravity and poor positioning in the presence of complete or severe flaccid paralysis
3. Associated malformations of the skeleton
4. Intrauterine positioning and lack of movement, which may be responsible for some deformities present at birth, seemingly inconsistent with the neurologic deficit.

Preventive orthotic treatment, when conscientiously applied, is most successful in deterring contractures that are related to faulty positioning. Braces alone are less effective in complete prevention of deformities caused by a significant muscle imbalance, although they may delay their appearance and progression. Fixed deformities present at birth or caused by underlying skeletal malformations do not respond to orthotic correction.[68]

With this particular diagnosis, the importance of standing with braces, regardless of the outlook for higher function, has to be stressed. Extensive flaccid paralysis is accompanied by significant osteoporosis. Osteoporotic fractures of the long bones tend to occur more often with minor unnoticed trauma after immobilization for surgical procedures and in the non-ambulatory group. These clinical observations suggest that weight bearing, even with passive support, may be beneficial in reducing osteoporosis at least to some extent.

The spinal cord malformation is usually not a well-defined transverse lesion; this situation leads to some variations in both motor and sensory findings. Such cases may permit the use of different orthoses than those required in complete lesion of a specific spinal segment. This possibility should be kept in mind when the role of orthotics will subsequently be discussed in relation to segmental levels of deficit.

Thoracic Lesions

Myelodysplasia in the thoracic segments spares the arms; variable degrees of trunk weakness and complete paralysis of the legs are seen.[74] Faulty positioning in supine and prone lying can lead to hip abduction, external rotation, and flexion contractures, with iliotibial band tightness and equinus deformity of the feet.[68] During infancy, these are preventable by exercises and do not require bracing. Unless hydrocephalus is significant or other neurologic complications occur, head control and upper extremity function develop as expected.

Sitting

These children can neither assume nor maintain active independent sitting. Eventually, they learn to sit up, pulling with their arms, and leaning on them for support while sitting in a kyphotic or lordotic position. Many children achieve this by 1 to 1 1/2 years of age.

A trunk corset or well-padded plastic shell can help to free up the arms for play in a proper seating arrangement.[74] This device merely serves as a support but does not prevent scoliosis. In thoracic myelodysplasia, paralytic scoliosis is an inevitable complication and requires early orthotic management. However, a TLSO is only a temporizing measure, and surgical stabilization of the spine eventually is needed. Orthoses for spinal deformities are discussed in Chapter 4. Scoliosis and the development of hip flexion contractures must be closely monitored after the child spends most of the day in sitting.

Standing

Children with thoracic level of paralysis require braces for standing and activities in the upright position. In most cases, standing with an orthosis is started between 12 and 18 months of age and is incorporated in daily activities of play and interaction. The standard HKAFO with spinal attachment, which was used in the past for standing children with thoracic level of paralysis, has been replaced by new devices.[67,77] Simplicity and versatility of design, application, and functional use make the new orthotic devices a preferred choice. Crutchless standing that requires less energy and frees up the arms for play and other functional activities is one of the most important universal advantages of the new breed of standing orthoses.

Parapodium

The parapodium was the first in this innovative and successful advancement of orthotic design for children with a high level of paralysis or severe generalized muscle weakness[67,77] (Fig. 6-5). This orthosis consists of a foot plate, tubular side bars, a back panel extending from the sacrum to the gluteal folds, and a padded anterior crossbar at the patellar tendons. An anterior chest panel, which extends up to the xiphoid process, completes the three-point principle of support. These components act as a continuous frame that ensures mediolateral and anteroposterior stability.

A unique constructional feature, different from the usual mechanical joints, is the mechanism for locking and unlocking the hips and knees. A pair of folding handles rotates the upright bars and with them the orthotic joints. When the joint axes are in the sagittal plane, the hips and knees are held in extension. Ninety degrees of rotation aligns them in the frontal plane and allows flex-

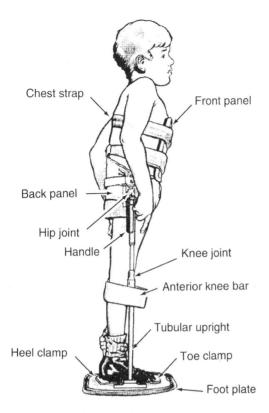

Chest strap

Front panel

Back panel

Hip joint

Handle

Knee joint

Anterior knee bar

Tubular upright

Toe clamp

Heel clamp

Foot plate

Fig. 6-5. Parapodium.

ion at both joints. The shoes are not attached permanently to the footplate but are secured in place by tight-fitting clamps. For this reason and because there are no straps and buckles, donning and removing this orthosis takes 1 to 2 minutes instead of the usual 10 to 15 minutes required for a standard HKAFO with a spinal attachment.

Numerous adaptations can be added to the basic design for increasing hip and knee stability or to accommodate contractures, leg-length discrepancy, or postural asymmetry. An AFO can be worn with the parapodium for unstable flail ankles. The standard back panel is adjustable to relieve pressure over the uneven surface of a large spinal lesion. A body jacket or TLSO can be used instead of the back and chest panel for scoliosis and pelvic asymmetry. The parapodium is available in the form of modular kits. It comes in various sizes adjustable for growth. One model has two posterior extensions and converts the orthosis to a chair on which the child can also sit.

Limitations

Young children can use the parapodium not only for standing but for ambulation with the aid of a walkerette or crutches. Forward progression is achieved by pivoting, drag, or swing-type gait. Although the parapodium is recommended for adolescents and adults, its usefulness and safety are limited by increasing body size. A principal factor for maintaining stability in the upright position is the surface area of the supporting footplate in relation to height and weight. In spite of larger footplate dimensions, stability tends to decrease when adult stature is approached and in obese children. Moreover, the bulky footplate required for taller patients is awkward for sitting in a wheelchair. These problems arise around adolescence, when the orthosis is usually abandoned if it was used only for standing.

Another standing orthosis that uses biomechanical principles similar to the parapodium is the Verlo orthosis.[78,79] Unlike the parapodium, it cannot be used for sitting, because it has no provision for hip and knee flexion.

The Orlau swivel walker is a modification of the parapodium[80,81] (Fig. 6-6). It has been used for some time in England and is now available in the United States. The swivel walker is propelled by a special footplate that converts lateral trunk movements to forward propulsion. The energy requirement for walking is lower with this device than with the parapodium.[82] The Orlau orthosis can be used only in erect position because it has no provision for hip and knee flexion. Ambulation with the parapodium, Orlau, and Verlo orthoses is with a nonreciprocal gait.

Reciprocal Gait

Orthotic devices that assist in a reciprocal gait pattern represent a relatively recently revived trend with an expanding scope of application in the management of low thoracic to upper lumbar segmental myelodysplasia and in disabilities with significant muscle weakness around all lower extremity joints.[77,83,84] The reciprocating gait orthosis (RGO) has undergone several changes in its mechanical construction. This device is discussed in the following section entitled "Upper Lumbar Lesions."

The hip guidance orthosis[85] (developed in England) uses the following principles: (1) ball-bearing hip joints to reduce rotational constraint and loss of efficiency; (2) rigid extremity and body components; (3) a fixed 5 degree hip adduction angle; (4) hip flexion limited to 5 to

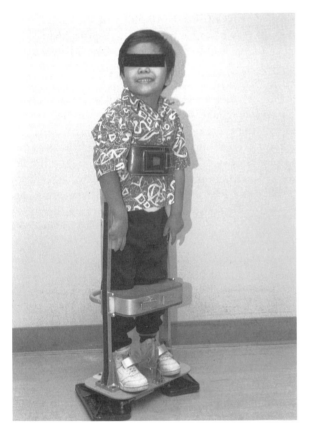

Fig. 6-6. Orlau swivel walker. Rotating footplates generate forward propulsion from trunk tilt to the side. Child with upper thoracic paraplegia.

ambulate in this manner varies greatly, depending on their physical and mental attributes. The range extends from 3 to 10 years, with peak incidence of accomplishment around 5 to 7 years.

As the child grows, the increasing size of the footplate makes floor clearance more difficult or impossible. Therefore, it is well to bear in mind that the parapodium and similar orthoses that may be a suitable walking device for younger children can hardly serve this purpose later. Ambulation as an exercise is attained by a few youngsters with upper thoracic deficits, and its likelihood increases in lesions below T6.[68,73] Some children in the latter group are household ambulators while young, most likely those with T10–T11 segmental lesion. Functional community ambulation is not expected.

As a rule, both the child and parents are inclined to abandon nonfunctional ambulation by the end of the early school years. Some children with a lesion in the lower thoracic segments show continuing promise of maintaining some degree of nonfunctional ambulation beyond that age. In these cases, a reciprocating gait orthosis can be a more suitable choice.

Achievement and maintenance of limited ambulation can be expected only if the child has well-developed upper extremity strength, lean body build, a stable spine, and no significant lower extremity contractures. Progressive hip flexion contractures are the principal mechanical cause of gradual regression of ambulation. In thoracic lesions, a wheelchair is needed for functional mobility at all ages.

10 degrees, and (5) provision for lateral rocking movements by the addition of rocker soles. The child achieves forward progression by pressing down on one arm, using crutches or a walkerette. This maneuver raises the foot, which is then moved forward by gravity. Enhanced functional level and physiologic efficiency of ambulation were reported with the use of this orthosis in children of 6 to 15 years of age who had T11–L3 neurologic deficits.

Optimal Age of Training

In extrapolating the results of a study on 53 normal children ages 11 to 36 months, who were trained to walk with a walkerette and Verlo orthosis, Taylor and Sand suggested that ambulation with these types of devices can be learned most expeditiously at approximately 24-month developmental level.[86] The chronological age when children with thoracic myelodysplasia can learn to

Upper Lumbar Lesions

A lesion between the first and third lumbar segments leaves the hip flexors and adductors partially or completely innervated. There may be partial knee extensor activity and weak knee flexion performed by the gracilis muscle. Hip abductors and extensors do not function, and the paralytic muscle imbalance leads to contractures and early hip dislocation.[68,70,87]

There is general agreement that unilateral hip dislocation requires surgery to prevent pelvifemoral asymmetry, which will initiate or enhance scoliosis. Surgery for bilateral hip dislocation is controversial in view of the limited ambulatory potential in upper lumbar paralysis.[87] A hip abduction brace is used at night as a temporizing measure until surgery is performed[68] (Fig. 6-4). The ankles are flail, and equinus foot deformities develop as a result of faulty positioning or may be present at birth.[15]

Active trunk control and hip flexion enable these children to sit, usually between 12 and 18 months, provided that their medical course is uncomplicated.[74] The characteristic sitting position is that of increased lordosis.

In L1 lesions, developmental and functional achievements requiring upright posture are similar to those in deficits of the lowest thoracic segments. In this group, however, unopposed hip flexion makes standing even more important. Standing and nonreciprocal gait orthoses are prescribed with the same considerations as in thoracic lesions.

The reciprocal gait orthosis (RGO) is a very appropriate device for upper lumbar paralysis in which active hip flexion is preserved[77,83,84] (Fig. 6-7A-E). The design of the RGO has undergone several changes over the years. The two early versions had a cord and pulley, or a cable with a gear box for the activating mechanism.[77] Eventually, a single cable replaced these components. A further modification was the Louisiana State University (LSU RGO) dual cable type.[83] Isocentric RGO (IRGO)[88] is the latest design; in this orthosis, the cable is substituted by a pelvic band attached to the posterior surface of the molded thoracic section. Pivoting around its central point of attachment, the pelvic band functions as a reciprocal activating mechanism.

In all types of RGOs, coupling of the cables or the pivoting pelvic band to both hip joints provides mechanical assistance to hip extension, prevents bilateral simultaneous hip flexion, and thereby helps to maintain stability and balance in standing position.[89] Unilateral hip flexion enhances extension moment at the contralateral joint through increased cable tension or through the lever arm of the pivoting pelvic band. In this manner, the orthosis permits and assists the patient in taking reciprocal steps. Forward stepping is achieved by active hip flexion, lower abdominal muscles, and /or trunk extension. In both the RGO and the IRGO, a latch disengages the reciprocal activating mechanism, which then allows bilateral hip flexion for sitting. The IRGO has two additional options: (1) a "preselected" hip joint that has a two-step release mechanism to prevent sudden collapse in hip flexion when the orthosis is unlocked in preparation for sitting; and (2) a hip abduction joint to eliminate the need for removing the orthosis for diaper change or catheterization, a great convenience in the care of children with spina bifida.[88] The molded thoracic section can be constructed as a spinal orthosis for children with scoliosis in both the cable and isocentric types of RGO. Advantages of the IRGO are a less bulky appearance and apparently a reduction of mechanical energy loss as a result of cable friction in the RGO. Most studies indicate increased efficiency of ambulation with any RGO compared with other

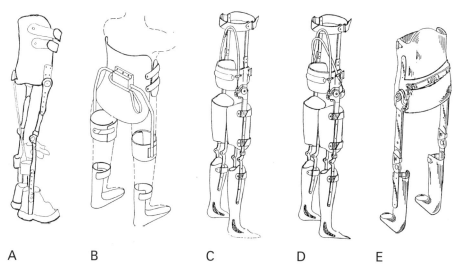

A   B   C   D   E

Fig. 6-7.   Development of different types of RGO. **(A)** Cord and pulley type (Motloch). **(B)** Gear box type (Motloch). **(C)** Single cable type. **(D)** Dual-cable Louisiana State University. **(E)** Isocentric type RGO. (The isocentric type RGO is registered by the Center for Orthotic Design Inc., Redwood City, CA). (Courtesy of Mr. Wallace Motloch.)

types of orthoses or nonreciprocal gait pattern.[85,90–95] A recent report demonstrated significantly lower physiologic cost index[96] with the IRGO than with the RGO, but there were no differences of importance in any other physiologic or gait parameters measured.

Although mild hip and knee flexion contractures do not exclude using an RGO[91], full range of motion facilitates a reciprocal gait. Severe fixed hip flexion contractures interfere with activating the reciprocating orthotic mechanism. Plantigrade foot alignment is an important requirement. Judicious consideration of surgical correction of the presenting muscle imbalance is recommended prior to fitting children with these orthoses.[92,97]

In most cases, the outcome of ambulation with RGO and walkerette is on household or exercise level.[91,98] Children over 3 years of age with low thoracic or upper lumbar segmental paralysis caused by myelodysplasia or spinal cord injury can generally learn to walk with an RGO.[83,97] As preparation, the parapodium or ORLAU swivel walker may be tried first for training to develop standing tolerance. Since physical and/or psychosocial factors may prevent successful use of an RGO,[91] careful selection of candidates is advisable. In a long-range perspective, the majority of children discontinue using the orthosis after 10 years of age[91] in favor of more functional wheelchair mobility.

Children with L2 and particularly with L3 innervation have the advantage of active knee extension, which enables them to maintain a straight knee position when they pull to stand. Most youngsters accomplish this milestone between 18 and 24 months. Unassisted standing and walking are not possible in the absence of active hip extension and abduction.[68] Crutches or canes will be needed.

Differences in orthotic management are probably the greatest in this group, both with respect to the extent of bracing and the age when it should be initiated. One approach is to use an HKAFO when the patient is about 1 year old.[72] This is used as a standing device to prevent contractures. Ambulation training with a walkerette or crutches begins later, its onset depending on developmental and medical status. Bracing is decreased to a KAFO, preferably after cessation of growth, when deformities are less likely to develop, and they are retained as definitive orthoses in most cases.

Another viewpoint is that children with L2 and L3 lesions use crawling or scooting as the primary mode of mobility in early years, and extensive orthoses interfere with these activities.[74] Therefore, orthotic fitting should

be deferred until after 2 years, when walking with upper extremity assistive devices becomes a more realistic functional goal. Exceptions are made, if warranted, by threatening hip flexion contractures when standing position with an orthosis is used for stretching. The tendency in this approach is to emphasize the functional rather than the preventive role of orthoses from an early age on. An HKAFO is not recommended, and stabilization is attempted by orthoses acting distal to the knee joint.

No rigid rules can be set about the approach one should follow, because clinical findings and course exhibit considerable diversity. In some cases, however, an HKAFO cannot be avoided as a result of hip instability, and children who need this extent of orthosis will be limited ambulators regardless of the type used.

In L2 segmental innervation, quadriceps strength is generally sufficient for stationary standing but not necessarily for counteracting the peak knee flexion torques that occur at certain points of stance phase on ambulation. Hip extensor weakness also jeopardizes proximal stabilization for the knees, and progressive hip flexion contractures lead to further compromise. Children with an L2 lesion therefore need a KAFO.

When mechanical control of hip alignment is poor, an HKAFO is required. This may be the case when a child first begins to walk; improved coordination and strength on practicing ambulation should eventually allow using KAFOs. Depending on the degree of knee control, offset joints, drop ring locks, or step locks may be used.[99] In the latter instance, ambulation can be practiced with alternatingly opened knee joints.

In selected cases, a KAFO with a pretibial shell or a supracondylar KAFO is adequate to enhance knee extension.[27,29] Hinged ankle joints with 5 to 10 degrees of plantar flexion will decrease knee flexion torque from heel strike to midstance and assist in knee stability.

In L3 lesions, knee extensor strength in the fair range is expected. There is a good possibility that these children can eventually walk using only AFOs.[68] In both L2 and L3 segmental weakness, orthotic needs should be periodically reassessed. One should be prepared to make changes and reduce the extent of orthoses as the child becomes more experienced with walking. Full passive range of motion at all lower extremity joints and the capability to maintain a near-vertical trunk–hip alignment with crutches are favorable clinical signs for considering reduction of orthotic support.

Genu recurvatum is encountered sometimes with preserved quadriceps function when hamstring weakness deprives the knee of its posterior support. Stabilization at the knee joint or from the ankle are two approaches to this problem. For mediolateral knee instability, a KAFO with biomechanical features appropriate for the presenting problem should be provided.

In L1–L3 lesions, the ankles are flail and assume a valgus attitude on weight bearing.[15,68] The ankle–foot components should be constructed to correct this problem in addition to controlling drop foot. Equinus deformity may be present at birth or is acquired from inadequate prevention. Talipes equinovarus is seen in congenital foot deformities.

Fitting of orthoses and shoes requires special care with sensory deficit in the feet. Abnormal foot alignment greatly increases the incidence of decubiti over areas of excessive pressure. Proper shoe fitting needs as much attention and time in these cases as a complex orthosis. This effort is worthwhile, because orthoses and plans for standing or ambulation cannot be implemented if the child has pressure sores on his feet.

Children with L2 or L3 lesions usually cruise by holding on for support around the age of 2 to 3 years.[74] They learn crutch walking with KAFOs around 5 years of age if the lesion is at L1, and at 3 to 4 years if the deficit is one or two segments lower. In a long-range perspective, about half of the patients become functional household or limited community ambulators.[68,73] Recurrent medical problems and progressive musculoskeletal complications are responsible for failure to attain, or regression of, ambulation. Hip dislocation is the most frequent complication in the group with mid-to-upper lumbar lesions[87] and is a serious hindrance to ambulation. Unilateral dislocation leads to severe pelvifemoral asymmetry and spinal deformities. In these situations, a standing orthosis and exercise ambulation may be the most appropriate, regardless of the exact segmental level of paralysis.

Low Lumbar Lesions

In L4 lesions, the knee extensors are strong; there is slight abductor and knee flexor function. Ankle dorsiflexion and inversion are largely unopposed. If the deficit spares the fifth lumbar segment, hip extensors, abductors, and knee flexors are gaining in strength; foot evertors are working but plantar flexion remains weak. Hip flexion contractures and dislocation are still possible threats and may require surgical treatment. In L4 lesions, knee exten-

sion contracture occurs from the strong quadriceps and weak flexors. Calcaneovarus foot deformity indicates an L4 lesion, while a calcaneus foot is more characteristic of L5 deficits.[14,68,87]

Children in this group have the physical capabilities of pulling-to-stand and cruising at an age close to the expected time.[74] Independent standing and walking tend to be delayed but are generally accomplished by 2 years. Triceps surae weakness makes stationary stance unstable. Gait deviations are gastrocnemius limp and gluteus medius lurch. Some children need upper extremity assistive devices when they start walking because of partial weakness around the hips. In most cases, they eventually discard the crutches. Despite the high energy cost of walking, children with a low lumbar lesion maintain functional ambulation.[73] Hip dislocation is less likely and occurs later than in upper lumbar lesions. It is a preventable complication.

In infancy, stretching and thermoplastic anterior ankle splints decrease the progression of calcaneus deformity. An orthosis is prescribed when the child pulls to stand. The main concern is ankle stabilization, which can be achieved by an AFO. Total-contact anterior shell is necessary to restrict the unwanted dorsiflexed ankle position. Partial hip extensor weakness and calcaneus foot tend to promote hip and knee flexion attitude. The floor reaction orthosis, which increases knee extension moment, is a good alternative for these postural deviations, provided the calcaneus deformity is not fixed.[48,49,74] With calcaneus attitude of the foot, recurrent heel decubiti and chronic osteomyelitis of the os calcis can develop. Careful and consistent monitoring is needed to prevent these complications.

In sacral lesions, various degrees of pes cavus deformity are present. Shoe modifications and soft-sole shoes relieve excessive pressure and discomfort at the prominent metatarsal heads and on the dorsal and plantar surfaces of claw toes.

OTHER NEUROMUSCULAR DISEASES

Duchenne Muscular Dystrophy

Duchenne muscular dystrophy affects boys and is the most frequent and severe type among the myopathies. It leads to wheelchair existence usually by adolescence and demise in the third decade of life. Symptoms appear in early childhood with predominant proximal weakness, most marked in the musculature of the shoulder and pelvic girdle. Characteristics of stance and gait are increased lumbar lordosis and trunk extension, hip and knee flexion, broad supporting base, gluteus medius and maximus gait, and toe walking.[100–103] These changes occur both as a result of and as compensation for muscle weakness and eventually lead to contractures.

In the past, orthoses have not been used in Duchenne muscular dystrophy. Recently, however, it was suggested that as weakness progresses and deformities occur, the compensatory biomechanical changes described above will reach a point when maintenance of upright posture is no longer possible.[102–106] Percutaneous tenotomies were recommended to release hip flexor, tensor fasciae latae, and triceps surae contractures if weakness is not severe enough to exclude ambulation. Surgery is followed by early mobilization and orthosis.[106] Because surgical releases eliminate the previously used biomechanical compensation, KAFOs are needed to provide a stabilizing system for the lower limbs.[106] Upright position is maintained by sitting on the orthotic support. The KAFO has the knee joints aligned in 5 degrees of flexion and the ankles held in neutral position, and an additional upper gluteal contoured thigh cuff is included. Careful fitting is needed for proper length adjustment of the orthosis. Slumping and falling forward occurs if the orthosis is too long, and backward tilt with severe compensatory kyphosis develops if it is too short. Because weight is an important consideration in the presence of severe weakness, high-strength polypropylene ischial weightbearing KAFOs are used. There are reports of successful application of swivel walker in muscular dystrophy.[107]

It should be noted that there are as many enthusiastic advocates as opponents of the combined surgical–orthotic intervention in Duchenne muscular dystrophy. This approach has been reported to prolong ambulatory status by several years.[105] To date, however, no controlled clinical studies compare the results of this method as opposed to conservative management.

Regardless of which approach is followed while the child is ambulatory, attempts should be made to slow the progression of deformities that often develop rapidly once the patient has become wheelchair bound.[103] It is important, therefore, at this stage to try preventing the deformities by a system of resting orthotic devices, with careful attention to recheck their fit as the child grows and joint configurations change. Development of severe equinocavovarus foot deformities in a wheelchair-bound child would eventually preclude wearing shoes. Preventive application of AFOs may delay the appearance of foot deformities. If a fixed deformity is already present, orthoses should be aligned in a tolerable position of correction.

Hip and knee flexion contractures inevitably develop if the child is allowed to sit for prolonged periods with his legs dependent in the wheelchair. Resting splints made of thermoplastic materials will keep the knees in extension and the feet in neutral position to prevent contractures at these joints. In advanced stages of the disease, flexion and abduction deformities of the hips make lying in bed very uncomfortable. Splints extended over the hips are not effective or tolerated. A soft contoured mattress insert or pad is useful in relieving discomfort. Hip abduction deformities also present difficulties while these children sit in a wheelchair. Contoured seat and back inserts are necessary to maintain optimal posture and comfort. Scoliosis, an inevitable complication in Duchenne type muscular dystrophy, is treated with TLSO or surgery.

Other Myopathies

The application of braces has not been recommended in limb girdle or fascioscapulohumeral types of muscular dystrophy. For the predominantly proximal distribution of muscle weakness, no satisfactory orthoses are available, and shoulder girdle weakness excludes the possibility of crutch walking.

In the less severe and more slowly progressive forms of congenital myopathies, orthoses can be of benefit for specific biomechanical problems. Standing orthosis, the Orlau swivel walker, hip guidance orthosis, or an RGO should be considered when warranted by generalized muscle weakness.[108]

Muscular Atrophies

Infantile progressive muscular atrophy, Werdnig-Hoffmann disease, is the most severe form of these degenerative disorders. Prognosis is usually poor, and death is anticipated in preschool age. However, more benign variants of this disease have longer survival.[108] In these cases, proper measures, including orthoses, should be instituted to prevent contractures and to assist in mobility, limited though it may be. This is particularly indicated because these children are bright and alert. Orthotic approach and selection are similar to that mentioned in congenital myopathies.[108] In Kugelberg-Welander disease, the juvenile form of spinal muscular atrophy weakness is predominantly proximal in distribution and creates biomechanical abnormalities similar to Duchenne or limb girdle dystrophy. Proximal weakness is not readily amenable to orthotic intervention, and HKAFO does not provide functional benefit.

In the various forms of hereditary polyneuropathies of childhood, orthoses to improve function are selected on the basis of developmental considerations and biomechanical abnormalities. Prescription of preventive splinting or orthoses is guided by anticipation of musculoskeletal complications.

ARTHRITIS AND COLLAGEN DISEASES

In the acute and subacute stages of juvenile rheumatoid arthritis and other collagen diseases associated with pain and weakness, splinting is the generally applied method for protective support and for maintaining and increasing range of motion.[109] Shoe modifications or shoe inserts alleviate the discomfort from joint inflammation in the foot.

Orthoses are not indicated for functional purposes in juvenile rheumatoid arthritis. In an extremely rare case, a KAFO may be considered as an adjunct to other treatment methods for severe knee flexion contracture in the chronic phase. Several special knee joints are available to control flexion and extension range and for assisting extension. The polycentric knee joint with a spring to assist extension exerts continuous stretching.[1] Placement of the mechanical joint must be most carefully determined so that its position corresponds to the axis of rotation of the anatomic joint. The dial lock restricts motion in one direction.[28] It can be set and adjusted at different degrees of extension and allows free movement through the rest of the range. The fan lock[28] does not permit motion, but it can also be adjusted to different joint positions. Posterior subluxation of the tibia is a contraindication to orthotic stretching of knee flexion con-

tractures. Hemophiliac arthropathy with knee flexion contracture was more frequent in the past.[109] Replacement therapy for the deficient clotting factor eliminated this problem. Acute hemarthrosis is treated with a knee immobilizer splint.[109]

DISORDERS OF THE SKELETAL SYSTEM

For congenital hip dislocation in patients under 3 months of age, the treatment is a Pavlik harness, abduction splint, or pillow.[15,64,110]

Legg-Calvé-Perthes disease or juvenile coxa plana is an avascular necrosis of the femoral capital epiphysis, which often occurs bilaterally.[15] The treatment of this disease has undergone several changes over the years. Originally, it consisted of nonweight bearing until the stage of regeneration was complete. In bilateral involvement, this meant bed rest, at times as long as 1 to 2 years. In unilateral cases, nonweight bearing was achieved by crutch walking and using a waist belt with a sling loop that held the affected extremity suspended in flexion.[111]

Subsequently, KAFOs were developed with ischial weight bearing to relieve pressure on the femoral head.[112] In the first model, an ischial ring seat was incorporated. By virtue of a shoe extension platform, the leg was freely suspended within the brace. The child could walk with crutches wearing this orthosis on one or both legs. In a unilateral case, a shoe lift was added on the unaffected side to compensate for the leg length difference created by the platform. The ischial ring was eventually replaced by a quadrilateral socket with ischial seat.[112] Current treatment is ambulation in an abduction orthosis after the synovitis and pain have subsided. The walking orthosis maintains the hip in 45 degrees of abduction and 20 degrees of internal rotation[113–115] (Fig. 6-7). This position provides concentric coverage of the femoral head and promotes spheric reossification as regeneration occurs. The simplest device was the Petrie cast, consisting of long-leg plaster cylinders abducted by a broomstick.[116] The casts were not removable but could be adjusted.

A number of walking abduction orthoses are available for bilateral hip pathology using similar principles of design[113–115,117] (Fig. 6-8). All have two medially situated upright bars, which are held in the desired position of abduction and internal rotation by two cross bars. One

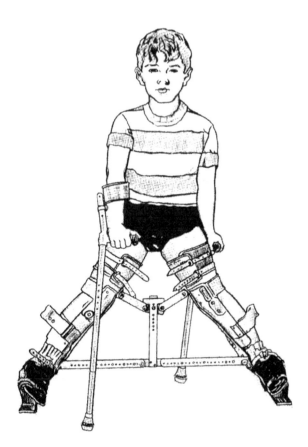

Fig. 6-8. Walking abduction orthosis for bilateral Legg-Perthes disease.

cross bar is located at the ankle and the other at the knee or at the proximal end of the upright bars. Shoe platforms or wedges provide a flat weightbearing surface. An important consideration when using these orthoses is to avoid stress on the medial collateral ligament and the development of genu valgum. The trilateral socket hip abduction orthosis has a quadrilateral plastic-laminated ischial weight-bearing rim and a metal upright with a walking heel. Weight bearing is transmitted through the medial upright. In children over 7 years of age or with more severe involvement, the orthopedic surgeon may elect operative rather than conservative treatment. Various designs of hip abduction walking orthoses include the Newington,[114] the Toronto,[113] and the Scottish Rite[115] braces.

Osteogenesis imperfecta is a rather rare disease but should be mentioned because of orthotic interest.[118,119] Light plastic orthoses that encase the lower extremities

both anteriorly and posteriorly may prevent bowing of the long bones caused by weight bearing. The principles of fracture bracing may be useful in the orthotic management of these children (see Ch. 2).

Genu varum, and particularly genu valgum in a mild form, are developmental phenomena in normal children. Spontaneous correction occurs by 5 to 7 years of age. In the absence of neuromuscular impairment, severe knee deformities can be caused by generalized primary or secondary metabolic diseases of the skeletal system, localized pathologic processes, or injuries and syndromes associated with ligamentous laxity.[15] Progressive deformities occur because epiphyseal growth is uneven, as a result of asymmetric compression forces. Progression becomes especially fast when the weight-bearing line passes either medial or lateral to the knee joint. Support for mediolateral knee instability can be incorporated in a standard KAFO with free knee joints using varus or valgus condyle pads or a puller.[1,6,28] A KAFO with an appropriately placed single medial or lateral bar is lighter in weight, but it may not provide adequate support for obese children.[120] Supracondylar KAFOs with free knee joints are biomechanically appropriate, but a snug fit allows limited accommodation for growth.[27,29] In selecting the most suitable orthosis, one should remember that these children are not neurologically impaired, that they are very active, and grow at a normal pace.

Foot deformities occur sometimes in otherwise healthy infants and may necessitate the use of corrective orthosis, either by itself or as an adjunct to other treatment modalities.[14] Rotational deformities of the tibia or the femur and metatarsus adductus are generally managed with bilateral shoe clamp foot orthoses with a spreader bar and footplate attached to the sole of the shoes during sleep.[14] The length of the bar determines limb abduction. Axial limb rotation can be varied by the position of the footplate on the bar. If the bar is curved with its apex proximally or distally, the foot will be in varus or valgus position, respectively.

UPPER EXTREMITY ORTHOSES

The need for functional upper extremity orthoses seems to arise less frequently in children than in adults. Clinical experience also suggests that these devices are not well accepted by youngsters. Children appear to prefer substitutive patterns of their own choice and reject interference with sensory feedback. Resting splints during sleep are better tolerated and are used in a variety of conditions for preventive purposes. Hand orthoses have certainly not gained significant application in the treatment of upper extremity impairment in neuromuscular deficits of early onset. An exception is cervical spinal cord injury where functional indications and biomechanical principles are identical to those in adults. A thumb abduction splint is often tried but has limited success in spastic cerebral palsy. Construction and proper fitting of orthoses or splints are often difficult for a small hand size, particularly the more complex types used for functional assistance in adults. If these practical problems are eliminated, application at an early age may give better results, similar to the experience with prostheses in congenital upper limb deficiency.

REFERENCES

1. Bunch WH (ed): Atlas of Orthotics. American Academy of Orthopedic Surgeons. 2nd ed. CV Mosby, St. Louis, 1985
2. Perry J: Kinesiology of lower extremity bracing. Clin Orthop 102:18, 1974
3. Campbell J, Ball J: Energetics of walking in cerebral palsy. Orthop Clin North Am 9:374, 1978
4. Molnar GE (ed): Pediatric Rehabilitation. 2nd Ed. Williams & Wilkins, Baltimore, 1992
5. Bobath KA: A neurophysiologic basis for the treatment of cerebral palsy. Clin Dev Med 75: 1984
6. Deaver GG, Brittis AL: Braces, crutches, wheelchairs. In: Rehabilitation Monograph No. 5. New York University, New York, 1953
7. Deaver GG: Cerebral palsy, methods of treating the neuromuscular disability. Arch Phys Med Rehabil 37:363, 1956
8. Garrett A, Lister M, Bresnan G: New concepts in cerebral palsy bracing. J Am Phys Ther Assoc 46:728, 1966
9. Guess VS: Control of lower extremity movement in cerebral palsy. In Perry J, Hislop JH (eds): Principles of Lower Extremity Bracing. American Physical Therapy Association, New York, 1967
10. Winters TF, Gage JR, Hicks R: Gait patterns in spastic hemiplegia in children and young adults. J Bone Joint Surg [Am] 69:437, 1987
11. Rosenthal RK: The use of orthotics in foot and ankle problems in cerebral palsy. Foot Ankle 4:195, 1984
12. Bleck EE: Orthopedic Management in Cerebral Palsy. 2nd Ed. Cambridge University Press, NY, 1987
13. Samilson RL, Perry J: The orthopaedic assessment of cerebral palsy. In Samilson RL (ed): Orthopaedic Aspects of Cerebral Palsy. Clinics in Developmental Medicine No. 52/53. JB Lippincott, Philadelphia, 1975
14. Tachdjian MO: The Child's Foot. WB Saunders, Philadelphia, 1985
15. Tachdjian MO: Pediatric Orthopedics. 2nd Ed. WB Saunders, Philadelphia, 1990
16. Root L: Varus and valgus foot in cerebral palsy and its management. Foot Ankle 4:174, 1984
17. Wu KK: Foot Orthoses. Williams & Wilkins, Baltimore, 1990
18. Middleton EA, Hurley GRB, McIlwain JS: The role of rigid and hinged polypropylene ankle-foot orthoses in the management of cerebral palsy: A case study. Prosthet Orthot Int 12:129, 1988
19. Ford C, Grotz RC, Shamp JK: The neurophysiological ankle-foot orthosis. Clin Prosthet Orthot 10:15, 1986
20. Bennett GC, Rang M, Jones D: Varus and valgus deformities of the foot in cerebral palsy. Dev Med Child Neurol 24:499, 1982
21. Sarno JE, Lehneis HR: Prescription considerations for plastic below knee orthoses. Arch Phys Med Rehabil 52:503, 1971
22. Dolan CME, Mereday C, Hartman G: Evaluation of NYU Insert Brace. New York University, New York, 1969
23. Krebs DE, Edelstein JE, Fishman S: Comparison of plastic/metal and leather/metal ankle-foot orthoses. Am J Phys Med Rehabil 67:175, 1988
24. Rosenthal RK, Deutsch SD, Miller W et al: A fixed ankle below-knee orthosis for the management of genu recurvatum in spastic cerebral palsy. J Bone Joint Surg [Am] 57:545, 1975
25. Lee KH, Johnston R: Bracing below the knee for hemiplegia: biomechanical analysis. Arch Phys Med Rehabil 54:466, 1973
26. Lee KH, Johnston R: Effect of below knee bracing on knee movement: biomechanical analysis. Arch Phys Med Rehabil 55:179, 1974
27. Cassvan A, Wunder KE, Fultonberg DM: Orthotic management of unstable knee. Arch Phys Med Rehabil 58:487, 1977
28. Heizer D: Bracing design for knee joint instability. In Perry J, Hislop HJ (eds): Principles of Lower Extremity Bracing. American Physical Therapy Association, New York, 1967
29. Lehneis HR: New developments in lower limb orthotics through bioengineering. Arch Phys Med Rehabil 53:303, 1972
30. Cusick BD: Progressive Casting and Splinting for Lower Extremity Deformities in Children With Neuromuscular Dysfunction. Therapy Skill Builders, Tucson, 1990
31. Norlin R, Odenrick P: Development of gait in children with spastic cerebral palsy. J Pediatr Orthop 6:674, 1986
32. Sutherland DH: Gait Disorders in Childhood and Adolescence. Williams & Wilkins, Baltimore, 1984

33. Murphy SB, Simon SR, Kijewski PK et al: Femoral anteversion. J Bone Joint Surg [Am] 69:1169, 1987

34. Sutherland DH, Cooper Z: The pathomechanics of progressive crouch gait in spastic diplegia. Orthop Clin North Am 9:143, 1978

35. Ingram TTS: Paediatric Aspects of Cerebral Palsy. ES Livingstone, Edinburgh, 1964

36. Ada L, Scott D: Use of inhibitory weight-bearing plasters to increase movement in the presence of spasticity. Aust J Physiother 26:57, 1980

37. Hayes NK, Burns YR: Discussion on the use of weight bearing plasters in the reduction of hypertonicity. Aust J Physiother 16:108, 1970

38. Sussman MD, Cusick B: Preliminary report: the role of short-leg, tone-reducing casts as an adjunct to physical therapy of patients with cerebral palsy. Johns Hopkins Med J 145:112, 1975

39. Zachazewski JE, Eberle ED, Jefferies M: Effect of tone-inhibiting casts and orthoses on gait. Phys Ther 62:453, 1982

40. Bertoti DB: Effect of short leg casting on ambulation in children with cerebral palsy. Phys Ther 66:1522, 1986

41. Stills M: Clinical experience with the "solid ankle" orthosis. Orthot Prosthet 30:13, 1976

42. Duncan WR, Mott DH: Foot reflexes and the use of "inhibitive casts." Foot Ankle 4:145, 1983

43. King HA, Staheli LT: Torsional problems in cerebral palsy. Foot Ankle 4:180, 1984

44. Lehman JF, Warren C, DeLateur BA: A biomechanical evaluation of knee instability in below knee braces. Arch Phys Med Rehabil 51:688, 1970

45. Evans EB: The knee in cerebral palsy. In Samilson RL (ed): Orthopaedic Aspects of Cerebral Palsy. Clinics in Developmental Medicine. No. 52/53. JB Lippincott, Philadelphia, 1975

46. Perry J: The cerebral palsy gait. In Samilson RL (ed): Orthopaedic Aspects of Cerebral Palsy. Clinics in Developmental Medicine. No. 52/53. JB Lippincott, Philadelphia, 1975

47. Harrington ED, Lin RS, Gage J: Use of anterior floor reaction orthosis in patients with cerebral palsy. Orthot Prosthet 37:34, 1983

48. Yang GW, Chu DS, Ahn JH et al: Floor reaction orthosis: clinical experience. Orthot Prosthet 40:33, 1986

49. Satiel JA: One piece laminated knee locking short leg brace. Orthot Prosthet 23:68, 1969

50. Warren CG, Lehmann JF, DeLateur BJ: Pelvic band use in orthotics for adult paraplegic patients. Arch Phys Med Rehabil 56:221, 1975

51. Waters RL, Lunsford BR: Energy expenditure of normal and pathologic gait: application to orthotic treatment. In Bunch WH (ed): Atlas of Orthotics. 2nd Ed. CV Mosby, St. Louis, 1985

52. Mital MA, Belkin SC, Sullivan MA: An approach to head, neck, and trunk stabilization and control in cerebral palsy by use of the Milwaukee brace. Dev Med Child Neurol 19: 198, 1976

53. Drennan JC: The role of the thoracic suspension orthosis in the management of myelomeningocele deformities. Inter-Clinic Inform Bull 17:6, 1979

54. Tardieu C, Huet De La Tour E, Bret MD, Tardieu G: Muscle hypoextensibility in children with cerebral palsy. I. Clinical and experimental observations. Arch Phys Med Rehabil 63:97, 1982

55. Tardieu G, Tardieu C, Colbeau-Justin P, Lespargot A: Muscle hypoextensibility in children with cerebral palsy. II. Therapeutic implications. Arch Phys Med Rehabil 63:103, 1982

56. Tardieu C, Lespargot A, Tabary C, Bret MD: For how long must the soleus muscle be stretched each day to prevent contracture? Dev Med Child Neurol 30:3, 1988

57. Booth FW: Physiologic and biomechanical effects of immobilization on muscle. Clin Orthop Rel Res 219:15, 1987

58. Tabary JC, Tabary C, Tardieu C et al: Physiological and structural changes in the cat soleus muscle due to immobilization at different lengths by plaster casts. J Anat 127:469, 1978

59. Otis JC, Root L, Kroll MA: Measurement of plantar flexion spasticity during treatment with tone reducing casts. J Pediatr Orthop 102:18, 1974

60. Watt J, Sims D, Harckham F et al: A prospective study of inhibitive casting as an adjunct to physiotherapy for cerebral palsied children. Dev Med Child Neurol 28:480, 1986

61. Gunsolus P, Welsh C, Houser C: Equilibrium reactions in the feet of children with spastic cerebral palsy and of normal children. Dev Med Child Neurol 17:580, 1975

62. Harris SR, Riffle K: Effects of inhibitive ankle-foot orthosis on standing balance in a child with cerebral palsy: a single subject design. Phys Ther 66:663, 1986

63. Hinderer KA, Harris SR, Purdy AH et al: Effects of "tone-reducing" vs standard plaster casts on improvement of children with cerebral palsy. Dev Med Child Neurol 30:370, 1988

64. Ilfeld LW: The management of congenital dislocation and dysplasia of the hips by means of a special splint. J Bone Joint Surg [Am] 39:99, 1957

65. Nakamura T, Ohamu M: Hip abduction splint for use at night for scissor leg of cerebral palsy patients. Orthot Prosthet 34(4):13, 1980

66. Sharrard WJW: The hip in cerebral palsy. In Samilson RL (ed): Orthopaedic Aspects of Cerebral Palsy. Clinics in Developmental Medicine. No. 52/53. JB Lippincott, Philadelphia, 1975

67. Motloch W: The parapodium: an orthotic device for neuromuscular disorders. Artif Limbs 15:36, 1971

68. Badell-Ribera A: Myelodysplasia. In Molnar GE (ed): Pediatric Rehabilitation. Williams & Wilkins, Baltimore, 1985

69. Freeman JM: Practical Management of Myelomeningocele. University Park Press, Baltimore, 1974

70. Shurtleff DB (ed): Myelodysplasias and Extrophies. New York, Grune & Stratton, 1986

71. Stark GD, Baker GCW: The neurologic involvement of the lower limb in myelomeningocele. Dev Med Child Neurol 9:732, 1967

72. Badell-Ribera A, Swinyard CA, Greenspan L, Deaver GG: Spina bifida with myelomeningocele: Evaluation of rehabilitation potential. In CA Swinyard (ed): Comprehensive Care of the Child With Spina Bifida Manifesta. Rehabilitation Monograph 31. New York University, New York, 1966

73. Hoffer MM, Feiwell E, Perry R et al: Functional ambulation in patients with myelomeningocele. J Bone Joint Surg [Am] 55:137, 1973

74. Bunch WH, Cass AS, Bensman AS, Long DM: Modern Management of Myelomeningocele. WH Green, St. Louis, 1972

75. Carroll N: The orthotic management of the spina bifida children. Clin Orthop 102:108, 1974

76. Heizer D: Brace design for flaccid paralysis. In Perry J, Hislop HJ (eds): Principles of Lower Extremity Bracing. American Physical Therapy Association, New York, 1967

77. Motloch WM: Device design in spina bifida. In Murdoch G: Advances in Orthotics. Williams & Wilkins, Baltimore, 1976

78. Taylor N, Pemberton DR: The Verlo: an orthosis for children with severe motor handicaps. Arch Phys Med Rehabil 53:534, 1972

79. Taylor N, Sand P: Verlo brace use in children with myelomeningocele and spinal cord injury. Arch Phys Med Rehabil 55:231, 1974

80. Stallard J, Major RE, Poiner R et al: Engineering design considerations of the Orlau swivel walker. Engin Med 15:3, 1986

81. Lough LK, Nielsen DH: Ambulation of children with meningomyelocele: parapodium vs parapodium with ORLAU swivel modification. Dev Med Child Neurol 28:489, 1986

82. Nene AV, Orth D, Patch JH: Energy cost of paraplegic locomotion with the ORLAU parawalker. Paraplegia 27:5, 1989

83. Douglas R, Larson PF, D'Ambrosia R, McCall RE: The LSU reciprocation gait orthosis. Orthopedics 6:834, 1983

84. Yngve DA, Douglas R, Roberts JM: The reciprocating gait orthosis in myelomeningocele. J Pediat Orthop 4:304, 1984

85. Rose GK, Stallard J, Sankarankutty M: Clinical evaluation of spina bifida patients using hip guidance orthosis. Dev Med Child Neurol 23:30, 1981

86. Taylor N, Sand P: Verlo orthosis: experience with different developmental levels in normal children. Arch Phys Med Rehabil 56:120, 1975

87. Menelaus M: The Orthopaedic Management of Spina Bifida Cystica. Churchill Livingstone, New York, 1980

88. Motloch W: Principles of orthotic management for child and adult paraplegia and clinical experience with the Isocentric RGO. International Society for Prosthetics and Orthotics II:28, 1992

89. Ogilvie C, Messenger N, Bowker P, Rowley DI: Orthotic compensation for non-functioning hip extensors. Zeitschrift fur Kinderchirurgie 2 (suppl. 43):33, 1988

90. Hirokawa S, Grimm M, Thanh L et al: Energy consumption in paraplegic ambulation using the reciprocating gait orthosis and electrical stimulation of the thigh muscles. Arch Phys Med Rehabil 71:687, 1980

91. Guidera KJ, Smith S, Raney E et al: Use of the reciprocating gait orthosis in myelodysplasia. J Pediatr Orthop 13:341, 1993

92. McCall RE, Schmidt WT: Clinical experience with the reciprocal gait orthosis in myelodysplasia. J Pediatr Orthop 6:157, 1986

93. Mazur JM, Sienko-Thomas S, Wright N, Cummings RJ: Swing through vs reciprocating gait patterns in patients with thoracic level spina bifida. Zeitschrift fur Kinderchirurgie 1 (suppl):23, 1990

94. Flandry F, Burke S, Roberts JM et al: Functional ambulation in myelodysplasia: the effect of orthotic selection on physical and physiologic performance. J Pediatr Orthop 6:661, 1986

95. Williams LO, Anderson AD, Campbell J et al: Energy cost of walking and of wheelchair propulsion by children with myelodysplasia: comparison with normal children. Dev Med Child Neurol 25:617, 1983

96. Winchester PK, Carollo JJ, Parekh RN et al: A comparison of paraplegic gait performance using two types of reciprocating gait orthoses. Prosthet Orthot Int 17:101, 1993

97. McCall RE, Douglas R, Rightor N: Surgical treatment in patients with myelodysplasia before using the LSU reciprocation-gait system. Orthopedics 6:1983

98. Charney EB, Melchionni JB, Smith DR: Community ambulation by children with myelomeningocele and high level of paralysis. J Pediatr Orthop 2:579, 1991

99. Lister MJ: Bracing the unstable knee in flaccid paralysis. In Perry J, Hislop HJ (eds): Principles of Lower Extremity Bracing. American Physical Therapy Association, New York, 1967

100. Johnson EW: Pathokinesiology of Duchenne muscular dystrophy: implications for management. Arch Phys Med Rehabil 58:4, 1977

101. Johnson EW, Kennedy JH: Comprehensive Management of Duchenne muscular dystrophy. Arch Phys Med Rehabil 52:110, 1971

102. Siegel JM: Pathomechanics of stance in Duchenne muscular dystrophy. Arch Phys Med Rehabil 53:403, 1972

103. Dubowitz V: Progressive muscular dystrophy: prevention of deformities. Clin Pediatr 3:323, 1964

104. Siegel JM, Miller JE, Ray RD: Subcutaneous lower limb tenotomy in treatment of pseudohypertrophic muscular dystrophy. J Bone Joint Surg [Am] 150:1437, 1968

105. Vignos PJ, Archibald KC: Maintenance of ambulation in childhood muscular dystrophy. J Chronic Dis 12:273, 1960

106. Siegel JM: Plastic molded knee-ankle-foot orthosis in the treatment of Duchenne muscular dystrophy. Arch Phys Med Rehabil 56:322, 1975

107. Gilbert JR, Williams SV et al: Swivel walker in Duchenne muscular dystrophy. Arch Dis Child 62:741, 1987

108. Eng GD: Diseases of the motor unit. In Molnar GE (ed): Pediatric Rehabilitation. Williams & Wilkins, Baltimore, 1985

109. Koch B: Rehabilitation of the Child with Joint Disease. In Molnar GE (ed): Pediatric Rehabilitation. Williams & Wilkins, Baltimore, 1985

110. Mendes DG: A night splint for congenital dislocation of the hip. J Bone Joint Surg [Am] 52:588, 1970

111. Snyder CH: Sling for use in Legg-Perthes disease. J Bone Joint Surg 29:524, 1947

112. Russek A, Eschen F: Ischial weight bearing brace with quadrilateral wood top. Orthop Prosthet Appl J 12:31, 1958

113. Bobechko WP, McLaurin CA, Motloch WM: The Toronto orthosis for Legg-Perthes disease. Artif Limbs 12:36, 1968

114. Curtis BH, Gunther SF, Gossling HR, Paul SW: Treatment of Legg-Perthes disease with the Newington ambulatory abduction brace. J Bone Joint Surg [Am] 56:1135, 1974

115. Purvis JM, Dimon JH et al: Preliminary experience with the Scottish Rite Hospital abduction orthosis for Legg-Perthes disease. Clin Orthop 150:49, 1980

116. Petrie JG, Bitenc J: The abduction weight-bearing treatment in Legg-Perthes disease. J Bone Joint Surg [Br] 53:54, 1971

117. Tachdjian MO, Jouett LO: Trilateral socket hip abduction orthosis for the treatment of Legg-Perthes disease. Orthot Prosthet 22:49, 1968

118. Morel G: Un nouveau type d'appareillage orthopedique: L'appariellage á atteles pneumatique. Rev Clin Orthop 57:409, 1971

119. Silber M, Chung TS, Varghese G et al: Pneumatic orthosis: a pilot study. Arch Phys Med Rehabil 56:27, 1975

120. Nietschke RO: A single bar above knee orthosis. Orthot Prosthet 25:20, 1971

Appendix 6-1
Orthotic L Codes

L Code	Orthosis
L0380	Thoracic–lumbar–sacral orthosis, anterior and posterior and lateral regional support with extensions
L0420	Thoracic–lumbar–sacral orthosis, two-piece, molded to patient model with interface
L0810	Halo procedure incorporated into jacket vest
L0860	Add: MRI-compatible system
L1000	Cervical–thoracic–lumbar–sacral orthosis, Milwaukee
L1500	Thoracic–hip–knee–ankle–foot orthosis, mobility frame (Newington Para Type)
L1520	Thoracic–hip–knee–ankle orthosis, Swivel Walker
L1620	Hip orthosis, Pavlik Harness
L1640	Hip orthosis, static, pelvic band or spread bar with thigh cuffs
L1680	Hip orthosis, Dynamic, pelvic control, adjust Rancho hip action (?) type
L1710	Newington type
L1720	Trilateral (Tachdihan type)
L1755	Patten bottom type
L1834	Knee orthosis, without knee joint, rigid, molded to patient model
L1960	Ankle–foot–orthosis, plastic, posterior solid ankle, molded to patient model
L1970	Ankle–foot–orthosis, plastic, with ankle joints, molded to patient model
L1970	Ankle–foot–orthosis, plastic, with ankle joints, molded to patient model

L Code	Orthosis
L1990	Ankle–foot–orthosis, double upright, free ankle joint, solid stirrup below-the-knee orthosis
L2020	Knee–ankle–foot orthosis, double upright, free knee joint, ankle joint, double-bar ankle–knee orthosis
L2030	Knee–ankle–foot orthosis, double upright, no knee join, ankle–knee orthosis
L2036	Knee–ankle–foot orthosis, full plastic, double upright, molded to patient model
L2040	Hip–knee–ankle foot orthosis, bilateral rotation straps, pelvis band/belt
L2050	Hip–knee–ankle foot orthosis, bilateral torsion cables, hip joint, pelvic band
L2060	Hip–knee–ankle foot orthosis, bilateral torsion cable, ball bearing hip joint
L2070	Hip–knee–ankle foot orthosis, unilateral rotation straps, pelvic band/belt
L2080	Hip–knee–ankle foot orthosis, unilateral torsion cable, hip joint, pelvic band
L2090	Hip–knee–ankle foot orthosis, unilateral torsion cable, ball bearing hip joint
L2200	Limited motion ankle joint, each joint
L2210	Dorsiflexion assist ankle joint, each joint
L2220	Dorsi- and plantar flexion assist/resist, each joint
L2250	Foot plate, molded to patient model, stirrup attachment
L2270	Varus/valgus correction T strap

L Code	Orthosis	L Code	Orthosis
L2275	Adduction: Varus/valgus correction, plastic modification	L2620	Hip joint, heavy duty, each
L2300	Abduction bar, jointed, adjustable (bilateral hip involvement)	L2640	Pelvic band and belt, bilateral
L2340	Pretibial shell, molded to patient model	L2650	Gluteal pad, each
		L2660	Thoracic band
L2375	Torsion control ankle joint, half solid stirrup	L2670	Paraspinal uprights
L2380	Torsion control, straight knee joint, each joint	L2680	Lateral thoracic support uprights
L2385	Straight knee joint, heavy duty, each joint	L2810	Knee control, condylar pad
L2405	Drop lock, each joint	L2999	Adductor: miscellaneous anterior clamshell
L2510	Quadrilateral brim, molded to patient model	L3140	Rotation positioning device, including shoe(s)
L2580	Pelvic sling	L3254	Nonstandard size or width
L2600	Hip joint, Clevis type, or thrust bearing, free, each	L3255	Nonstandard size or length
		L3257	Additional charge for split size
L2610	Hip joint, Clevis or thrust bearing, lock, each	L3310	Lift heel and sole, neoprene, per inch

Appendix 6-2
Diagnostic ICD9 Codes

ICD9 Code	Diagnosis
24.00	Spastic equinus of the ankle
335.00	Werdnig-Hoffmann disease
335.10	Spinal muscle atrophy, juvenile
335.11	Kugelberg-Welander disease
343	Cerebral palsy diplegia
343.1	Cerebral palsy hemiplegia
343.2	Cerebral palsy quadriparesis
333.7	Athetoid-Dyskinetic
343.9	Cerebral palsy spastic
343.10	Hemiplegia, congenital
344.90	Motor paralysis
356.90	Polyneuropathies
359.10	Duchenne's muscular dystrophy
436.00	Hemiplegia, acquired
714.31	Juvenile rheumatoid arthritis, acute
718.40	Internal hip rotation, contracture (acquired)
718.46	Knee contraction
728.85	Hypertonicity (muscular)
728.89	Hamstring contracture
728.90	Hypotonicity (muscular)
732.10	Legg-Calvé-Perthes disease
732.10	Juvenile coxa plana
735.00	Hallux valgus (acquired)
736.20	Inversion foot (acquired foot deformity)
736.30	Hip joint deformity, acquired
736.41	Genu valgum, acquired

ICD9 Code	Diagnosis
736.42	Genu varum, acquired
736.50	Genu recurvatum, acquired
736.60	Deformity of the knee, acquired
736.75	Varus foot (cavovarus)
737.20	Lumbar lordosis (acquired)
741.00	Arnold-Chiari malformation
741.90	Spina bifida
741.90	Meningocele
742.30	Aqueductal stenosis (with spina bifida, congenital)
742.59	Myelodysplasia
754.20	Scoliosis (congenital)
754.30	Hip dislocation, congenital
754.32	Hip subluxation, congenital
754.40	Genu recurvatum, acquired
754.69	Pes planovalgus, congenital
755.60	Rotational deformities of tibia, congenital
755.61	Coxa valga (congenital)
755.63	Femoral anteversion (neck, congenital)
755.64	Genu varum, congenital
756.14	Hemivertebrae
756.19	Kyphosis (congenital)
756.51	Osteogenesis imperfecta
779.80	Atonic (congenital)
781.20	Ataxic (gait)
835.03	Hip dislocation, anterior
919	Hemarthrosis, acute

Wheelchairs and Wheeled Mobility

Ann H. Gettel
John B. Redford

7

While not considered an orthosis in the truest sense of the word, a wheelchair may be the ultimate orthotic device; it provides a unique combination of mobility aid, positioning device, and functional aid for the whole person. In addition to providing a means for mobility, its features are chosen with the individual's needs, goals, and abilities all incorporated into the wheelchair prescription. The wheelchair may include features to reduce muscular exertion or provide access to communication devices or a surface for activities of daily living. The quality of life for many a disabled person virtually depends on the wheelchair.

No longer can a single type of wheelchair be expected to meet the needs of most people. Chair design options have evolved over the years to meet those needs. From the person with tetraplegia and ventilator dependency to the highly functioning wheelchair athlete, the individual's needs and goals must be analyzed. This often requires a multidisciplinary team approach to wheelchair prescription.

All ages may need mobile seating devices, from infants to the very elderly; specific seating principles apply to each age group. Understanding the principles of seating and the biomechanics that underlie an appropriate wheelchair prescription is crucial when one considers the myriad of diagnostic groups with special seating needs.

An estimated 1.2 million Americans use wheelchairs as their primary source of mobility, including nearly a quarter million people with spinal cord injury (SCI), nearly half a million nursing home residents, and the rest with other mobility limiting conditions, such as amputations, severe arthritis, neuromuscular disease, multiple sclerosis, encephalopathy, and cerebral palsy.[1,2]

This chapter outlines basic wheelchair components, the biomechanics of seating and propulsion, principles of wheelchair prescription, interventions by age group, and problem solving, including the use of specific principles and modifications for various diagnostic groups.

BASIC WHEELCHAIR COMPONENTS

Certain features of wheelchair design are fairly universal. Wheelchair components can logically be broken down into sections: the frame, propulsion unit, seating section, the extremity positioning components, and safety features (Fig. 7-1). Using a consistent approach to client evaluation and prescription, one can choose features in each of these sections or units, specialized where neces-

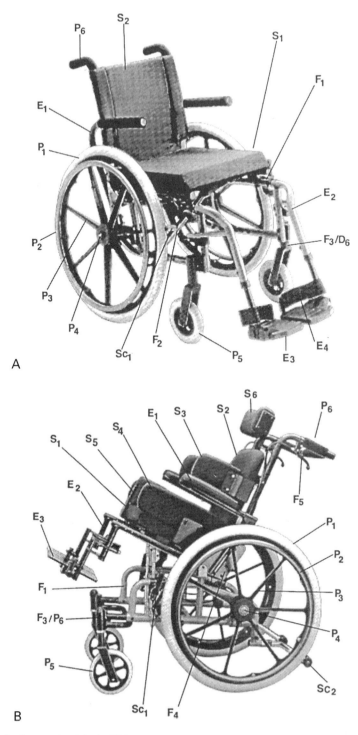

Fig. 7-1. **(A)** Standard-type wheelchair. **(B)** Tilt-in-space wheelchair. *Frame components:* F1, frame; F2, crossbar; F3, castor housing; F4, tilt-in-space frame; F5, tilt-in-space control. *Seating system components:* S1, seat; S2, back; S3, lateral thoracic support; S4, lateral pelvic/thigh support; S5, medial thigh support; S6, posterior head support. *Extremity control components:* E1, arm support; E2, front rigging; E3, foot plate; E4, heel support. *Propulsion system:* P1, rear tire; P2, hand rim; P3, mag wheel; P4, rear axle; P5, castor; P6, castor housing; P6, push handles. *Safety components:* SC1, wheel locks; SC2, pelvic belt (not shown); SC3, anti-tip bars. (Courtesy of Invacare, Addmaker.)

Table 7-1 Terms for Wheelchair Componants

Unit	Type Component	Subtype	Special Features
Frame	Manual	Folding	Standard Hemi-height Recline One-arm drive
		Rigid	Sports Tilt-in-space
	Power	Standard	Recline Tilt-in-space Standing
		Hybrid	Power on folding, Manual base Power base with choice of seating platforms
Propulsion	Wheels	Spoke Laced spoke Mag Composite	
	Rims	Standard Contoured	Coated Quad pegs Textured
	Tires	Pneumatic Solid Combo	
	Castors	Pneumatic Solid	
	Axle	Fixed Adjustable	
	Hangers		Specify angle
Seating System	Seat	Sling Solid Dropped Adjustable tension Custom	
	Cushion	Foam Contoured foam Gel Air-filled Combo	Contour-U Silhouette Vacuum-molded Others

Continues

Table 7-1 *(Continued)*

Unit	Type Component	Subtype	Special Features
Seating System Cont'd	Positioning	Antithrust design Pelvic well Medial thigh support Lateral thigh supports Lateral pelvic support Anterior pelvic support Thigh troughs Knee-block	
	Back	Solid Sling Adjustable tension Custom	
	Positioning	Lumbar support Lateral thoracic Supports Sacral support Biangular design	

Extremity Positioning	Arm Supports	Primary
		   Height adjustable
		   Removable
		   Tubular
		   Desk length
		   Full length
		   Absent
			Secondary
			   Padding
			   Anterior shoulder
			    support
			   Posterior shoulder
			    support
			   Superior shoulder
			    support
			   Balanced forearm
			    orthosis

	Arm trough, tray	Primary
		   Standard
		   Clear
		   Wooden
			Secondary mounting for
			   Communication system
			   Computer
			   Elbow blocks

	Leg rests	Standard Elevating Swing-away Removable Angle adjustable Spring dampening	
	Rigid	Sports Platform	Foot straps

Continues

Table 7-1 *(Continued)*

Unit	Type Component	Subtype	Special Features
Extremity Positioning Cont'd	Positioning aids	Posterior calf supports Foot support Foot positioner Anterior knee support Anterior leg support	
Safety Components	Positioning/harnessing	Pelvic stabilizer Anterior trunk support Subaxis pads/bar Pelvic belt Safety belt Foot/leg straps	
	Headrests	Flat Curved Three piece Occipital support ATNR Block Circumferential collar Horseshoe collar Headband	
	Grade-aids Anti-tip bars		
	Brakes	Standard mount Low mount Extensions	

sary to meet individual needs. With this approach, components are not inadvertently omitted.

The prescription should always refer to frame type, whether folding or rigid, manual or power, recline, or tilt-in-space. It should specify size and growth capabilities, if necessary. One should make a general assessment of the needed chair weight based on the strength, build, and diagnosis of the chair user.

The prescription of the propulsion system should include not only the wheels and casters, but also axle design (i.e., adjustable vs. fixed), tire type, and hangers for casters. With regard to wheel position and caster type, the importance of biomechanical principles of propulsion cannot be overlooked.

The seating systems may be the most crucial unit of the wheelchair, with design features chosen not only to aid in posture and positioning but also to act as a base of support for the rest of the seating prescription. The seating system selected should maximize wheeling efficiency, help control tone, provide optimal support and postural repositioning, and maintain or promote skin integrity. Specialized wheelchair cushions are usually required to meet such needs. For overall wheelchair seating, support of the pelvis is crucial to ensure that other design features of the wheelchair function effectively.

Table 7-1 summarizes the various terms used in describing wheelchair components.

BASIC PRINCIPLES OF SEATING SYSTEMS

Because the seating system is the cornerstone for successful positioning, seat design, and seat cushioning material are of crucial importance. Cushions for wheelchair seats and backs may be fabricated of many kinds of materials and in several distinct styles. No single system meets the needs of all persons who use wheelchairs regularly.[3] Often, several different cushion types can adequately meet the medical and positioning needs of a client. The following sections describe the variety of seats and cushions currently available.

Sling Seat

The simplest seat design is the sling seat. While acceptable for limited distances and uncomplicated circumstances, it has many drawbacks. For one, the sling design cannot adequately stabilize the pelvis. The wheelchair user without excellent trunk control and pelvic stability tends to list to one side, further compromising posture. The sling seat encourages a posture of posterior pelvic tilt, pelvic obliquity, internal rotation, and adduction at the hips (Fig. 7-2). In children, and in adults following hip surgery, this position may increase the risk for hip dislocation. Vital capacity and other pulmonary function measures are demonstrably worse for children with cerebral palsy in a sling seat compared with more supportive seating.[4]

The sagging sling property can be eliminated easily by the addition of a firm foam insert, with a convex lower surface and a flat upper surface, with a cushion on top, or alternatively, a cushioned plywood base.

Linear-Planar Design

The next most common seating system is the linear-planar design, which consists of a firm, flat foam seat and a firm, flat foam back. It is suitable for those with good sitting balance, a level pelvis, and low risk of skin breakdown, especially if it is needed for longer distance mobility for the user who can walk limited distances. Prefabricated components are generally available.

Slab or flat foam cushions be be used in the system or added to any firm chair seat requiring a little more padding. A very popular variety is the viscoelastic foam cushion (T foam and others) that has the property of compressibility; it has the ability to decrease in volume and absorb energy on impact, with stiffness dependent on the rate of loading. However, foam cushions have memory, returning to their original shape once the

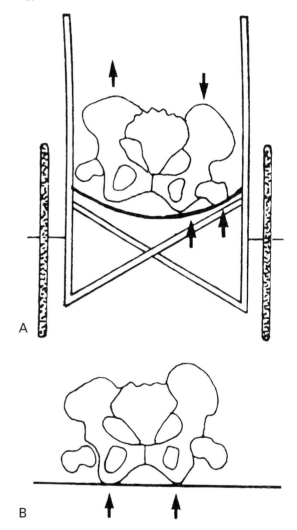

Fig. 7-2. Views of pelvis in front plane in setting. **(A)** Sitting in a wheelchair with sling seat. The sling seat encourages poor posture and impairs pelvis stability, causing an increased incidence of hip adduction, hip internal rotation, posterior pelvic tilt, and pelvic obliquity. **(B)** Sitting on a firm seat concentrates stabilizing forces at the ischial tuberosities for a level pelvis.

load has been removed. Cushions with memory may be less effective at reducing peak interface pressures than those that are fluid-filled, air-filled, or custom-contoured cushions. With repeated loading, inexpensive foams lack durability and must be monitored for bottoming out.

Modular

Modular seating also uses a linear-planar design with firm, generally flat foam surfaces. However, adjustable positioning components—such as lateral thoracic supports and hip and thigh supports to reduce hip abduction and adduction tendencies—allow a modular seating system to produce stabilizing forces for the person who lacks sufficient postural control to maintain balance. Modular positioning aids also can help retard the progression of some deformities caused by excessive hip adductor tone, hip muscle imbalance, or mild pelvic obliquity. They may also provide a more functional position for persons with scoliosis. Prefabricated, easily adjustable components are available from many companies.

Contoured Foam

Contoured foam is often favored over flat foam for seating systems. Foam cushions can be extensively modified to best meet a wheelchair user's specific needs. A firm, noncontoured cushion can compress soft tissues. However, that very deforming ability limits a flat cushion's usefulness in optimal seating, especially for the user with increased risk for skin breakdown. Chow has demonstrated that matching a cushion to buttock shape results in lower skin-to-cushion interface pressures and less tissue distortion than a flat cushion.[5,6] Pressure distribution over the skin was also better using soft foam than stiffer foam. Generally, softer, more compliant foams demonstrate better envelopment of the buttocks. Enveloping results from the ability of foam to decrease in volume during compression. Unlike a flat cushion, a good enveloping cushion will give a more uniform pressure distribution and stable sitting surface. Contoured foam also seems to reduce the potentially damaging effects of external loading, and so may be appropriate for many heavy wheelchair users. However, when the cushion materials deform excessively, whether flat or contoured, the risk of bottoming-out increases. Therefore, appropriate cushion selection needs a balance between enveloping and bottoming-out.[7]

Contoured cushions can be used for the individual with uncomplicated seating needs in place of linear-planar design. Contoured modular foam components can be added to meet more complex seating and positioning needs. Many foam cushions that match normal ana-tomic contours are commercially available, but more difficult seating problems may need custom contouring.

Special Pressure-Relief Cushions

Wheelchair cushions designed to decrease the risk of skin pressure come in a variety of forms. Most are either foam; air-, fluid-, or water-filled bladders; plastic enclosed gels and fluids; or combinations of several different materials. These cushions are designed either for total contact to equalize or redistribute weight bearing over a maximal surface area, or for specific pressure relief achieved by carving out the cushion under bony prominences, or for a combination of these principles.[8] Stress, defined as force divided by the area over which it acts, is an important factor in choosing an appropriate wheelchair seating system. Localized areas of increased stress are inevitable in seating and, if ignored, can lead to major skin problems. Two main types of stresses are encountered in wheelchair usage. First, those that act perpendicular to the skin, also referred to as normal stresses or, commonly, as pressure, and second, those that act parallel to the skin, or shear stresses or forces.

Air- and fluid-filled cushions are commonly used as pressure-relief cushions for the at-risk wheelchair user. Principles of gel or fluid use include provision of postural stability and concentrating pressure relief under pressure-sensitive areas, including the sacrum and ischial tuberosities, with movement of the gel or fluid to accommodate the position shifts of the user. Fluids are moderate conductors of heat and have a high heat capacity.[9] For energetic wheelchair users, the thermal property of the fluid helps to dissipate metabolic heat; overheating the skin surface adds to the risk of skin breakdown. Gel or fluid cushions are also beneficial in warm environments if effective water vapor and sweat removal can be ensured. However, in cold environments or for weak individuals who have difficulty keeping warm, these cushions make additional demands on the metabolic system. Also, the cushions can be quite heavy—from 8 to 35 pounds—which can present problems for ease of transport. The Jay, or now, the J2, cushion is one of the more widely used cushions, though other companies have adopted some of the basic features of Jay's original design. It uses a contoured foam base that can incorporate medial and lateral thigh and hip support, with a fluid-filled pad, which pockets into the depression created for the ischial tuberosities, covered with a washable cover. Users of cushions featuring gel- or fluid-filled components at times have difficulty with transfers, because of the contouring that it provides. Bottoming-out of the fluid was previously a problem, but this has been alleviated by partitioning the fluid or overfilling the cushion.[10] The conforming properties of fluid, and the lack of memory of this substance, helps to decrease peak pressures over bony prominences.

The ROHO, an air-filled cushion consisting of multiple balloon-like bladders, is a frequently prescribed, effective pressure-relief cushion. Air cushions lie between fluid and foam cushions in controlling heat and moisture collection. Their effectiveness and usage to prevent skin breakdown have been well documented, and comparison studies are available in the literature.[3,10,11] Users of ROHO cushions may feel unstable or may have difficulty transferring to another surface, especially when first using this cushion or if they have decreased lateral stability that is due to trunk weakness.[10] Skin protection and stability depend on correct inflation and ongoing maintenance of the air-filled cushion.

Foam materials can be used in pressure-relief cushions, either by distributing weight bearing over maximal surface area using a custom-contoured design, or by relieving pressure by cut-out design in the areas underlying bony prominences. The fabrication and usage of custom-molded, total-contact cushions are discussed elsewhere in this chapter.

In addition to cushion type, lower limb positioning also plays an important role in improving the distribution of pressure over the sacrum and ischial tuberosities.[12] In an upright seated position, the forces produced at the weight-bearing surfaces of the buttocks are equal to the body weight minus the supporting forces provided by the footrests or floor. The most prominent and least compressible components of the weight-bearing surface are the ischial tuberosities. Raising the foot rests too high places undue pressure beneath the ischial tuberosities, whereas placing them too low increases the pressure at the relatively pressure tolerant distal thighs but increases the chance for posterior pelvic tilt. Optimal positioning should balance out the weight distribution between the lower limbs and the weight-bearing surfaces of the pelvis.

Devices that measure the pressure between the skin and the cushion can identify regions of localized pressure and can indicate how well a cushion can distribute those forces. The device may involve single or multiple sensors with single or continuous measurement. These measurements are generally assessed in the static rather than in the dynamic state and may not reflect pressure present during propulsion of the wheelchair.[13] Although such devices in a seating clinic setting help the team to choose the best and safest features in a wheelchair cushion, by augmenting or confirming clinical judgment, they should not provide the sole criterion for cushion selection.

Custom-Molded Seating

Custom-molded seating may be indicated for the wheelchair user with very complex seating and positioning needs, such as persons with fixed deformities, pronounced muscle tone, poor postural control unresponsive to conventional management, or a combination of these difficulties. The many kinds of custom-molded seating systems vary in cost, comfort, and effectiveness. Computer assisted design and computer assisted manufacture (CAD-CAM) are valuable recent innovations in provision of custom seating for complex problems. In general, custom-molded systems give total contact at weight-bearing surfaces and often encompass pelvis, trunk, limb, and head control within a single unit, molded for the individual.

People with severe, fixed deformities with or without increased muscle tone who cannot be adequately positioned in conventional modular systems may benefit from CAD-CAM technology for customized seating. A simulation chair is used to obtain the initial mold. The simulator is generally adjustable in width, depth, angulation, and position in space and is coupled with preshaped modular vacuum bags. Once the optimal simulator seatings are achieved, the air is extracted from the vacuum bags to create a mold of the user's seating surface. During the vacuum-molding process, other supportive features can be added, including lateral thoracic supports, a headrest, and features for pelvis and thigh positioning, such as wedges, pommels, and components for pelvic obliquity accommodation or correction. Once the best positioning is achieved, and the vacuum process is complete, the shape of the resultant mold is transferred into a computer by a process known as digitizing. Based on electromagnetic principles, the system uses a stylus or linear potentiometer to capture the shape information. The data can be fine-tuned or modified as it is transferred to the computer, including adjustments of the seat to back angle, seat depth, width and height, and accentuation of pressure-relief areas. The computer image of the final product can be viewed in three dimensions and from any angle. This information is then transmitted via modem or disc to the manufacturer, who then generates a positive mold, with which the final product is fabricated, using a computerized milling machine. The finished cushions are sent to the wheelchair vendor, who mounts the cushion on the wheelchair base. Initial fitting, which provides information regarding minor modifications, is followed by a trial usage period, during which careful follow-up by the vendor and the seating team is required, with emphasis on seating tolerance, comfort, and skin integrity.[14]

Custom-molded seating is largely accommodative, furnishing good positioning and support for body asymmetries and fixed deformities, but little correction even for minor deformities. A custom-molded system primarily aids function by providing the best, most consistent support possible, with comfort as a crucial adjunct to this end.[14]

The custom seating system must not interfere with function. One must not overlook visual interactions, or access to communication or computer systems. Although aligning windswept hips, knees, and pelvis to achieve a "straight" posture is often tempting, a scoliotic patient may be accommodating for other deficiencies. For example, a seating system that straightens the head in an impaired person may disrupt the visual gaze pattern, decreasing visual function and awareness. Accommodation to the deformities without trying to correct them will preserve function and increase sitting tolerance in such a patient.

Not all custom-molded methods or cushions have been covered in this discussion. Table 7-2 summarizes many of the available cushions and custom-molded systems.

BIOMECHANICS OF WHEELCHAIR USE

The ideal human portrayed in biomechanical diagrams sits in a typically balanced position of opposing forces. Figure 7-3 shows the forces involved in seating. Rarely is a 90-degree position at the hips, knees, and ankles entirely feasible or desirable.[8] Nondisabled individuals seldom find this position comfortable for prolonged periods of time. The human form does not naturally assume

Table 7-2 Types of Cushions and Specialized Seating

Polyfoam
  Plain, up to 4 inches thick, different densities
  Serrated
  Viscoelastic (multidensity)
  Precontoured molded foam
Fluid flotation
  Air
  Air cell (ROHO)
  Water flotation
  Elastomeric gel
Combination or hybrid using above
Customized specialized seating
  Vacuum forming of sheet plastics
  Resin-bonded vacuum consolidation of glass or styrofoam beads
  Matrices made of lockable plastic components
  Foam molding around a user
  CAD-CAM products

this angular position, but some tend to use this as the nearly ideal position of seating. If this position is the aim, multiple frustrations soon follow, which lead to the addition of numerous seat belts, chest harnesses, bolsters, and so forth to make the person fit the chair instead of from the outset just fitting the chair to the person. Approximating the natural contours of the body and providing adequate control at the pelvic level will give comfortable, upright posturing without resorting to excessive secondary support devices.

Multiple factors may prevent or hinder the achievement of an ideal posture for a given individual (Table 7-3).

Positions of Function

An active wheelchair user, especially one who has decreased sensation in the area of weight bearing, assumes three major positions at different times.[15] The first is the readiness position, which is marked by a forward and upright posture; this position facilitates reach, alertness, and participation in activities. The second, is the resting posture, which is generally relaxed and supported posteriorly and may be slightly reclined relative to the readi-

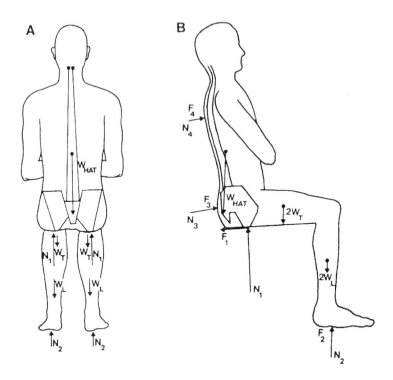

Fig. 7-3. Forces encountered with sitting, with the lower extremities supported. **(A)** The sagittal plane. **(B)** The coronal plane. W_{HAT} is the combined weight of the head, arms, and trunk. W_T is the weight of the thigh. W_L is the weight of each leg and foot. N is the normal force, and F is the resultant force vector. (From Letts,[8] with permission.)

ness position. A third position is the weight-shift position, determined for each user after assessing specific needs and abilities. The clinician observes, for example, the client's ability to perform a wheelchair push-up or side-to-side weight shift or to relieve pressure by leaning

forward over the thighs and whether the patient depends on other people or technology to achieve weight shift. The seating system must be designed to allow the person to shift weight by the most appropriate and effective method; the seat must not be so restrictive that it prevents safe and regular weight shifts.

Biomechanics of Seating

Pelvis

A key goal in wheelchair seating is to stabilize the pelvis. During upright seating, 80 percent of the trunk weight is borne directly through the pelvis.[8] A level, stable pelvis is required to optimize trunk control and upper extremity functioning. On examining the pelvic area during evaluation for a seating system, note must be made of the range of motion of the spine and hip, any pelvic asymmetry or obliquity, the pelvic tilt and degree of its flexibility, any associated windswept deformity or hip dislocation, and

Table 7-3 Factors Interfering With Postural Control

Spasticity
Paralysis
Joint contractures
Scoliosis
Altered neurologic reflexes
Pelvic obliquity
Poor head or trunk control
Impaired cognitive function
Other sensory impairment (visual, auditory, and insensate weight-bearing surfaces, etc.)

whether the noted deformities are fixed or flexible. Assessment of the integrity of the weight-bearing surface should take place early in the evaluation, with attention to soft tissue coverage, bony prominences, and skin sensation.

Posterior pelvic tilt is very frequent, even in able-bodied individuals[16a] (Fig. 7-4). Tilting the pelvis posteriorly moves the center of gravity posterior to the ischial tuberosities; this in turn increases weight bearing through the sacrum and the force borne by the lumbar spine during sitting. Shearing force over the pelvis and spine is also increased with a posterior pelvic tilt.

Sitting on flat surfaces tends to be more uncomfortable than on contoured surfaces because high pressures develop under bony prominences. However, a firm seat stimulates trunk extension better than a soft surface because it promotes pelvic stabilization. A sling seat, in contrast, tends to produce posterior pelvic tilt and pelvic obliquity. Because the ischium represents the primary bony contact in sitting, it provides pelvic stabilization

and proprioceptive feedback for balance. But this stabilization must be counterbalanced with sufficient relief under the ischial area to avoid skin breakdown in high-risk patients.[16,17]

Sitting on a flat horizontal surface increases the tendency toward posterior pelvic tilt. Because of soft tissue compression, the distal thighs are set lower than the proximal thighs, and forces that encourage slouching or sliding off the seat are increased. The relative elevation of the proximal femur, coupled with a pivotal point produced by the distal thigh's contact with the seat edge, results in lifting the anterior pelvis, which then rocks the pelvis into a posterior tilt.[18] A posterior slope of the seat (or use of an anterior wedge) helps prevent the occupant from sliding forward in the chair, which is due to the effect of gravity. Because it helps to stabilize the pelvis against forward excursion, the posterior slope decreases the shearing forces on the weight-bearing surfaces (or reverses the shear forces from forward to rearward.[12] However, the flat surface still facilitates a posterior pelvic tilt,[16] and the anterior wedge may increase the tendency toward loss of trunk stability, resulting in increased slumping.[19] Figure 7-5 provides a sequence of pictures that demonstrate these concepts.

Contouring the seat to create pelvic depression to contain ischial tuberosities provides a horizontal position for the femurs and supports the pelvis in a neutral position, thereby helping to prevent posterior pelvic tilt and sliding. This may be coupled with a slight anterior wedge to further anchor the pelvis into a supported position, or alternatively, the use of slight posterior wedging along with the ischial contouring may facilitate spine extension[18] (Fig. 7-6).

In the user with good trunk stability, the combination of a lumbar support, slight physiologic contouring of the seat, and a 95-degree thigh-to-trunk angle may be enough to improve the pelvic position. These modifications, coupled with a high back, allow for more comfort and less intensive bolstering in less active users who require more stability. This configuration removes some pressure from the ischial tuberosities and redistributes it over a greater surface area on the lower back. Inactive users, and users with decreased trunk control, find this seating design is particularly suitable. A pelvic belt mounted at 80 to 90 degrees to the horizontal can help keep the user from sliding forward.[19] A belt mounted anterior and inferior to the greater trochanters helps to stabilize the pelvis in the corrected position, by bringing

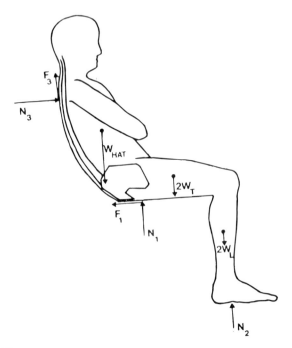

Fig. 7-4. Sagittal view of sitting with pelvis tilted posteriorly. Posterior pelvic tilt results in sacral sitting, with a significant shift of the center of gravity posteriorly, approximated by W_{HAT}, with a compensatory thoracic kyphosis, loss of lumbar lordosis, and increased normal and shear forces over the thoracolumbar spine and the sacrum. (Adapted from Letts,[8] with permission.)

the line of pull under the axis of rotation of the pelvis[20] (Fig. 7-7). A seat belt with the line of pull superior to the greater trochanters may facilitate posterior pelvic tilt. A rigid anterior pelvic support, or sub-ASIS (anterior superior iliac spine) bar, can likewise be used to stabilize the pelvis.[21]

In contrast to the less active user, energetic users tend to increase their pelvic stability by increasing hip flexion or by slightly increasing posterior pelvic tilt. This posture, coupled with a subscapular back height, permits active, maximal upper body usage and the most efficient propulsion. For these active users, contouring the seat in the pelvic area creates increased pelvic stability. This

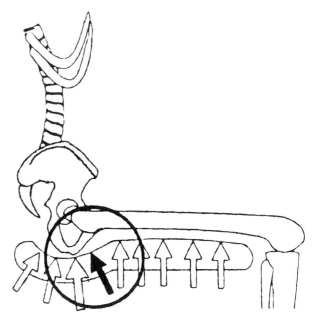

Fig. 7-6.   Lateral view of a contoured seat. Contouring the seat anchors the pelvis by blocking the forward rotation of the ischial tuberosities and distributes weightbearing evenly over the buttocks and thighs. Shear forces are diminished. (From Engstrom,[16] with permission.)

avoids excessive posterior pelvic tilt and gives the advantage of stability while escaping the disadvantage of a posteriorly tilted pelvis and potential skin breakdown.

Fixed pelvic deformities should be accommodated for by the seating system, with the goal of balancing trunk and head position. Flexible deformities can be addressed using unilateral seat buildups under the lower ischial tuberosity. Note, however, that with fixed deformities, this buildup only accentuates the deformity.[19]

Lower Extremities

The lower extremities are positioned in neutral rotation at the hips. The hip flexion, or trunk–thigh angle may be slightly less than 90 degrees if extensor tone is a problem, though a posterior pelvic tilt and a forward slumping tendency may then be produced, especially with more acute hip flexion angles.[19,21] Active users often prefer a more acutely flexed angle at the hips for pelvic stabilization, comfort, balance, and efficient propulsion. On the other hand, opening the hip flexion angle can help rock the pelvis forward and may facilitate spine extension. If the hamstrings are tight, a knee flexion angle more acute than 90 degrees may be necessary, and secondarily, the

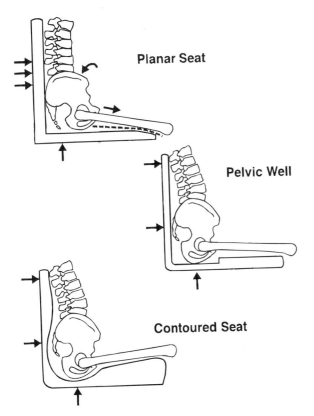

Planar Seat

Pelvic Well

Contoured Seat

Fig. 7-5.   Three lateral views of seating with effects on posture. The *planar seat* facilitates posterior pelvic tilt, with the distal thighs lower than the proximal. The resultant tendency is for the user to slide forward in the seat, with increased shear forces over the sacrum and spinous process. The *pelvic well* will allow gravity to keep the pelvis back in the seat; it may lead to increased thoracic kyphosis and loss of pelvic control. A *contoured seat* supports the ischial tuberosities and therefore, the pelvis, in a stable posture in the chair. (Courtesy of Jay Medical, Boulder, CO.)

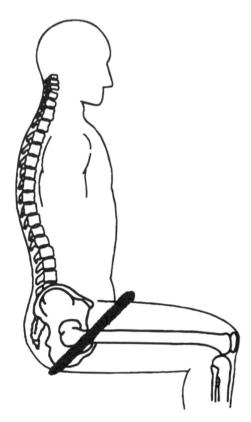

Fig. 7-7. Position for pelvic belt. The greater trochanters represent the axis of rotation for the pelvis. The line of pull of the pelvic belt should be directed anterior and inferior to this axis, to stabilize the pelvis. (Courtesy of Jay Medical, Boulder, CO.)

seat to back angle may need to be opened beyond 90 degrees to take the stretch off the hamstrings.[19]

The client with a tendency toward hip adduction should be positioned in hip abduction, especially if the client has an increased risk for hip dislocation of subluxation. If a medial thigh support is used, it should be placed distally, at the medial thigh just above the knee to avoid stimulating even more hip adduction.

The feet are positioned in a neutral position at the ankle. If needed, a 45-degree ankle strap can maintain the foot position. Straps over the arch of the foot, directed downward, may facilitate the positive supporting reaction in some clients with spasticity, and should be avoided. Angle-adjustable foot plates may be indicated with ankle and foot deformities, and the available range of motion will dictate proper position. Ankle–foot orthoses (AFOs) may be needed as part of the wheelchair prescription, to optimize lower extremity support.

Trunk

The trunk should be upright and centered over the midline of the wheelchair. The amount of support required to achieve and maintain this position varies greatly, depending on the abilities and build of the wheelchair user. The active person with excellent trunk control will use a low-profile back; the person without trunk control will need a high back with extensive lateral thoracic supports and possibly an anterior chest support.

The user with flexible scoliosis or kyphosis may need to have support provided to minimize abnormal biomechanical and gravitational forces and their effects on posture. Scoliosis management from a seating perspective involves a three-point support technique: A lateral thoracic support used as a scoliosis pad is placed under the apex of the curve; another is offset high on the opposite side, with bilateral pelvic supports (Fig. 7-8). Any at-

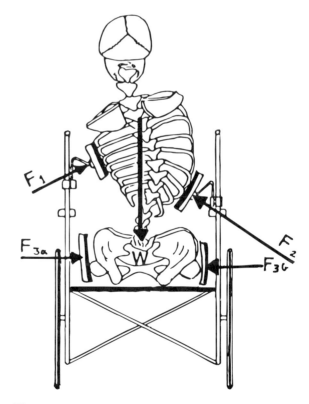

Fig. 7-8. Three-point stabilization used for flexible scoliosis. F2 is the major correcting support, directed upward under the apex of the curve, with opposing supports offset high on the opposite side (F1) and bilaterally at the pelvis (F3A&B). (Adapted from Letts,[8] with permission.)

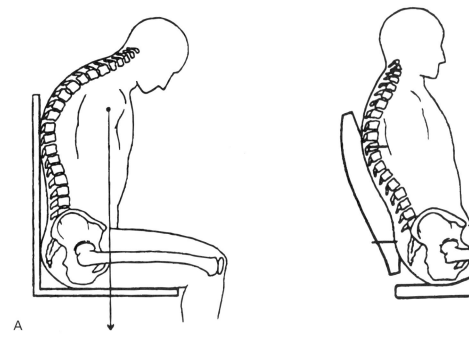

Fig. 7-9. Lateral views of a fixed thoracic kyphosis. **(A)** Using an upright back for an individual with a fixed kyphosis results in a flexed posture, with a forward head and neck position, and a downward gaze at rest. **(B)** Opening the seat-to-back angle, with appropriate seat contouring to prevent sliding forward, facilitates spine extension for the individual with flexible thoracic kyphosis. This may be coupled with a biangular back or a lumbar support to maintain an upright posture. (Courtesy of Jay Medical, Boulder, CO.)

tempts at correction should be tempered with the need to maintain comfort. Usually, some posterior tilting of the seat to back complex is used, to reduce the effects of gravity on the curve. If the curve is fixed, seating needs are accommodative, aiming to maximize function and comfort. Seating systems have not been shown to significantly alter the natural course of scoliosis.[19]

Users with a flexible kyphosis may benefit from a custom-contoured back and an anterior support, if needed. Opening the seat-to-back angle and using a lumbar support or a biangular back may help facilitate spine extension. Fixed kyphosis requires accommodative measures to maintain a functional posture and to optimize visual orientation[16,19] (Fig. 7-9).

Upper Extremities/Head

Armrests assist in avoiding poor postures in the seated position, by helping with trunk control and reducing fatigue. Proper arm support can help unweight the ischial tuberosities by 25 to 35 percent. Many active users re-

move the armrests, to avoid any interference with propulsion or transfers.

In users with spasticity, shoulder protraction may be needed to improve midline arm positioning and to reduce extensor tone. This is accomplished by adding protractor pads to the upper back or on the lap tray.

Abnormal reflexes, such as asymmetric tonic neck reflex (ATNR), symmetric tonic neck reflex (STNR), or tonic labyrinthine supine reflex may interfere with head positioning. Headrest position and design may help to inhibit these undesirable reflexes, using occipital support to stabilize the head in the sagittal plane and using lateral attachments for rotatory control.

Headrests may be used with or without a collar and may incorporate occipital support, ATNR pads, head straps, or chin straps. Head and neck supports need to be used with care and monitored diligently, because they may affect tone, neck position, respiratory function, and swallowing. If improperly used, head/neck rests, straps, and anterior chest and trunk supports can be dangerous;

that is, they can cause pain, choking, and difficulty breathing or swallowing.[19]

In someone with a forward flexed position at the neck—with cerebral palsy, for example—the prescriber's impulse may be to tilt the chair backward, maintaining a steady seat-to-back angle, in an attempt to relax the neck and improve positioning. This often results in an even greater tendency for the client to pull forward, with an attendant increase in trunk and extremity tone. By decreasing the compounding effects of gravity on the position, a slight tilt may help if there is general truncal hypotonia, neck hyperextension, and increased thoracic kyphosis.

In some centers, seating simulators have been advocated to determine the optimal position for a wheelchair user and the effect of using biomechanical principles to improve seating. Simulators can alter angles at the hips, knees, and ankles, as well as change seat and back length, width, and height. This allows the seating clinic team to create a mock-up of the proposed seating components to preview the potential success of the seating and positioning system. A simulator cannot take the place of sound clinical judgment, however.[19,22]

Biomechanics of Wheelchair Propulsion

The biomechanics of wheelchair propulsion entail how a wheelchair user transmits power to the wheels. The design and construction of a wheelchair can crucially affect performance, durability, and energy consumption or efficiency during propulsion. Because gross mechanical efficiency of upper limb propulsion is relatively low—less than 10 percent efficient—wheelchair designers have made great efforts to improve this efficiency.[23] Although studies show that lever or crank propulsion can be more energy efficient than propulsion with standard hand rims, practical considerations have restricted their use. Alternative and innovative designs, as they currently exist, add cost, weight, and complexity to wheelchair design, and they may be mechanically difficult to maintain. McLaurin and Brubaker have designed a single-action lever system; that is, a lever system that produces a driving force only in one direction, which overcomes the problem of older models.[24,25] Linden and coworkers suggest that reverse wheelchair ergonometry, for which the movement required simulates a rowing motion, is physiologically more efficient than conventional methods of propulsion.[26]

In standard wheelchair users, seat position with respect to the hand rims considerably affects efficiency because of the mechanics of arm use during power stroke and recovery. Efficient arm use, in turn, is affected by the position of the axle in relation to the center of gravity of the person sitting in the chair[27] (Fig. 7-10).

Seat position relative to the main wheel axle determines stability, maneuverability, efficiency, and safety. Moving the center of gravity of the wheelchair user forward relative to the axle reduces the chair's forward stability and increases its rear stability; moving it backward has the opposite effect.[28] In determining the position of the axle, a balance must be struck between stability and efficiency, because the more energy-efficient configurations are generally not the most stable. Height, weight, build, and functional abilities of a person are determining factors in axle placement, but safety must always be considered. Serious wheelchair accidents occur in 3.3 percent of wheelchair users each year. Falls and tipping over account for the majority of these accidents. As with other wheelchair features, the crucial balance between safety and maneuverability must be selected for each individual wheelchair user. An inappropriate axle position relative to the center of gravity caused the majority of these accidents.[29–31]

Wheelchair Design and Ergonomics

Ergonomics is described as the science of optimizing human work conditions with respect to human capabilities, taking health, safety, comfort, and efficiency into consideration.[23] The vast majority of wheelchairs prescribed are manually propelled. Older wheelchair designs have been significantly modified using technology from sports chair design to meet demands for better performance in daily use and recreation. New, light, durable metals have allowed fabrication of lightweight and ultralightweight designs. Previously labeled as "sports" chairs, ultralightweight models have become very popular and useful for daily use in nonathletes. They are especially useful for active users, athletes, frail users, and children. The lightweight design can greatly improve propelling efficiency.[27,32]

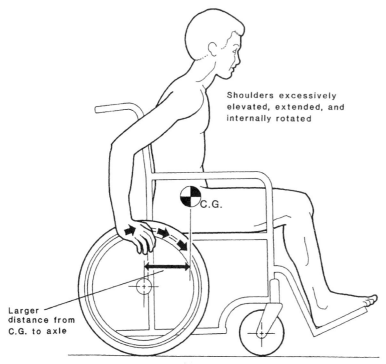

Shoulders excessively
elevated, extended, and
internally rotated

C.G.

Larger
distance from
C.G. to axle

A

Fig. 7-10. A comparison between conventional and lightweight design. **(A)** Conventional wheelchair alignment, demonstrating inefficient propulsion biomechanics and suboptimal active posture. Note the longer distance between the center of gravity and the axle. **(B)** Lightweight configuration, with biomechanically favorable posture for propulsion. The center of gravity and the rear axle are closer together than in the convention configuration. (From Brubaker,[27] with permission.)

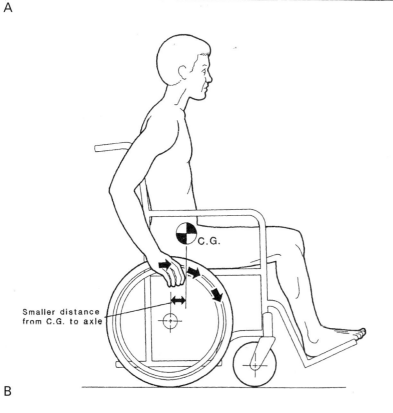

C.G.

Smaller distance
from C.G. to axle

B

Persons who plan to transport the chair independently by car can have either a folding or rigid ultralight frame designs; the ultralightweight design not only assists with independent propulsion and a wider range of mobility, but also helps the user regain independence in the community. Although these lighter and more efficient chairs are in many ways technologically superior, they are not the best choice for every wheelchair user; further, not every user can afford them. Prescription of heavier, conventional chairs is still warranted when the need is largely for temporary use, short-distance dependent mobility, for obese individuals, or for some part-time users who have some walking ability. The difference in weight is significant: around 50 pounds for a conventional wheelchair, up to 40 pounds for a lightweight chair, and between 15 and 25 pounds for an ultralightweight model.

In addition to the difference in weight, conventional and ultralightweight wheelchairs differ in axle placement relative to the seat. The axle is mounted under the seat back in the conventional model, forward, more under the center of gravity of the user in the ultralightweight models. The newer models feature more axle positions and most "sports" chairs, and many lightweight designs have adjustable axle positions to achieve ideal placement. They also feature adjustability in the back design, variations in push handles and armrests (or lack thereof), and different castor hanger, front rigging, and footrest designs.[33]

Although the relatively forward position of the axle shifts the weight balance and creates a greater tendency toward tipping backward, shortening of the wheel base is a positive feature associated with this change. The shorter wheel base produces greater maneuverability, and the position of the wheel relative to the upper limb strengthens the wheeling stroke and favorably affects energy usage.

On the basis of rearward dynamic stability, many clinicians choose the longer wheel base chair, believing it to be safest for the client. Although this may be the ideal solution for some clients, the increase in rolling resistance, downhill turning tendency, and the increased force required for turning all compound the difficulty for the users with marginal propulsion ability.[34]

The amount of energy or work required to propel a wheelchair depends on the wind resistance and the terrain, including ramps and side slopes. Other ergonomic factors will be described individually.

Rolling Resistance

The inherent resistance of rolling is affected by the weight distribution between the front and the rear wheels. In the conventional wheelchair, approximately 60 percent of the body weight is supported over the rear wheels, and 40 percent over the front casters. Moving the seat and, consequently, the center of gravity rearward, results in weight redistribution that reduces rolling resistance. Moving the rear axle forward accomplishes the same favorable result. This may be important for the wheelchair user with marginal self-propulsion ability. Even one degree of misalignment of the wheels can double rolling resistance.[35] However, changing camber, or tipping the wheels inward at the top, has little or no effect on rolling resistance or mechanical efficiency, but gives some advantage to stability and maneuverability.[36] Although pneumatic tires are preferred to solid rubber from the standpoint of rolling resistance, comfort, and weight, synthetic tires are superior in wear resistance and are not subject to flats from slow leakage of punctures. Newer designs may be more durable, cheaper, lighter and have a rolling resistance equivalent to pneumatics. New designs with springs and shock absorption systems have the potential to reduce rolling resistance and improve comfort.

Downhill Turning Tendency

Wherever there is a lateral incline, there is a downward turning tendency, also known as a side-slope effect, which must be compensated for by the wheelchair user. This is ever prevalent, because virtually all improved outdoor surfaces have a 1- to 2-degree slope to aid in drainage. The effort required to overcome this tendency is significant; a 2-degree slope results in a nearly twofold increase in energy required for forward propulsion. But the effort can be reduced by moving the seat and center of gravity rearward relative to the rear wheel axle.[37]

Yaw Axis Control

The yaw axis is involved with maneuverability, or ease of altering the direction of the chair, by overcoming the polar moment of inertia of the wheelchair. The higher the moment of inertia, the greater the difficulty with a change in direction. This moment of inertia is reduced by moving the sear rearward, thereby decreasing the distance from the main axis to the center of gravity (in a sense, by providing a shorter lever arm) and making it easier for the user to wheel in a straight line.[37]

Pitch Axis Control

The *pitch axis* refers to rotation at the axle in an anterior and posterior direction. It affects how easily a chair tips backward during propulsion. The ability of a wheelchair user to safely perform "wheelies" is essential for independence with higher level community mobility skills, such as curb negotiation. Control for wheelies is improved by a rearward seat position, although tipping tendency is increased. Trunk control is important for maintaining pitch axis control, and the skilled user will lean forward to counterbalance the backward tipping force encountered with wheelies.[37]

Propulsion Efficiency

Propulsion efficiency is related to the factors already noted, but it is improved by minimizing energy consumption in the recovery phase of the propulsion cycle. To grab the rim for the next stroke of the wheel, conventional wheelchair positioning requires excessive internal rotation, extension, and elevation of the shoulders during the recovery phase. If the user is positioned more rearward, the recovery phase is aided by gravity, and return to stroke-initiation position is relatively effortless. In the conventional axle position, the propulsion stroke is predominantly downward, but when positioned with the center of gravity closer to the axle, the stroke is more efficient and horizontal.[25,27,34]

Static Stability

Static stability refers to the tipping angle in the forward to rear and side-to-side directions, without the chair moving, both with and without the wheels locked. The static stability increases with a longer distance between the rear wheel axle and the center of gravity, that is, by placing the seat in a relatively forward position. Conversely, static stability decreases with a rearward seat position. If there is any concern about stability, antitip devices can be added, though most active users master balance control without them.[37]

In general, it is easier for a wheelchair user to recover from an unstable position with a rearward seat configuration, because of the improved pitch axis control and the decreased angular displacement afforded by this more rearward position. So, despite the attendant decrease in static stability, the overall safety and stability of the wheelchair are increased, especially for the active user with good trunk balance and control.

Weight/Portability

The actual weight of the wheelchair has surprisingly little effect on the propulsion or performance of the wheelchair on level surfaces. However, if the wheelchair user must propel over graded surfaces, or transport the chair in and out of a vehicle independently, weight is a crucial factor in its usefulness. Focusing attention on weight distribution in the chair and efficiency of propulsion will have a greater impact on function than will simply considering the overall weight of the system.[37]

Table 7-4 summarizes the preceding information on wheelchair design and ergonomics.

WHEELCHAIR PRESCRIPTION

Before initiating a wheelchair prescription, one should first determine the client's goals and, when appropriate,

Table 7-4 Wheelchair Ergonomic Factors

Principle	Rearward/Shorter Wheel Base	Forward/Longer Wheel Base
Rolling resistance	Improved	Increased
Downhill turning tendency	Improved	Increased
Yaw axis control (Maneuverability)	Increased/decreased	Decreased
Pitch axis control (wheelie control/dynamic stability)	Improved	Decreased/increased
Propulsion efficiency	Improved	Decreased
Static stability	Decreased	Improved
Weight/portability	Usually better	Varies

those of the care givers. Intentions for seating may be simply mobility—dependent or independent—but for many, goals may include improved comfort, postural stabilization, and skin protection.[38] The client may need stabilization or accommodation of orthopedic abnormalities and modifications to meet medical needs. More active clients may desire involvement in sports. An appealing cosmetic design is frequently a desired feature for many clients. All wheelchair users need comfortable seating. Those with very limited function may benefit greatly from improved positioning to increase awareness, head control, and ultimately, function. Specialized chairs may facilitate health maintenance; using the tilt-in-space design decreases shear forces, assists weight shifts, and provides an optimal position for feeding or suctioning. Clients may choose wheelchairs to allow educational and academic pursuits or employment. More often than not, the client and care giver may have numerous goals for seating. A combination of wheelchair features is frequently necessary to meet or approximate all goals. To avoid unnecessary cost, the wheelchair prescribed should have only those features that promote optimal function.

The Team Approach

The team approach to wheelchair prescription generally will ensure the best approach and closest match to the client's needs.[18] A different perspective is presented by each team member. Although, for a straightforward case, only a two- or three-person team may be necessary, a full team may include a physician, an occupational therapist, a physical therapist, an orthotist, a rehabilitation engineer, a rehabilitation technology supplier (RTS), the client, and the care givers. Others such as a social worker, an educator, a vocational counselor and a speech pathologist may play an advisory role.

Examples of some activities of various team members follow:

1. Physician: reviews all medical problems, goals, plans, and technical aspects of the case, including attention to a progressively worsening or improving course. The physician then makes recommendations based on medical issues, such as orthopedic, neurologic, or cardiopulmonary disorders. The physician is frequently the team leader and the liaison with the RTS and payer.

2. Occupational therapist (OT): assesses upper limb function and overall functional potential, including positioning strategies for head, trunk, and upper limbs, and upper extremity strength and function. This therapist is skilled in goal setting and problem solving and might recommend modifications for manual propulsion, powered mobility, a lap tray, balanced forearm orthosis, or a communication system. The OT may evaluate transfers in the home or work setting and weight shifting maneuvers.

3. Physical therapist (PT): assesses overall functioning strength and positioning, including documentation of range of motion limitations that may interfere with seating. Recommendations include means of propulsion and modifications to improve seating posture, transfer abilities, and lower limb positioning. This therapist might recommend elevating leg rests, removable arm rests, and safety features. There may be considerable overlap of the roles of the PT and OT depending on the team composition and clinic policy. Both the OT and the PT are involved in training the wheelchair user and advocating for funding.

4. The orthotist and the rehabilitation engineer: become involved with the more complex case needing special attention to biomechanical or ergonomic issues. They may advise on construction of special contoured seating, specialized wheelchair modifications, or orthotic devices that may need to be added to optimize function.

5. Rehabilitation technology supplier: The reliable RTS, whose integrity and expertise further add to the assessment by the other team members, should be included in the initial and follow-up evaluations. This individual can be a good resource on the newest and best equipment on the market.

The Wheelchair Prescription

Before the wheelchair prescription, a history and physical examination are performed. Certain information is essential before the chair is prescribed, and this is summarized in Table 7-5.

The actual prescription incorporates the principles outlined in the section on biomechanics. Specific inter-

Table 7-5 Information Gathering for Wheelchair
Prescription

History of disability, progressive or improving
Medical/surgical history
Review of systems (pulmonary cardiac, neurologic, gastrointestinal)
Life-style
Current function
Goals, clients, and/or care giver's
Home architecture/accessibility
Employment or school history
Work or school environment
Availability of transportation
Special needs, such as standing, sports
Expected use over a varied terrain

ventions for individual diagnoses and established seating problems are discussed in later sections. In general, wheelchair prescription follows a routine sequence that should start with the pelvis and work upward. When the pelvis is firmly anchored, feet and thighs are positioned to form a base of support. This is followed by choosing back and head supports, finishing up with the arms. Selection of appropriate seating and positioning in some centers is helped by use of simulators. These are sufficiently adjustable to simulate a range of different seating configurations. After making the adjustments, the required seat is then selected or manufactured to provide optimal configuration.[19] In the clinic without a simulator, it is very desirable for the team to have a good selection of chairs and cushions on hand to try out various preliminary recommendations.

For the severely impaired person, positioning strategies focused on the pelvis, head, and trunk may be required to inhibit undesirable muscle tone and reflexes. For communication and cognition, head positioning is crucial for participation in learning and conversation with others. Appropriate seating may actually improve vocal quality by reducing abnormal tonal influences and may overcome spasticity, which may interfere with speech. Also, positioning for optimal breath support for speech should be considered. If necessary, a communication system can be mounted on the wheelchair.

For a patient with a brain or spinal cord injury, a major issue in seating may be the spasticity control afforded by the chair. If uncontrolled, this can seriously impair function and safety. In some cases, surgical correction of deformities may be necessary before any special prescription is attempted.

Easy weight shifts may be needed for those with insensate skin who are at risk for skin breakdown. Clearly, after a spinal cord injury, immediate change in position is necessary for the management for autonomic dysreflexia or orthostatic hypotension.

A sample prescription form/letter of medical necessity is given in Appendix 7-1. Using this scheme for prescrip-

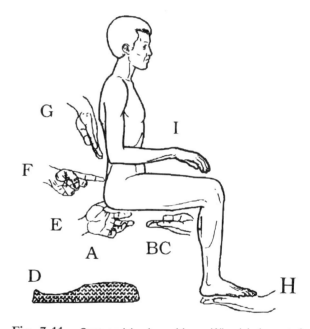

Fig. 7-11. Seat and back positions. Wheelchair seat *A,* Allow at least 1 inch for clearance on either side; seat height must allow for addition of a cushion. *B, C,* Front part of seat must be flat and firm; from front of seat must be slightly lower than front for comfort under ischial area. *D,* A contoured cushion with a firm base is the best choice for pressure relief and to prevent person from sliding forward. *H,* Feet need firm support and freedom to move—especially if the feet are needed for propulsion. Back support: *E,* Adequate room is required for lower part of pelvis to be seated all the way to the back of seat. *F,* Good support is needed to the lower lumbar area; additional support from cushion may be necessary. *G,* Height, shape, and angle of the upper part should be adjusted to adapt comfortably to dorsal kyphosis and to give more lateral support if needed. *I,* Armrests take pressure off the spine and pelvis. Top surfaces should be 1 inch higher than the olecranon processes of the elbows when the arms are released.

tion involves many of the biomechanical principles previously discussed.

The Wheelchair Checkout

When the chair arrives and the user is seated, certain assessments should always be made. These include checking the seat width, depth, and height (Fig. 7-11). The height of the arm rests should be adjusted if set too high or too low. The eyes and shoulders should be level, as should the pelvis. One should assess the support of the spinal curvature that is normal for that individual. Other assessments of the chair should include the height of footrests: The legs should be supported independently of the thighs for comfort and protection of skin over the ischial area. The arm position should be that best suited to reach the wheels; the position of the wheel axle should be that best providing optimal propulsion and safety (Fig. 7-12).

If control of spasticity is a goal, the team evaluates the effectiveness of the strategies used in positioning the client. Correct positioning may retard or slow the progression of deformities. Positioning can also improve respiratory function, allow suctioning, and facilitate pulmonary toilet in general.

The self-propelling client must have good access to the wheels for propulsion and the wheel locks for safety. The position of the axles relative to the seat must be optimal for energy-efficient propulsion. A functional assessment should review actual chair propulsion, transfers, and safety. Therapists generally evaluate the client's readiness to learn higher level skills, such as wheelies, curb climbing, and negotiation of ramps and uneven terrain. The physical therapist should be involved in training when the user is ready to learn these higher level skills.

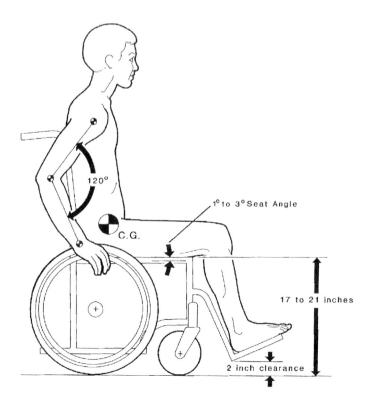

Fig. 7-12. Posture and propulsion. The elbow is flexed 60 degrees from 0 when the hand rim is grasped at the highest point. The seat angle or incline slopes posteriorly 1 to 3 degrees from the horizontal. Footrests clear the ground by 2 inches. The height of the front seat is most commonly 17 to 21 inches. (From Brubaker,[37] with permission.)

The wheelchair may need additional features for fine tuning of the seating. This is particularly true for the person with very complex seating issues; optimal positioning may require several adjustments, additions, or modifications.

In the final analysis, the wheelchair checkout should determine whether the goals originally outlined have been met. The client or care givers participate in this analysis, and discrepancies are explained or corrected. The RTS and the therapists teach proper care, maintenance, and disassembly for transportation, and arrange for any future wheelchair needs, questions, and follow-up.

WHEELCHAIR NEEDS BY AGE GROUP

Interventions at each age group depend on the normal developmental stages and unique needs for that age. For children, the focus is on the normal developmental stages appropriate for each age, with interventions and prescriptions designed to meet the normal developmental milestones. And for children and for adults, the focus is on achieving the best functional potential in the face of residual disability. Specific needs for each age group are reviewed in the sections that follow.

Birth to 12 Months

Normal developmental milestones at each stage should be paralleled by seating system considerations. For example, normal babies begin to explore their environment beginning at around 6 to 8 months. Development progresses in an orderly sequence toward the acquisition of higher level mobility skills, such as cruising, pulling to stand, and walking. Seating goals, even for this very young group, should begin to address independent mobility. A wheelchair or wheeled cart that is low to the ground at an age-appropriate peer level encourages socialization, stimulation, and independent transfers in and out of the chair. Future stability with wheelchair seating depends on maintaining a stable, symmetric pelvis, even in this young age group. Certainly, the cognitive status of each child should be carefully considered, and expectations and time frames adjusted accordingly. Several very small-frame designs are available commercially. If developmental or cognitive problems make only dependent mobility suitable, one may order a modified stroller system or a modular seating system with supportive features that can be withdrawn as the baby's skills improve.[8]

Twelve Months Through Preschool Years

Developmental considerations should continue to define seating and positioning interventions. In general, seating systems for children should encourage a level pelvis and a relatively abducted position at the hips to promote acetabular development. For the child with increased tone, consistent heel cord and hamstring stretching programs should begin early, and timely use of orthopedic procedures is indicated.

Positioning of young children should lend to the development of normal spinal curves and to prevention or delay of orthopedic deformities. The primary thoracic kyphotic curve present at birth is followed later by the development of secondary cervical and lumbar lordotic curves. In children with moderate or severe gross motor delays, these secondary curves frequently fail to develop. This failure may be compounded by poor head and trunk control and by abnormal muscle tone interfering with independent sitting.[39]

The child must sit upright to interact with the environment and with peers; sitting increases sensory input received, even in a child without independent head control, and upright positioning helps to normalize tone and thereby increase upper extremity function. For increased environmental awareness, some young children also need devices such as standing frames, swivel walkers, and parapodium designs.

The early focus is on minimizing deformity and promoting normal skeletal development. For example, sitting with hip abduction promotes acetabular development; contouring the seat improves postural control and development of spinal curves. Pursuing spinal alignment too vigorously is dangerous because postural deviations may be accentuated and not helped. For example, lumbar supports frequently push children forward, increasing thoracic kyphosis. Though judiciously used, a biangular back design may help to stabilize the pelvis in a neutral position and may assist with subsequent spinal alignment. A biangular back is characterized by a two-piece cushion, connected at an axis located just superior to the

ASIS, in which both the superior segment and the inferior segment are angled posteriorly relative to the vertical, and can be used to support the back and pelvis.[8]

Head support should by approached with care, because pressure over the occiput may stimulate abnormal reflex activity in the child with spasticity, including the tonic labyrinthine reflex, which significantly interferes with seating.[19]

In children, chairs must be readily transported, lightweight, easy to propel, and have built-in growth potential. Many seating devices marketed for this age group are made to be colorful, washable, and lightweight. Some, however, do not provide support in an optimal position; they may actually promote a posterior pelvic tilt and retard development of normal spinal curves. Although these devices may be successfully used for feeding or therapeutic activities, they should not be used as definitive seating systems unless properly designed to prevent unsatisfactory positioning.

A therapist can frequently modify commercially available strollers to provide adequate seating for dependent mobility as an adjunct to independent wheelchair propulsion. Advantages of strollers over wheelchairs are their lighter weight, easier transportability, and frequently, a more pleasing appearance. Foam wedges, towels, or a combination of additions as bolsters can be removed as the child's need changes over time or as better postural control develops. Umbrella or sling strollers should be avoided; they promote sacral sitting, a kyphotic thoracic spine, and inadequate pelvic support. This is true in any age group, but particularly in infants and young children. Sitting in these strollers tends to increase spastic hip internal rotation and adduction in young children with cerebral palsy, spinal cord injury, or head injury, thus increasing the risk of hip subluxation.

Many commercially available car seats are appropriate for children with disabilities or can be modified to be suitable. The seating team should assess car safety at the seating clinic visit and review this with the family.

Childhood

For the school-aged child, there must be continued focus on preventing or slowing the development of fixed orthopedic deformities by providing a seating system that provides support while allowing optimal function. During these years, children develop spinal curves, including

lumbar lordosis. The lumbar region needs support, though excessive bolstering should be avoided.[8]

Slouching, with a flexible thoracic kyphosis, and posterior pelvic tilt may be seen during childhood, and the child may have spasticity or fixed deformities that require accommodation. The specific strategies for management of these issues by the seating team is discussed elsewhere in this chapter.

Mobility aides for children must be durable for play and rough use but readily transportable and lightweight to promote independent propulsion. The frames should grow with the child by adjustment of the position of the rear upright supports and push canes. Clinicians fitting the child's chair may start with a relatively forward sitting position, then move it backward as the legs grow longer. Other methods to achieve chair growth include starting with a thick back cushion that can be removed or pared down later or extending the posterior part of the seat under the back cushion for 2 to 3 inches, then moving the seat forward to lengthen it as the child grows. Jay has designed a cushion that grows with the child, which has favorable practical and financial implications.

Axle position adjustability for children's chairs is crucial. In a chair that is designed to grow, an adjustable axle may mean the difference between independent and dependent mobility. When the axle cannot be brought forward, the child who has been moved forward in a relatively large chair may not be able to reach the push rims for independent propulsion. As in adults, optimal axle position improves wheeling efficiency.[37]

Peer acceptance is important and is more likely with a pleasing cosmetic design, aided by the child's choice of colors. Many companies will add special monograms or logos, and children should be encouraged to personalize their own chair.

Adolescence

Rapid growth is a major feature of adolescence. If fixed deformities have not been previously addressed orthotically or surgically, seating may become even more challenging during these years. Pain may become an issue in adolescents with joint contractures and persistent spasticity. Young people with spina bifida have an increasing tendency toward skin breakdown, mainly in the mid and late teen years, when decreasing ambulation and increasing weight add an increased risk of skin breakdown. The consistent need for weight shifting becomes even more evident during this period.

During adolescence, wheelchair focus is still on function, comfort, and support, but more emphasis is placed on future expectations, such as vocational considerations and whether independent car transfers and driving are reasonable goals. Peer acceptance and favorable cosmetic appearance are most important during this time, as teenagers are developing their personal identity.

Adulthood

The wheelchair prescription for adults should take into consideration the person's goals, diagnosis, functional impairment, previous vocational and avocational history, and other factors already covered elsewhere in the chapter. Growth in length is no longer a consideration, but wheelchair adjustability for changes in girth or with disease progression may be needed.

Obesity can present major difficulties on seating in all age groups, but particularly in adults. It is best to fit as narrow a seat as comfortably possible so the user can enter more narrow door ways or maneuver in smaller spaces. Lightweight wheelchairs are not recommended for persons over 250 pounds, and heavy-duty chairs are the rule for any chairs that are 20 inches or more in width.

Back pain is commonly seen in adults with prolonged sitting. It may be postural and involve compressing nerve roots from suboptimal spinal posture, but the cause is often obscure. It may be possible with cushions or special seating to promote postures to reduce the pain; sometimes only trial and error can determine the right combination for relief. Pain may also be helped by frequent shifting of weight in the chair and exercises to stretch tight structures around the pelvis and knees. The widespread prevalence of pain in long-term adult wheelchair users suggests that the person prescribing the initial and subsequent seating systems must emphasize postural support, before poor seating habits and postures become established.

In adults, prolonged sitting may contribute to the development of leg edema, because the venous pump from muscle activity is weak or inadequate. This tendency is further aggravated by concurrent circulatory disorders. People with postural, dependent edema may benefit from elevating leg rests or the use of compression garments.

For some conditions affecting mobility in adults, detailed descriptions are given in the final section.

The Elderly

The older we get, the more we sit. Many elderly people spend most of their waking hours in a seated position, especially in nursing homes. Therefore, it is no surprise that the largest group of wheelchair users are the elderly. Fenwick has reported that 67 percent of adult users in wheelchairs in England and Wales are more than 60 years old, and in the United States, an estimated 850,000 persons over 65 are regular users.[40] Determining the special needs of this age group, therefore, has great social and economic significance.

To determine the problems with elderly wheelchair users, Shaw and Taylor studied the occurrence of seating problems in a nursing home population.[41] The most prevalent problems of wheelchair users, in order of occurrence, were discomfort, poor posture, loss of mobility, and decubitus ulcer formation. The more dependent the person, such as a patient disabled by a stroke or Parkinsonism, the greater the seating problems. Seat discomfort was more prevalent than back discomfort. Sliding down or out of the seat and leaning to the side were the most frequent postural problems. Hindered mobility seemed largely based on the use of small wheels or bulky chairs that were not appropriate for the users. Bedsores and lack of pressure relief were the least prevalent problems. Clearly, any study in which this problem was assessed would bring to the attention of care givers the risks of skin breakdown. Nevertheless, the risk of skin breakdown from improper seating in the elderly should generate more concern than in any other age group, because decubitus ulcers seriously affect longevity, as well as function, and quality of life. In the elderly, careful attention by care givers and the seating team to preventive strategies is critical.

From this study by Shaw and Taylor,[41] it is clear that seating comfort must be the primary consideration in prescribing for the elderly. Therefore, the wheelchair prescriber must carefully attend to the contour of the seat and back and to the height of the seat, armrests, and footrests. Because of the hammocking effect of upholstery in most folding wheelchairs, comfortable seating often means using cushions contoured to flatten out the seat or fit the back to accommodate spinal problems.

Elaborate systems for postural control are rarely necessary except in the very severely disabled spastic elderly.

One main difference between wheelchair use in the elderly compared with other disabled users is the much higher prelevance of cognitive and emotional impairment. Various disorders producing dementia are prevalent, frequently making the simplest tasks of wheelchair operation difficult or impossible. Comfortable seating and ease of operating the wheelchair by care givers must be the primary consideration in elderly users with cognitive impairment. A motorized wheelchair, although often requested by anxious relatives, is out of the question for many elderly with faulty cognition.

Generally, elderly wheelchair users can be considered to fall in one of the following groups[42]:

1. Nonmobile and dependent
2. Mobile, nonambulatory
3. Ambulatory but with special wheelchair needs

The nonmobile and dependent elderly mostly live in nursing homes and often have secondary contractures and other complications. Newer model dependency chairs offer more comfort and adaptability to users than older so called "geri-chairs." Equipment companies are now marketing adult postural seating systems with multiple position adjustments, many modular features, and a variety of accessories at reasonable cost. One company has a model that converts from attendant-propelled to self-propelled by having large front wheel that snap on and off the chair. For the hard-to-fit elderly user, elaborate modular systems are available featuring both a reclining and tilting system of seating.[42]

Cost may be an overriding consideration in nursing homes. Whenever possible, seating needs should be based on simple criteria. The chairs must be readily available and easily repaired or adjusted. They should be waterproof (sanitation), promote reduced restraint use (legal and psychological), reduce fall frequency (safety), and decrease the risk of skin breakdown. Ease of use is critical for staff acceptance; for example, cushions should be labeled with user's names and directions written on them, such as *top, bottom, front,* and *hand wash.*

Mobile nonambulatory wheelchair users represent the largest group of the elderly. Electric mobility is discussed elsewhere, but a motorized chair may be a good choice as long as transportation for the chair is available and the user has been tested for cognitive deficits or safety

precautions. In general, the same principles pertain to the elderly as to other adults regarding self-propulsion, but a few specialized features may be considered. As a rule, wheelchairs should be as lightweight as possible. Mag wheels are easy to maintain and safer for older users, who tend to catch their fingers in spoked wheels. The standard height of conventional cross-framed wheelchairs is 20 inches, which makes it hard to fit users of short stature, especially elderly women with severe osteoporosis, who frequently have fixed thoracic kyphosis. The low seat hemichair, particularly suited to individuals with hemiplegia, who can drive the chair with one arm and one leg, is also good choice for short elderly users. The rearward axle position in conventional wheelchairs frequently results in propulsion inefficiency for the elderly, especially for the short, elderly woman with thoracic kyphosis. This has been described elsewhere in this chapter. The back design may need to accommodate fixed thoracic kyphosis, and contouring helps to maintain posture and visual interactions. Lever drive wheelchairs are very helpful for people with hemiplegia who cannot master propulsion with one arm and leg. Bilateral lower limb amputations are common in this age group; wheelchairs with no front rigging and an axle located several centimeters behind the usual site help to ensure safety and balance.

The lighter the wheelchair, the easier it is to wheel or transport—an important feature if the care giver is also elderly. Although rigid ultralight wheelchairs are more energy-efficient during propulsion than conventional folding frame chairs, they are not as easily transported and provide a stiffer ride; thus, they have not been popular among the elderly. Most standard folding wheelchair models come in lightweight forms that are 24 pounds or less, but they cost more than standard-weight chairs. Financing them may be a difficult issue for many families.

With a care giver who cannot lift a manual chair into an automobile, the simplest aid is to transport a Tilt-and-Tote carrier that attaches to a trailer hitch. Portable ramps or motorized lifts are expensive but are the only options for transporting powered wheelchairs for the elderly. If power mobility is prescribed, transportation becomes a major constraint. It must be decided from the start whether the wheelchair will be used outdoors frequently, so provisions can be made for transporting it.

Ambulatory users who mainly use a wheelchair to travel distances outside the home can be fitted with less expensive folding chairs with fixed arm and footrests. They may need no special prescription considerations. However, wheelchair users with cardiac conditions and other medical problems causing lower limb edema may need to be evaluated for compression garments and the use of elevating removable leg rests. But in some cases elevating leg rests may actually worsen the edema problem. When tight hamstrings are present, the resultant posterior pelvic tilt and increased kyphosis cause slumped posture, which in turn increases intra-abdominal pressure, which may impede venous and lymphatic circulation.

Elderly users with decreased endurance benefit from lightweight chairs with features such as removable armrests and footrests. Chairs with these features are more expensive but can be lighter and propel more easily than the conventional chair. A firm seat and thick cushion, 3 or 4 inches in height, enable the user to rise from the chair more easily than from a low seat. Users with arthritis of the hips or knees appreciate higher seats.

For elderly users who tend to slide out of the chair or who cannot maintain an upright position because of muscle weakness, sustaining stable seating can be problematic. Solutions involving contouring of the seat and back cushions to diminish the forces that result in sliding and facilitate upright posture are discussed in the section on biomechanics. Contoured or wedged cushions can solve many postural problems, but more complex circumstances may need prescription of seats with tilting or reclining features. A wheelchair tray can provide arm support and help correct forward tilting of the trunk, as well as provide a supportive surface to aid in the completion of activities of daily living. Arm troughs or a hemitray can support paralyzed upper limbs of the individual with hemiplegia. Some situations require pelvic belts to anchor the pelvis firmly into the seat, but the belts need constant adjustment and consistent application. Pelvic belts must be set at a proper angle to the seat to counteract the tendency for some users to slip forward under the straps, with the angle of pull directed anterior and inferior to the axis of rotation of the pelvis.[20] Newer medial thigh support designs are available to accommodate adults, particularly those with hyperkinetic behavior (e.g., Pommel wedge, Alimed Inc., Dedham, MA). A padded foam support placed between the thighs will guard against hip adduction in those with hip fractures or hip joint replacements.

Involuntary restraining devices, such as Posey vests, must be eliminated to avoid increasing the agitation in cognitively impaired individuals and placing the client at risk for asphyxiation. A number of orthotic devices are marketed that are touted as thoracolumbosacral orthoses (TLSOs) for posture correction that have been custom fitted and attached to the chair, but these function more like restraining vests. The concerned clinician can treat undesirable postures and discomfort in more imaginative and less expensive ways by consulting members of a seating team or a reliable medical equipment vendor.

SKIN BREAKDOWN: PROBLEMS AND SOLUTIONS

Not only are decubitus ulcers a problem for the wheelchair user with regard to loss of mobility, time lost from work or school, and associated illnesses, but the annual cost of hospital management of decubitus ulcers is staggering. Recently, the cumulative costs of hospital treatment of pressure ulcers in spinal cord injury were estimated at greater than $66 million each year.[43] Thirty percent of all persons with spinal cord injury will develop at least one pressure sore within the first few years after injury. Complications of pressure sores account for 7 to 8 percent of deaths in the spinal cord injury (SCI) population.[44–46]

Pressure sores result from multiple factors. The most crucial are contact pressure and shearing forces, or those forces that are directed tangentially to the skin. Other factors include excessive moisture, local infection, excessive heat, poor nutritional status, and loss of adequate soft tissue coverage. Asymmetric anatomy, resulting in exaggerated bony prominences when sitting, increases risk of skin breakdown, because of the excessive direct pressure and shearing over a relatively small surface area. As moisture increases the risk for skin maceration and erosion by shearing forces, incontinence is a significant factor in seating safety. Incontinent-proof cushion covers and good bowel and bladder management are obvious solutions. Other strategies to reduce risks include controlling local infection; reducing heat at the seat–cushion interface; improving nutrition, which includes treating anemia; and ensuring appropriate lower extremity support.[19]

In sitting, approximately 65 percent of body weight is borne through the buttocks and thighs, especially the

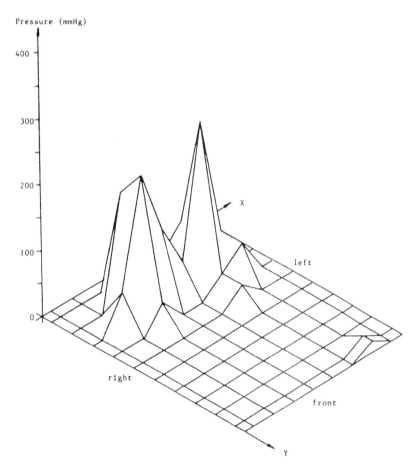

Fig. 7-13.   Sample printout obtained from pressure-sensor device, resulting in this three-dimensional diagram. Note the high pressures generated under the ischial tuberosities.

ischial tuberosities and, in sacral sitters, through the skin overlying the sacrum and coccyx (Fig. 7-13). The usual capillary arterial blood pressure of 30 mm Hg is easily occluded during normal sitting.[47] A person with normal sensation and mobility shifts weight unconsciously to avoid tissue ischemia and the discomfort that normally heralds it. Because people with poor sensation or motor function may not easily shift their weight, they are at an increased risk for skin breakdown.

Shearing forces interfere with normal blood flow. When they occur during sliding or poor transferring techniques, the risk of significant pressure sore formation increases even at pressures that under usual circumstances do not result in pressure sores.[47]

Groups of people who are at risk for pressure sores include those with the following characteristics:

1. Decreased sensation
2. Significant weakness or paralysis
3. Lack of awareness
4. Deformities, such as pelvic obliquity and/or hip dislocation, or scoliosis

The clinician prescribing a wheelchair should always analyze the risk factors for skin breakdown by assessing bony prominences, skin sensation, cognitive awareness, and reduced independent mobility in the wheelchair from any cause.

Wheelchair users and care givers need to realize that even the best wheelchair cushion cannot prevent skin breakdown without close attention to skin care. Forces exerted on the main weight-bearing body surfaces in seated individuals produce dangerously high pressures (more than 60 mm Hg), despite the use of special cushions. Clinicians should instruct the at-risk user or family in the most appropriate pressure-relief technique, or combination of techniques, such as pushups, forward leaning, side-to-side shifting, or tilting the back of the wheelchair to 65 degrees. Tilting the chair backward 35 degrees or less only results in minimal drop in pressures measured over the ischial tuberosities; however, 65 degrees of tilt decreases the pressure over the ischial tuberosities significantly but not to levels considered adequate for protection against skin breakdown.[46] Having the individual lean forward over the thighs is the best method to relieve pressures generated over the ischial tuberosities for those wheelchair users who lack the arm strength necessary to perform wheelchair push-ups.[46] Wheelchair

checkout should always include an assessment of the wheelchair user's understanding of and ability to safely perform pressure-relieving techniques.

TROUBLESHOOTING

At times, chair users will present with well-established unsatisfactory seating positions and postural deviations. These findings may alter the goals for better seating but should be evaluated systematically. Drastic seating changes may cause more problems than they fix. When a client presents with multiple long-standing problems with the current wheelchair, attempting to fix these problems with even the most optimal seating system may meet with unexpected and untoward results. For example, the visual system tends to accommodate to an unusual position in clients who have assumed a rotated, asymmetric head-tilted posture for a prolonged period. The compensations for the unusual posture feel and look

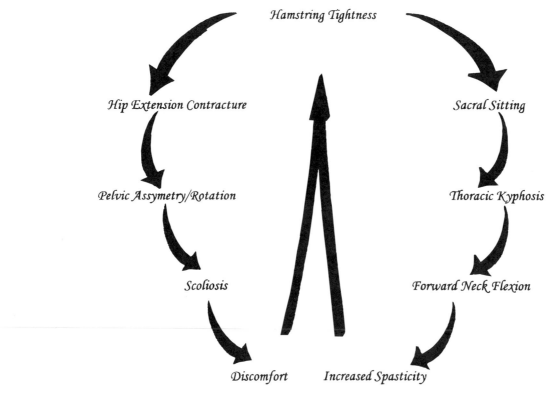

Fig. 7-14. The vicious cycle of hamstring tightness.

right to these individuals, and what we would call proper positioning feel infinitely wrong to them. Making stepwise changes over prolonged periods requires extreme patience on the part of the seating clinic team; but they are frequently preferred and in the long run better accepted by the client than fixing everything at once. People generally resist change, and that applies to wheelchair users who must first recognize the need for change before any alterations will be accepted. The use of adjustable seating is recommended to accomplish serial seating with one system.

Hamstring Tightness

Any discussion of troubleshooting in seating should start with muscles controlling the pelvis. In this regard, the hamstrings may be the most important muscle group for optional positioning, comfort, and function for the wheelchair user. Although tightness of the hamstrings is encountered with many diverse diagnostic groups, one applies similar strategies to correct the subsequent problems, regardless of cause.

Because this muscle group crosses two joints, tightness of the hamstrings can drastically change the position of the pelvis and the knees. Tightness can increase the tendency to tilt the pelvis posteriorly. This position increases the chances of bearing weight through the sacrum, or sacral sitting instead of the normal position of ischial sitting. Sacral sitting, in turn, increases the risk of skin breakdown over the sacral surface. A cycle then develops, with one detrimental factor leading to another, ending in fixed deformities and pain, which disrupt positioning, decrease sitting tolerance, and reduce function. Figure 7-14 outlines some of the features of that cycle.

Surgical releases of the tight hamstrings should be considered if the tension consistently interferes with seating and has not responded to physical therapy. If surgical intervention is neither desired nor feasible, one should consider increasing the amount of knee flexion allowed by the wheelchair, by positioning the feet more posteriorly than usual. In other words, positioning should accommodate for the deformity and contracture, rather than forcibly correct it. Attempts to increase hamstring range of motion by intentionally extending the knees beyond the comfortable resting length in the wheelchair only accentuates the seating problem. This increases the tendency to slide forward and produce posterior pelvic tilt. Chances are that the chair will then cause more discomfort, consequently reducing that person's sitting tolerance and eliminating the means of mobility and independence[19] (Fig. 7-15).

When footrest repositioning is not possible because of the chair or frame design, or if it is only partially effective, a posterior wedge may be used to open the seat to back angle relatively more than usual to take some of the stretch off the hamstrings. This usually needs to be accompanied by a pelvic well, or a depression built into the posterior aspect of the cushion that encompasses the sacrum and the ischial tuberosities and prevents the user from sliding out of the chair. An alternative choice is to tilt the now open seat–back unit posteriorly. Frequently, a combination of interventions focused on the tight hamstrings is needed to avoid the potentially disastrous cycle, and failure to respect the limitation of range of motion of this important muscle group will increase the difficulty in obtaining optimal seating.

Slouched Seating

An individual presenting in a personal wheelchair or for wheelchair evaluation with slouched seating should be evaluated to determine the cause. Then options for improvement of posture through modifications to the seating system should be considered. Potential causes include the following:

Tight hamstrings
Poor trunk control
Inadequate supportive surface at the pelvis
Hip extension contractures
Increased extensor tone
Back support too vertical
Combination of these factors

When tight hamstrings are implicated as the cause, management strategies and wheelchair modifications described in the preceding section should be pursued. If poor trunk control or poor pelvic support is the cause, the solution may be to ensure adequate pelvic and spine support by the appropriate choice of primary and secondary seat and back supportive features. The limited range from hip extensor contractures should be accommodated by the careful choice of the seat-to-back angle, to maintain support, comfort, and provide functional seating. If

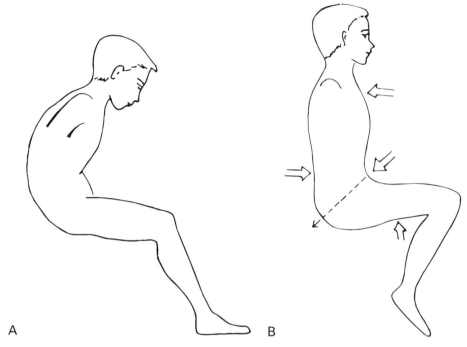

Fig. 7-15.   Seating for hamstring tightness. **(A)** Incorrect position: keeping the knees extended only causes increased pelvic tilt and a round back. **(B)** Correct position: permitting the knees to flex and applying supports *(arrows)* provides upright sitting.

increased extensor tone is present, measures to control the tone should be introduced. The simplest solution in many who present with slumped seating requires repositioning the back cushion into a less upright and more reclined position relative to the seat, accompanied by anatomic contouring of the back or seat.

Forward Head Position

If the user constantly sits with the head forward and the neck flexed, consideration should be given to tilting the seat and back posteriorly. If done correctly, this should maintain the optimal angle previously determined at the hips, ankles, and knees but reposition the head and back to afford visual interactions. Too much recline will frequently compound the problem. Head and neck supports, or anterior chest supports should be chosen carefully, and their use should be monitored to prevent misapplication. Concurrent use of a pelvic belt is indicated with any head, neck, or chest support.[19]

Asymmetric Spine

A fixed or flexible scoliosis may be due to abnormal muscle tone or asymmetric contraction of paraspinal and hip flexor muscles. It may be seen with pelvic obliquity, hemiparesis, and primary orthopedic deformities. Scoliosis is common in spastic quadriparesis and develops in nearly all childhood-onset high spinal cord injuries. It develops toward the end stages of Duchenne's muscular dystrophy. To apply preventive measures requires an understanding of risk factors and expected time frame of scoliosis development in various diagnostic groups. Although obtaining an ideal seating system is not likely to alter the natural course of scoliosis, it may improve function and is, therefore, worth the time and effort required. Furthermore, better timing of necessary surgery can be done when progression of the curve in nonambulatory children or adolescents is monitored serially.

If surgery is not an option, the seating team should attempt to address scoliosis associated with pelvic obliquity and ensure a stable and well-supported base for the wheelchair user. A three-point support system is used in wheelchairs for control of scoliosis. Lateral pads and other additions to the seating position will not correct the curves but may slow advancement and give adequate support for comfortable seating. A slight recline of the back, or tilt of the seat–back complex is often necessary to accommodate more severe scoliosis, by alleviating some of the effect of gravity on the curve.[19] A soft TLSO may be used if trunk stability is the main problem and if the deformity is flexible. In some cases, a total contact supportive seating orthosis (SSO) may be necessary, such as that developed by Gilette Hospital.[48] This may be the only solution for a very complex seating problem in which a user requires precise support that is due to fixed deformities with poor trunk and head control. The Gilette design features total contact throughout the weight-bearing surface to correct flexible deformities and to accommodate fixed deformities, yet provides good support for seating comfort. The rigid nature of this type of seating system may restrict movement that is needed for function, however, and a balance must be struck between support and function.

Windswept Deformity

The term *windswept hip deformity* refers to adduction of one hip, abduction of the opposite hip, and possibly, concurrent pelvic obliquity[49] (Fig. 7-16). It may also be associated with scoliosis or hip dislocation and can pose a major problem in seating. Studies by Lonstein and Beck recognized no cause-and-effect relationship between any of these conditions, that is, scoliosis and hip dislocation leading to the other deformities.[50] They are all caused by muscle imbalance and spasticity. Their studies did not support the assumption that the hip is usually subluxed on the high side of the pelvis; the subluxation can be either on the high or the low side relative to the obliquity. Letts and co-workers[51] describe subluxation leading to dislocation, the development of pelvic obliquity, and potential for scoliosis and the windswept deformity. The average age of hip dislocation is 6 to 7 years.[51]

Although aligning the hips to a corrected position is frequently a goal, this correction may actually induce or exacerbate other potential problems. For example, if the hips of a person with a fixed scoliosis or fixed pelvic obliquity are rotated so that they point forward, the

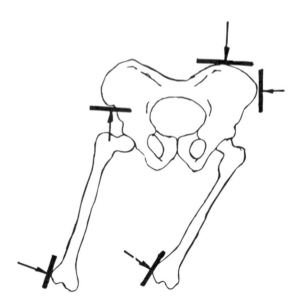

Fig. 7-16. Windswept hip deformity (skeletal pattern). Arrows show forces applied to seating system to counteract this tendency.

shoulders may then lie obliquely to the front of the chair. This attempt to correct the hip position may so disrupt the field of vision that suitable posture and function actually decrease. The art, then, is to furnish a balance of corrective forces that maximize comfort, positioning, and function. Unfortunately, attempts at corrective seating frequently lead to pain, increasing deformity, and to increased tendency toward scoliosis. The scoliosis is typically convex toward the nondislocated hip, but not always. Attempts at prevention of windswept deformity should be made by a combination of proper seating with early and timely orthopedic interventions. As always, prevention is preferred to accommodation in special seating, which may be the only option once this deformity is well established.

For windswept deformity, some authorities have advocated the use of anterior knee supports applied to the abducted limb, counterbalanced by a posterior pelvic support behind the adducted opposite limb. This, coupled with an adductor block for the adducted hip and a lateral thigh support for the abducted side, can at times be useful. However, this approach—specifically, the use of a knee support—should not be undertaken in young children, because it may actually promote hip dislocation.[52]

Hypotonic Child/Adult Collapsing Into Flexion

To solve the dilemma of the wheelchair user who sits in a totally relaxed and flexed posture may require a tilt-in-space wheelchair, and adjustable-tension seating system, or a combination of contouring the seat and using a posterior wedge to create a fixed tilting position. The latter is particularly useful in children. In a fixed frame chair, it is frequently possible to recline the seat–back–headrest complex up to 45 degrees, although extensive modifications may be required. Angle-adjustable back supports and seat cushions with appropriate contouring promote better postures and orient the user in such a way that he or she can relax into, instead of out of, the system.

The flexed, collapsed individual may respond to measures aimed at stabilizing the pelvis, including the use of a posterior pelvic support, or a biangular back. If these measures are inadequate, the seat-to-back angle may be opened to increase or stimulate spinal extension. In a person with mixed muscle tone, one might try a combination of antithrust, that is, a block placed just anterior to the ischial tuberosities on the seat, to inhibit extensor tone in the lower extremities along with slight opening of the seat-to-back angle to facilitate an upright position. This method creates a balance of two opposing forces to achieve the best positioning but must be accompanied by appropriate pelvic support and a contoured or biangular back. One should avoid merely opening the seat-to-back angle, because this may result in the loss of pelvic support and an increased tendency toward posterior pelvic tilt.

SPECIALIZED WHEELCHAIRS

Sports Wheelchairs

International competitions for the wheelchair athlete are now a major feature of the world of sports. Sports are helpful in improving the athletes' emotional state and physiologic function while improving long-term prognosis. Biomechanical engineers are contributing substantially to wheelchair sport. They have improved the design of competitive wheelchairs, which increases the mechanical efficiency of participants and helps to reduce the risk of injury. In fact, many improvements for the standard wheelchair in daily use originated in the design for sports chairs.[53]

Third-party payers will generally not pay for sports chairs, and a thorough discussion of these chairs is beyond the scope of this chapter. Manufacturers may sell racing wheelchairs directly to consumers or custom build them for an athlete's specific needs. The racing chair is ultralight and sturdy and generally has a rigid frame design to promote efficient transmission of energy to the wheels. The seat is low to the ground for maximal stability and often has either a cage seat or a bucket seat design, incorporating a nonadjustable box depth to help maintain the desired stiffness or lightness.[54] For racing, a long wheel base is more stable dynamically, while short-based chairs have superior performance in short races and tend to draft more effectively while racing.[55] Seats are usually of a sling design, with cloth or nylon straps to help position the athlete aerodynamically and ergonomically, while providing support to decrease extraneous motion, and a knees-up position improves arm swing and upper torso stability. The large (26- to 27-inch) cambered rear wheels, lie usually just under the axillae. The wheels often have interlocking spokes or are simply solid discs with relatively small hand rims. The number of spokes is generally small, often with trispoke or monospoke design to aid aerodynamically, by decreasing turbulence. Large front casters—around 12 inches—have spokes and a low friction hub with precision bearings. Steering handles and brakes may be attached to the front wheels. Alternately, a single front wheel helps to decrease rolling resistance and improves chair weight but tends to be less stable.[54] The front of the chair may be extensively modified or customized to decrease wind resistance. The most important seating consideration in racing or sports chairs, regardless of frame design, is body position relative to push-rim orientation for maximally efficient propulsion,[55] as described in the biomechanics section.[27]

Power Wheelchairs

Power wheelchairs are prescribed for people who cannot propel a manual wheelchair as a result of weakness, poor endurance, significant cardiac or respiratory limitations, or limb absence, paralysis, or deformity. Individuals who request power chairs must have the necessary cognitive function, judgment, and vision to safely direct them.

The seating principles in a power wheelchair are the

same as those described for manual chairs. However, positioning of the upper limbs becomes very critical for placement of the joystick, and if controls other than manual ones are necessary, trunk and head position must be very carefully evaluated.

Many power wheelchairs are based on manual chair design, but many specialized power bases are available, especially for outdoor use. Experimental and prototype designs in power chairs have specialized features, such as standing mechanisms, and chairs that can negotiate uneven surfaces and stairs. For the person using a manual wheelchair who is progressively losing strength, on option might be to add power to the manual chair. Several such add-on designs are available, but are not as effective as designs with built-in power, especially the new powered wheelchairs with direct drives through the wheels instead of belt drives.[56]

Selecting a powered wheelchair should be based on the same prescription principles described for manual ones. However, they present even more problems with safety and performance. The Rehabilitation Engineering Society of North America (RESNA) has established standards for power wheelchair performance.[57] A useful guide to evaluating powered wheelchairs based on these principles is available from the National Rehabilitation Information Center (NARIC) (Silver Spring, MD). The main point to consider when selecting such a wheelchair is overall weight and dimensions required for turning. This will largely depend on where the chair will be used. Short-based wheelchairs are better inside small houses because of the ease of turning in small spaces. For transport or storage, one may want to choose a folding wheelchair design. This involves removing batteries, which are heavy, and many care givers cannot manage them easily. A means of transportation must be found, which may involve purchasing a van and a lift. Environment barriers should be evaluated before power chair prescription, because extensive home modifications may be required, including widening doorways, providing ramps, and moving furniture.

Stability

Power wheelchairs tend to be more unstable than manual ones because of their speed, the higher position of the rider, and the somewhat narrower base. If the chair is to be used over door thresholds, on inclined surfaces, and over uneven terrain, extra features may need to be added. Antitip bars, a lower center of gravity, and wider wheels

on a longer wheel base may all be considered in the chair selection process.

Wheel Locks

Many power wheelchairs have two types of wheel locks: an electromechanical brake or lock that automatically holds the chair still when it comes to a stop and a manual brake or wheel lock. The former type may be adjusted to govern braking speed, a useful feature if the user has unsteady balance. The latter—just like all manual brakes—should not need so much force to engage them that they cannot be managed by user or care giver.

Battery Life

The range of the wheelchair—that is, the distance it will travel on a single charge—depends on many factors. Some of these involve the user's driving habits, such as driving fast or slow, use of frequent quick starts, covering rough terrain, and proper tire inflation. The batteries should be conveniently placed for removal and should have indicators showing when the charge is low so that the user never is stranded without a charged battery in a remote area.

Determination of Speed, Acceleration, and Deceleration

The more active the user, particularly outdoors, the more range may be covered, but a chair with very high acceleration or deceleration causes problems in persons with poor trunk control. Most chairs can be adjusted to control these factors. As a point of reference, typical walking speed is about 2.5 miles per hour, and jogging is 4 to 5 miles per hour.

Maintenance and Durability

Power wheelchairs are subject to much more stress than manual wheelchairs. For example, some riders jump curbs with them or travel over very rough terrain. Wheelchair components should be strong enough to allow lifting the chair with the rider; components should not pull out when chair is in midair. Potential users should only buy wheelchairs that have been approved as rough tested, but they should be aware of the mechanical limitations of all power chairs so that the wheelchair is not subjected to excessive stresses. Detachable accessories and components should be easily removed without tools. Inflating tires, tightening loose components, or replacing lost hardware should all be done regularly by the user. Major repairs, however, should be done by a skilled technician. This includes all electrical repairs of motorized chairs, which should meet the ANSI/RESNA wheelchair standards; unless these are met, a motorized wheelchair could present a real safety hazard.

Power mobility may be required only for longer distances for the individual who can ambulate or propel a manual wheelchair for shorter distances. Special control switches can be devised even for the individual with poor hand and arm function, profound weakness, or ataxia. Placement of the switch requires assessment of strength and coordination of a suitable muscle group—hand, shoulder, neck, face or tongue, or sip-and-puff design, for example. Significant advances in electronic switching and the use of integrated control systems allow the user to access a variety of functions including propulsion, communication, environmental control, and skills necessary for employment.[58]

Scooters

Three-wheeled scooters or carts—some have four wheels—differ from standard powered wheelchairs by their seat design and the use of a tiller control over the front wheel or wheels. The seat is usually a bracket type mounted on a central pedestal and can be easily adjusted in height. It may have a swivel action to ease entry or egress from the scooter.

Persons who use scooters must be cognitively aware and must have good trunk balance and arm control. Scooters are most useful for those who need a supplementary means for mobility, particularly outdoors and in urban environments. A comparative evaluation of scooters similar to one for evaluating powered wheelchairs has been described.[59] Most rehabilitation technology suppliers can provide details on the many models that are available.

SPECIFIC DISEASE PROCESSES WITH SPECIAL CONSIDERATIONS FOR SEATING

Neuromuscular Diseases

Muscle weakness that limits a person's strength and ability to maintain posture is characteristic of neuromuscular diseases, such as the genetically transmitted muscular

dystrophies, spinal muscular atrophy varients, and amyotrophic lateral sclerosis (ALS). The development of scoliosis is rarely a problem in these progressive diseases until walking ceases, and the patient depends largely or wholly on a wheelchair for mobility. Unfortunately, special seating cannot really halt progression of scoliosis, yet much more attention must be given to spinal support to compensate for loss of muscle power. Positioning can be critical for these individuals to minimize the demands on their musculature by promoting balanced postures.

Most of these diseases are slowly progressive. The seating team should consider the need for eventual head support when initially ordering a wheelchair. The individual with ALS, for example, will usually require support of the head and neck in the future to facilitate safety with swallowing. The need for power drive should be thought about early in the course of ALS rather than later switching to power from manual, because funding may be difficult to procure. Many people with neuromuscular diseases prefer a combination of manual and power mobility, with power wheelchair use increasing as functional abilities diminish.[60] The power drive system should be easily changed from joystick operation to an alternate method of control as needs change. Special bracketry for mounting respiratory equipment may be needed in the later stages of many of the neuromuscular diseases.

Multiple Sclerosis

Seating consideration for individuals with multiple sclerosis should be based on clinical course to date, cognitive changes, frequency and type of exacerbation/remissions, degree of recovery following relapses, and whether the condition shows a very slowly progressive course. The chair should be prescribed with clinical progression in mind and options for future adaptability, striving for a balance between function and support. Whenever possible, an ultralightweight frame type should be used for energy conservation. Head support may be especially useful when ataxic intention tremors of the head and neck interfere with posture. For clients who retain some walking ability, a motorized scooter or three-wheeled cart may be considered. Good trunk control, fairly good arm strength and good hand control are prerequisites for continued operation of a scooter.

For people with multiple sclerosis and similar conditions with decreased hand sensation, using gloves should be encouraged. Plastic-coated hand rims provide less exposure to temperature extremes, and mag wheels are better than spoked ones to prevent catching fingers in spokes. Heel loops prevent feet from getting caught behind the foot rests.

Use of highly contrasting colors on any pieces requiring removal or adjustment helps those with visual disturbances, who may also need modification of battery indicators. Cognition is clearly an issue, as is safety awareness. Judgment should be assessed before prescribing a power system.

Many people with multiple sclerosis need incontinent-proof cushion covers, as does anyone with the possibility of urinary incontinence. Cushion covers must be easily washable, and air circulation around the covers is crucial to keep the heat level down. Care must be taken with total-contact design because venting of the total-contact surface may be necessary to help prevent overheating.

In multiple sclerosis as in other potentially progressive conditions, the physician should explicitly detail the need for change to the third-party payer, for example, if a manual chair purchased the previous year requires a change to powered mobility a year later.

Spinal Cord Injury

The mobility needs for the person with spinal cord injury vary greatly with the level of injury. The seating system must be chosen with care, because problems with decreased sensation and incontinence are nearly universal. As with other wheelchair users, a balance must be struck between support and function. Some active and energetic spinal cord-injured persons will prefer a less stable seating system if it allows more flexibility and function. Spasticity, contractures, and neurogenic bowel and bladder dysfunction all require evaluation. The following general guidelines are based on the lowest levels of intact function:

Function at or above C3:
  Facial muscles, tongue, neck flexion/extension and rotation are partly spared.
  Assisted ventilation is required.
  Dependent on others for manual chair propulsion and transfers.
  Power system drive by head or mouth controls.
  Future possibilities: voice-activated mechanism.

Function at or above C4
  Sternocleidomastoids trapezius and upper cervical paraspinal muscles are also spared.
  Most spend majority of time free of assisted ventilation.
  Body English and changes in head position can be used for trunk position.
  Dependent on others for manual chair propulsion and transfers.
  Power system drive by head controls, sip and puff, pneumatic control, mouth control for propulsion, and tilt of electric chair.
  Future possibilities: voice-activated mechanisms

Function at or above C5
  Deltoid and biceps are also mostly spared.
  Oblique projections on the manual rims allow for short-distance propulsion on level surfaces.
  Some independence with modified weight shifts.
  Dependent for transfers and longer distance manual propulsion.
  Power mobility with modified joystick upper limb controlled.

Function at or above C6
  Shoulder girdle, elbow flexion, and radial wrist extension are also fully spared.
  Manual propulsion for longer distances possible.
  Many have independent modified transfers and weight shifts.
  May need power for long distances and difficult terrain.
  Vehicle modifications make driving possible.

Function at or above C7
  Triceps and extrinsic finger flexors and extensors are also spared.
  Independent transfers and push-ups for weight shifts.
  Independent mobility with manual propulsion.
  Functional independence may decrease with increasing age.
  Drives vehicles with manual control.

Function at thoracic levels
  Upper extremities, including hands, are also spared.
  Independent wheelchair mobility, transfers, and weight shifts.
  Independent driving with hand controls.

Function at lumbar levels
> Independent wheelchair use.
> May have some ambulation.
> Brackets to store gait aids may be added to wheelchair.

See Table 7-6.

Regardless of the level of residual neurologic function, certain considerations are necessary. Support should be provided appropriately, without being excessive. The seating system must be chosen with care because of insensate skin and potential for skin breakdown. Spasticity is frequently problematic and must be addressed by appropriate positioning for the lower extremities, including flexion angles at the hips, knees, and ankles that may need to be more acute than 90 degrees, with positioning components that produce minimal tactile stimulation, to reduce the frequency of spasms. Pneumatic tires may help prevent quick stretch of muscles when traversing varied terrain, thereby aiding spasticity control.

Meningomyelocele

In spina bifida or meningomyelocele, the strategies just described may apply, with crucial differences in the following areas. The major differences include a notable absence of spasticity in most individuals with spina bifida, a tendency toward longer trunk length relative to leg length, and the presence of hydrocephalus and brain stem abnormalities. Various structural abnormalities may be encountered, including gibbous deformity that requires accommodation, scoliosis, pelvic obliquity, and structural hip abnormalities, all of which must be addressed with the seating system, as described elsewhere in this chapter. Progression of the deformities and of the level of impairment is frequently noted with increasing age. Any rapid increase in scoliosis or development of spasticity may herald potentially reversible problems, including tethered cord, syrinx, or shunt malfunction. These should be excluded before proceeding with the seating prescription. In those with myelomeningocoele at lower levels, often a balance must be achieved between walking capacity, which may be quite limited, and wheelchair use. Discussions with the family should begin early concerning the potential benefits, both of ambulation, however limited and the need for wheelchair mobility. In children, Agre and co-workers found that those sub-jects who both walked and wheeled discovered wheeling much more energy efficient. Wheeling at 4.8 kilometers per hour was 11 percent more efficient than walking at 33 percent of that velocity.[60] Franks and co-workers demonstrated significant adverse effects on academic function that were due to fatigue from ambulation, and they caution that alternate means of mobility must be considered to promote overall development if assisted ambulation is not energy efficient, time efficient, or safe.[61] Families and individuals with spina bifida should be counseled to this effect. As adulthood is reached, the majority of those with spina bifida use wheelchairs as their primary means of mobility.[62]

Cerebral Palsy and Other Forms of Static Encephalopathy

Cerebral palsy is an abnormality of muscle tone and movement that is due to an insult or injury to the immature brain and is by definition nonprogressive. Other types of static or nonprogressive encephalopathies in older children or adults frequently result from head injuries, cerebral hypoxia, or sequelae from infection. These individuals may have abnormal muscle tone and movement patterns similar to those seen in cerebral palsy (or alternatively, to those seen after cerebral infarction). Interventions for seating vary with the type, features, and severity of cerebral dysfunction, regardless of cause. Most wheelchair goals for these persons encompass tone management, reflex inhibition, and facilitation of function in all areas. The management strategies for excessive tone, pelvic obliquity, windswept deformity, and other positioning dilemmas frequently encountered with cerebral palsy or other static encephalopathy are described elsewhere in this chapter and in the literature.[63]

Special circumstances must be considered in the severely involved adult with cerebral palsy. Many of the orthopedic deformities that are due to muscle imbalance and increased tone have already occurred and stabilized. However, pain that is due to deformities, dislocation, and spasticity often increases after adolescence. The clinic team must create a seating system that provides optimal support, function, and stability in the adult with cerebral palsy or head injury. To achieve the most appropriate therapeutic seating for the multi-impaired adult with a fixed central nervous system disorder requires particular

Table 7-6 Matching Mobility Needs to Levels of Spinal Cord Injury

Level	C3 or Above	C4	C5	C6	C7	C8–T12	L1–L4
Muscles spaced	Facial, tongue, neck flexion/extension some rotation	Also SCM, trapezius, upper cervical paraspinal	Also deltoids; biceps mostly spared	Also shoulder girdle, biceps, and radial wrist extension	Also triceps and extrinsic finger flexion/extension	Also upper extremity function fully spared, increasing trunk control with lower levels	Also lower extremity function increasing with lower lesion levels
Medical issues	Assisted ventilation AH, OH	Part-time ventilation AH, OH	AH, OH	AH, OH	AH, OH	AH risk to T6–T10, OH	Occasional OH
Positioning issues	Spasticity, skin at risk, tilt or recline	Same "body English" for trunk position	Spasticity skin at risk, focus on function	Same	Same	Same	Same, may need mounting for orthoses and gait aids
Manual chair use	Dependent	Dependent	Oblique projections for level—surface propulsion	Independent	Independent	Independent	Independent; may have some short-distance ambulation
Transfers	Dependent	Dependent	Modified weight shifts, mostly dependent	Many with modified independence for transfers and weight shifts	Independent	Independent	Independent
Power chair use	Head, mouth, sip and puff, tilt or recline, ECU	Same	Modified joy stick for mobility and weight shifts	May need power for long distance and difficult terrain	Most do not need power mobility	Generally do not need	Generally do not need
Driving	Dependent	Same	Usually dependent	Drive with vehicle modifications	Independent with hand controls, including transfers	Same	Some drive with minimal modification
Future potential	Voices-activated	Same	Same				
	Power chairs		Lighter, lever or geared manual chairs	Same	Same	Same	Same

Abbreviations: SCM, sternocleidomastoid; AH, autonomic hyper-reflexia; OH, othostatic hypotension; ECU, environmental control unit.

attention to the balance of anterior and posterior tilt of the pelvis and the position or angle of the back rest.[64]

Amputations

In sitting, the center of gravity in a person with bilateral lower extremity amputations, even when fitted with prostheses, lies further to the rear than in the nonamputee. Because this affects stability, the axles may need to be moved to the rear for optimal safety. A less satisfactory method is to add weights to the front of the wheelchair. Persons with hip disarticulation or hemicorpectomy require specialized seating; custom-designed air-filled or gel-filled cushions, CAD-CAM–generated foam cushions, and molded systems have all been successfully used.

Upper limb amputees who cannot walk or persons with hemiplegia may require specific chair modifications for independent mobility. The one-arm drive chair features interconnections of driving wheels, so that both can be operated from one side, through a dual set of hand rims. However, many persons with hemiplegia with cognitive deficits damage have difficulty operating such chairs. More commonly, hemiframe modifications are used; the frame itself is lowered, and the footrest on the sound side is removed so that the wheelchair can be propelled using the sound arm, aided by pushing with the sound foot. Electric mobility is also an option, but safety may be compromised by hemianopsia and unilateral neglect.

WHEELCHAIRS OF THE FUTURE

While technology of wheeled mobility will continue to advance, the trend from the past few decades has been that the large, commercial wheelchair producers have dictated what is generally available. For example, even though studies have demonstrated that alternate means of propulsion, such as lever- or crank-driven wheels, may be more energy-efficient than standard wheelchair propulsion, the cost of production and broad-scale distribution of these items would be prohibitive. With the restructuring of Medicaid and Medicare, with attendant decreases in reimbursements for durable medical equipment, major producers have responded by producing less expensive chairs. However, there is a distinct limit as to how far this trend can go, while still maintaining quality.

Lobbying to these funding agencies, as well as to third-party payers, may be needed to ensure that funding is available for those who need the equipment. Decreasing the allowables in the long run only hurts the end user.

Regarding chairs of the future, Brubaker emphasizes the need for wheelchairs that meet the needs and possibilities of the individual user and for design advances that are based on that premise.[27] Technology related to bicycle usage may be applied to future wheelchair design—specifically, incorporating geared systems into the propulsion system, allowing individuals with marginal strength to have greater power transmitted to the wheels. The provision of braking devices similar to hand brakes on bicycles would allow greater control with deceleration, especially on ramped surfaces, rather than using friction from the hands on the wheels to slow the chair. The addition of a shock absorbtion system would increase comfort, improving sitting tolerance, and as always, lighter, more durable structural components are desired and feasible for development.

Already chairs are available that can be used to negotiate varied terrains, including stair ascent and descent, through sand, and on off-road trails. Broader availability and increased knowledge about these options are needed. Standing chairs also show promise in better meeting the personal, vocational, and avocational needs of the wheelchair user.[65]

For the power chair user, the future promises further developments in switch accessibility including expansion of environmental control accessibility and communication and mobility with a single network of integrated switch controls. Infrared designs for drive control are already being used and are promising for the individual with limited movement.[66,67] As technology advances, more sophisticated interfacing systems may allow chairs to move where the user looks or even thinks.

Hybrid designs using power-assisted manual propulsion would allow the marginal manual chair user the benefit of upper extremity activity and self-propulsion, without resorting exclusively to power mobility, with dependence for manual chair needs. Cremers has been developing just such a design.[64,68]

An overall focus on matching the needs and desires of the individual with appropriate technological advances, with an eye on cost containment, promises that the wheelchairs of the future will provide greater independence and maximal function in the face of residual disability, truly representing the ultimate orthoses.

REFERENCES

1. Pope AM, Tarlov AR: Disability in America, towards a National Agenda for prevention. National Institute of Medicine, National Academy Press, Washington, DC, 1991
2. Phillips L, Nicosia A: An overview . . . with reflections past and present of a consumer. J Rehabil Res Dev Clin Suppl 2: 1, 1990
3. Post KM: From the field: clinical notes on cushion prescription. Am J Occup Ther 45:559, 1991
4. Nwaobi OM, Smith PD: Effect of adaptive seating on pulmonary function of children with cerebral palsy. Dev Med Child Neurol 28:351, 1986
5. Chow WW, Odell EL: Deformations and stresses in soft body tissues of a sitting person. J Biomech Engin 100:79, 1988
6. Chow WW: Mechanical properties of gels and other materials with respect to their use in pads transmitting forces to the human body. Doctoral dissertation, University of Michigan, 1974
7. Springle SH, Faisant TE, Chung KC: Clinical evaluation of custom-contoured cushions for the spinal cord injured. Arch Phys Med Rehabil 71:655, 1990
8. Letts RM: Principles of Seating the Disabled. CRC Press, Boca Raton, FL, 1991
9. Ferguson-Pell MW: Seat cushion selection. J Rehabil Res Dev Clin Suppl 2:49, 1990
10. Garber SL, Dyerly LR: Wheelchair cushions for persons with spinal cord injury: an update. Am J Occup Ther 45:550, 1991
11. Garber SL: Wheelchair cushions for spinal cord-injured individuals. Am J Occup Ther 39:722, 1985
12. Gilsdorf P, Patterson R, Fisher S: Thirty-minute continuous sitting force measurements with different support surfaces in the spinal cord injured and able-bodied. J Rehabil Res Dev 28(4):33, 1991
13. Bar CA: Evaluation of cushions using dynamic pressure measurement. Prosthet Orthot Int 15:232, 1991
14. St-Georges M, Valiquette C, Drouin G: Computer-aided design in wheelchair seating. J Rehabil Res Dev 26(4):23, 1989
15. Henderson JL, Price SH, Brandstater ME, Mandac BR: Efficacy of three measures to relieve pressure in seated persons with spinal cord injury. Arch Phys Med Rehabil 75:535, 1994
16. Engström B: Ergonomics Wheelchair and Positioning, 1993
16a. Bardsley G: Biomechanical Basis of Orthotic Management. Butterworth-Heinemann, Boston, 1993
17. Sprigle S, Chung KC, Brubaker CE: Reduction of sitting pressures with custom contoured cushions. J Rehabil Res Dev 27:135, 1990
18. Carlson JM, Lonstein J, Beck KO, Wilkie DC: Seating with children and young adults with cerebral palsy. Clin Prosth Orthot 11:176, 1987
19. Trefler E, Taylor SJ: Prescription and positioning: evaluating the physically disabled individual for wheelchair seating. Prosthet Orthot Int 15:217, 1991
20. Hetzel TR: Skin integrity: Concepts of control. In: Proceedings of the 10th International Seating Symposium. Vancouver, 1994
21. Margolis SA, Wengert ME, Kobarka: The Subasis bar. In: Proceeding of the 4th International Seating Symposium. University of Vancouver, 1988
22. Bardlsey GI, Taylor PM: The development of an assessment chair. Prosthet Orthot Int 6:75, 1982
23. van der Woude LH, Veeger HEJ, Rozendal RH: Ergonomics of wheelchair design: a prerequisite for optimum wheeling conditions. Adapt Phys Act Q 6:106, 1989
24. McLaurin CA, Brubaker CE: Lever drive system for wheelchairs. J Rehabil Res Dev 23(2):54, 1986
25. McLaurin CA, Brubaker CE: Biomechanics and the wheelchair. Prosthet Orthot Int 15:24, 1991
26. Linden AL, Holland GJ, Loy SF, Vincent WJ: A physiological comparison of forward vs reverse wheelchair ergometry. Med Sci Sports Exerc 25:1265, 1993
27. Brubaker CE: Wheelchair prescription: an analysis of factors that affect mobility and performance. J Rehabil Res Dev 23(4):19, 1986
28. Majaess GG, Kirby RL, Ackroyd-Stolarz SA, Charlebois PB: Influence of seat position on the static and dynamic forward and rear stability of occupied wheelchairs. Arch Phys Med Rehabil 74:977, 1993
29. Kirby US: Nonfatal wheelchair-related accidents reported to the National Electronic Injury Surveillance System. Am J Phys Med Rehabil 73:163, 1994
30. Kirby RL, Ackroyd-Stolarz SA, Brown MG et al: Wheelchair-related accidents caused by tips and falls among non-institutional users of manually propelled wheelchairs in Nova Scotia. Am J Phys Med Rehabil 75:319, 1994
31. Ummat S, Kirby RL: Nonfatal wheelchair-related accidents report to the National Electronic Injury Surveillance System. Am J Phys Med Rehabil 73:163, 1994
32. Masse LC, Lamontagne M, O'Riain MD: Biomechanical analysis of wheelchair propulsion for various seating positions. J Rehabil Res Dev 29(3):12, 1992
33. Ragnarsson KT: Prescription considerations and a comparison of conventional and lightweight wheelchairs. J Rehabil Res Dev Clin Suppl 2:8, 1990
34. Brubaker CE: Ergonomic considerations. Choosing a wheelchair system. J Rehabil Res Dev Clin Suppl 2:44, 1990
35. McLaurin CA: Current directions in wheelchair research. J Rehabil Res Dev Clin Suppl 2:88, 1990
36. Veeger D, van der Woude LH, Rozendal RH: The effect of rear wheel camber in manual wheelchair propulsion. J Rehabil Res Dev 26(2):37, 1989
37. Brubaker CE: Wheelchair prescription: an analysis of factors that affect mobility and performance. J Rehabil Res Dev 23(4):19, 1986

38. Behrman AL: Factors in functional assessment. J Rehabil Res Dev Clin Suppl 2:17, 1990

39. Zacharkow D: Posture, Sitting, Standing, Chair Design and Exercise. Charles C Thomas, Springfield, IL, 1988

40. Fenweck D: Wheelchairs and Their Users. Office of Population Census & Surveys, Social Survey Division, London, 1977

41. Shaw G, Taylor SJ: A survey of seating problems of the institutionalized elderly. Assist Technol 3:5, 1991

42. Redford JB: Seating and wheeled mobility in the disabled elderly population. Arch Phys Med Rehabil 74:877, 1993

43. Mawson AR, Riundo JJ, Jr, Neville P et al: Risk factors for early occurring pressure ulcers following spinal cord injury. Am J Phys Med Rehabil 67:123, 1988

44. Staas WE, Cioschi HM: Pressure sores—a multifaceted approach to prevention and treatment. In: Rehabilitation medicine. Adding life to years (special issue). West J Med 154: 539, 1991

45. Cooney TG, Reuler JB: Pressure sores. West J Med 140:622, 1984

46. Henderson JL, Price SH, Brandstater ME, Mandac BR: Efficacy of three measures to relieve pressure in seated persons with spinal cord injury. Arch Phys Med Rehabil 75:535, 1994

47. Dinsdale SM: Decubitus ulcers: role of pressure and friction in causation. Arch Phys Med Rehabil 55:147, 1974

48. Carlson JM, Winter R: The "Gillette" sitting support orthosis. Orthot Prosthet 32:4, 1978

49. Bleck EE: The hip in cerebral palsy. Orthop Clin North Am 11:79, 1980

50. Lonstein JE, Beck K: Hip dislocation and subluxation in cerebral palsy. J Pediatr Orthop 6:521, 1986

51. Letts M, Klassen D, Shapiro L, Jurenka S: The windswept hip phenomenon. J Bone Join Surg [Br] 64:257, 1982

52. Green EM, Nelham BL: Development of sitting ability, assessment of children with a handicap and prescription of appropriate seating system. Prosthet Orthot Int 15:203–16, 1991

53. Shephard RJ: Sports medicine and the wheelchair athlete. Sports Med 5:226, 1988

54. Cooper RA: Racing chair lingo . . . or how to order a racing wheelchair. Sports 'n Spokes, 13(6):29, 1988

55. MacLeish MS, Cooper RA, Harralson J: Design of a composite monocoque frame racing wheel. J Rehabil Res Dev 30: 233, 1993

56. Warren CG: Powered mobility and its implications. J Rehabil Res Dev Clin Suppl 2:74, 1990

57. The ANSI/RESNA wheelchair standards: sample evaluation and guide to interpreting test data for prescribing power wheelchairs. Health Devices 22:432, 1993

58. Hawley MS, Cudd PA, Wells JH et al: Wheelchair-mounted integrated control systems for multiply handicapped people. J Biomed Engin 14(3):193, 1992

59. Rehabilitation Engineering Center, Product Comparison and Evaluation: Scooters. National Rehabilitation Hospital, Washington, D.C., 1991

60. Lord JP, Lieberman JS, Portwood MM et al: Functional ability and equipment use among patients with neuromuscular disease. Arch Phys Med Rehabil 68:346, 1987

61. Agre JC, Findley TW, McNally MC et al: Physical activity capacity in children with myelomeningocele. Arch Phys Med Rehabil 68:372, 1987

62. Franks CA, Palisano RJ, Darbee JC: The effect of walking with an assistive device and using a wheelchair on school performance in students with myelomeningocele. Phys Ther 71(8):26, 1991

63. O'Connell DG, Barhart R, Parks L: Muscular endurance and wheelchair propulsion in children with cerebral palsy or myelomeningocele. Arch Phys Med Rehabil 73:709, 1992

64. Hundertmark LH: Evaluating the adult with cerebral palsy for specialized adaptive seating. Phys Ther 65:209, 1985

65. van den Berg JP, den Ouden A, Stam HJ: The Standmobile: a new, electrically powered, mobile stand up device for use in paraplegia. Case report. Paraplegia 32:202, 1994

66. Hawley MS, Cudd PA, Wells JH et al: Wheelchair-mounted integrated control systems for multiply handicapped people. J Biomed Engin 14:193, 1992

67. Choate MJ: Infrared wheelchair controls. Biomed Scie Instrument 26:107, 1990

68. Cremers GB: Hybrid-powered wheelchair: a combination of arm force and electrical power for propelling a wheelchair. J Medical Engineer Technol 13(1–2):142, 1989

Appendix 7-1

Seating Letter of Medical Necessity

I. Patient Information:

Patient Name: _____ Hospital #: _____ Date: _____

Case Manager: _____ Date of Birth: _____

Diagnosis: _____ Prognosis: _____ Age: _____ Sex: _____

Onset of Disability: _____ History of Present Illness: _____

II. Current Function:

a. **Ambulation:**
❑ None ❑ Limited ❑ Wheelchair needed to be mobile ❑ Type of gait aid needed _____

b. **Type of Transfer:**
❑ Indep. ❑ Partial Assist ❑ Dependent

c. **Amount of Assistance Needed (if any):**
❑ 1 Person ❑ 2 Persons ❑ Other _____

d. **Activities of Daily Living:**
❑ Indep. ❑ Partial Assist ❑ Dependent

e. **Current Wheelchair/When Obtained:** _____

f. **School/Employment:** _____

g. **Therapies:** ❑ PT ❑ OT ❑ SLP ❑ Other _____

h. **Architectural Barriers:** _____

i. **Special Circumstances:** _____ j. **Transportation:** _____

III. Physical Examination:

a. **General & Neurological Assessment:**
_____

b. **Sitting Balance:**
❑ Good - Hands-free with ability to weight shift   ❑ Fair - Hands-free only
❑ Poor - Propped with hand support   ❑ Dependent - Needs external support

c. **Self Propulsion Ability:** ❑ YES ❑ NO

d. **Sitting Posture on Mat Table:**

❑ Posterior Pelvic Tilt	❑ Fixed	❑ Flexible	_____
❑ Anterior Pelvic Tilt	❑ Fixed	❑ Flexible	_____
❑ Pelvic Obliquity	❑ Right	❑ Left	_____
❑ Pelvic Rotation Protracted Forward to	❑ Right	❑ Left	_____ °
❑ Kyphosis	❑ Fixed	❑ Flexible	_____
❑ Lordosis	❑ Fixed	❑ Flexible	_____
❑ Scoliosis Convex to -	❑ Fixed	❑ Flexible	_____ °
❑ Forward Head/Neck Hyperextension	❑ Fixed	❑ Flexible	_____
❑ Leg Abduction	❑ Fixed	❑ Flexible	_____
❑ Leg Adduction	❑ Fixed	❑ Flexible	_____
❑ Wind Sweeping	❑ Fixed	❑ Flexible	_____

❑ Other _____

e. **Tonal Influences/Reflexes in Sitting:**
❑ Extensor ❑ Flexor ❑ ATNR ❑ STNR
❑ Positive Support ❑ Ankle Clonus ❑ Other _____

f. **Lower Extremity Range of Motion; (Supine/Seated):**

Hip Flexion (Normal = 0° to 125°)   ❑ Normal _____   ❑ Abnormal _____
Knee Extension w/hip at 90°   ❑ Normal _____   ❑ Abnormal _____
Ankle   ❑ Normal _____   ❑ Abnormal _____

g. **Skin Breakdown - Location:**
❑ Ischial Tuberosities ❑ Coccyx ❑ Spine ❑ Other _____ ❑ Intact

h. **Upper Extremity Function:**
❑ Normal ❑ Abnormal _____

IV. *Wheelchair Evaluation:*

a. **Wheelchair Frame:**
- ❑ Rigid ❑ Tilt 'N Space ❑ Growth Potential ❑ Folding ❑ Recline/Semi Recline
- ❑ Adjustable Axle ❑ Ultra Lightweight ❑ Other _____
- Brand/Model: _____

b. **Arm Positioning:**
- ❑ Tubular ❑ Desk Special Features: _____
- ❑ Full Length ❑ Arm Pad _____
- ❑ Trough ❑ Height Adjustable _____
- ❑ Removable ❑ Upper extremtity support surface ❑ None ❑ Other _____

c. **Foot Positioning:**
- ❑ Swing-Away ❑ Angle Adjustable Special Features: _____
- ❑ Platform ❑ Rigid _____
- ❑ Elevating ❑ Shoe Holders _____
- ❑ Foot Straps _____

d. **Seating System:**
- ❑ Jay/Jay GS ❑ Custom Foam ❑ Roho ❑ Silhouette/System 2000
- ❑ Foam _____ ❑ Avanti Personal ❑ Contour U ❑ Pelvic Well
- ❑ Anti-thrust ❑ Hip Guides Special Features: _____
- ❑ Thigh Guides ❑ Abduction Wedge _____
- ❑ Physiologic Contour ❑ Adjustable Tension _____

e. **Back Cushion:**
- ❑ Jay II/Jay GS ❑ Contour U Special Features: _____
- ❑ Custom Foam ❑ Biangular _____
- ❑ Sling ❑ Avanti Personal _____
- ❑ Adjustable Tension ❑ Other _____

f. **Headrest/Support:**
- ❑ Ottobock ❑ Whitmeyer/ATNR Special Features: _____
- ❑ Extended ❑ 3 Piece _____
- ❑ 1 Piece Curved ❑ Other _____

g. **Restraint System:**
- ❑ Pelvic Belt ❑ Padded Special Features: _____
- ❑ Dual Pull ❑ 2 Point ❑ 4 Point _____

h. **Tires, Wheels & Brakes:** _____

i. **Additional Comments:** _____
_____
_____

V. *Reason for Medical Necessity:*
- ❑ Independent Mobility ❑ Dependent Mobility
- ❑ Improve Posture ❑ Posture Relief
- ❑ Accommodate Deformity ❑ Accommodate Joint Limitations
- ❑ Relieve Pain ❑ Increase Sitting Tolerance
- ❑ Reduce Tonal Influences ❑ Improve Functional Level
- ❑ Improve Head Position/Visual Field ❑ Allow for Growth/Weight Gain
- ❑ Improve Appearance ❑ Meet Caregiver Goals
- ❑ Meet Transportation/Vocational/School Needs ❑ Safety for feeding/swallowing
- ❑ Adjustability for medical problems (seizures, suction, _____).
- ❑ Other _____

VI. *Vendor Assignment:* _____

VII. *Copies to:*
- ❑ Referring MD _____
- ❑ Family _____
- ❑ Other _____

_____ Date: _____
Physician's signature certifies the above represents her judgment of the patient's medical need for the above prescribed equipment.

Measurement Guide

DEALER NAME_____ PHONE: (_____) _____

P.O.# _____ DATE:_____

PATIENTS NAME:_____

CHAIR MAKE:_____ MODEL:_____

CONSTRUCTION WIDTH:_____DEPTH:_____BACK HEIGHT:_____

UPHOLSTERY COLOR:_____FRAME COLOR:_____

A. SEAT TO TOP OF HEAD _____

B. SEAT TO SHOULDER _____

C. CALF TO BUTTOCKS _____

D. LEG LENGTH _____

E. CHEST DEPTH _____

F. AXILLA TO AXILLA _____

G. HIP WIDTH _____

H. SEAT TO AXILLA _____

I. SEAT TO ELBOW _____

J. SHOULDER WIDTH _____

1. _____
2. _____
3. _____
4. _____
5. _____
6. _____
7. _____
8. _____
9. _____

Numeric Codes Used for Basic Chair Designs

K0001   Standard wheelchair
K0002   Standard hemi (low seat) wheelchair
K0003   Lightweight wheelchair
K0004   High-strength, lightweight wheelchair
K0005   Ultralightweight wheelchair
K0006   Heavy-duty wheelchair
K0007   Extra heavy-duty wheelchair
K0008   Custom manual wheelchair base
K0009   Other manual wheelchair base

MOTORIZED/POWER WHEELCHAIR BASE

K0010   Standard-weight frame motorized/ power wheelchair
K0011   Standard-weight frame motorized/ power wheelchair with programmable control parameters for speed adjust- ment, tremor dampening, acceleration control, and braking
K0012   Custom motorized/power wheelchair base
K0014   Other motorized/power wheelchair base

Note: Options and accessories for wheelchairs require the addition of a KO code number. If the following criteria are met, they may be covered by insurance:

1. The patient's condition is such that without the use of a wheelchair, he would otherwise be bed- or chair-confined (an individual may qualify for a wheelchair and still be considered bed-confined.

2. The options/accessories are necessary for the pa- tient to perform one or more of the following ac- tivities:
   a. Function in the home.
   b. Perform instrumental activities of daily living.

Adaptive Driving Modifications

Herbert Kent
John B. Redford

This chapter informs physicians and health professionals of different types of adaptive driving equipment available for people with physical disabilities. It also should serve as a source of information about the availability of such equipment.

An unimpaired driver operating a car with manual transmission requires continuous coordination of the upper and lower limbs; the hands and feet are used to shift gears, steer, and apply brakes. During operation of the vehicle, it may become necessary to turn on the headlights, switch from low to high beam, operate the windshield wipers and, at times, adjust the heater or air conditioner. Most of these operations of driving are done routinely. The left hand normally steers, the right hand shifts gears; the left foot operates the clutch, and the right foot depresses the accelerator. Thus, driving a vehicle is a complex task, particularly when one has to concentrate on the roadway, view the dashboard dials, and operate the automobile safely.

A visual, cognitive, or physical disability can affect driving skills. Automotive improvements, such as automatic transmissions, have made it easier for someone who has lost a limb to drive. A left leg below-knee amputee generally operates both the accelerator and brake pedals with the right leg. When a hand is lost, shifting is less frequent, and the steering wheel can be controlled with one hand with the use of adaptive driving equipment. On the other hand, people with spinal cord injuries or bilateral amputations cannot always depend on simple modifications. People with physical disabilities that affect their ability to operate a motor vehicle should have an evaluation with qualified professionals to determine their ability to operate a motor vehicle safely and the types of adaptive driving equipment needed.

With advances in technology, the van has become extremely popular; it has helped serve people previously unable to drive, including those with quadriplegia, multiple sclerosis, muscular dystrophy, and postpolio syndrome, who often demonstrate dependence in transfers to and from the wheelchair. Modern vans enable them to drive from the position of their wheelchair.

To protect the patient and public, federal agencies are making a systematic effort to require that vehicles and adaptive equipment conform to minimum standards of safety and quality. Also, it is recognized that national requirements for licensure of the disabled will eventually be necessary. Federal standards setting minimum levels of acceptable safety and quality for adaptive driving equipment have been published in the *Federal Register*.[1] Appendix 8-1 provides additional source materials.

219

ADAPTIVE DRIVING EQUIPMENT

Whether modifications are required for drivers who have little or no use of their lower limbs, impaired function of the upper limbs, or a combination of both (as in quadriplegia), it is essential to match the available equipment with the person's functional abilities. Throughout this chapter, various types of adaptive driving equipment are listed and described along with their implications for use.

Hand Controls for Acceleration or Braking

The hand control—either right or left—usually consists of a lever attached to a bracket on the steering column with rods connected to the brake and accelerator pedals. A cam or gear is added to the lever so that the operating force can be changed from the accelerator to the brake pedal. There is a mechanical advantage built into the system. The ratio is 1:3 as a rule. These hand control systems may have one of three different shaped handles: straight bar type, knob, or yoke end. The straight bar and knob handles require a functional grip. The yoke-shaped handle can be used for people with quadriplegia to assist with wrist stabilization when using the hand control.

The Horn and Dimmer Switch Buttons
The horn and dimmer switch buttons are generally located next to the handle for ease in operating these functions without removing the hand from this device. Three types of hand controls are available:

1. *Push–pull:* Braking is achieved by pushing the horizontal hand lever away from the driver and parallel to the steering column. Acceleration is achieved by pulling the hand lever toward the driver (Fig. 8-1).
2. *Push–twist:* Braking is achieved by pushing the horizontal hand lever away from the driver and parallel to the steering column. Acceleration is achieved by clockwise (forward twisting) rotation of the handgrip, similar to motorcycle operation.

3. *Push–right angle pull:* Braking is achieved by pushing the horizontal hand lever away from the driver and parallel to the steering column. Acceleration is achieved by pulling the hand lever in a direction perpendicular (at right angle) to the steering column and down toward the driver's lap.

All three types of hand controls have the same braking action, that is, forward, by a pushing motion. If the car stops suddenly, the driver is thrown forward, transferring his weight to the hand control lever, which activates the brakes.

Most hand controls are usually installed on the left side, because the gear shift and ignition are located on

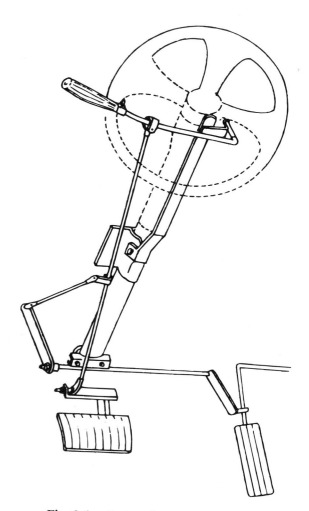

Fig. 8-1. Push–pull type of hand control.

the right. However, they can be installed on either the right or left side of the steering column.

Steering Aids

Steering devices in the following list can be used when only one upper extremity can perform the steering function, whether resulting from limited hand control or a functional limitation of the involved upper extremity.

1. A knob that can rotate is commonly used as a spinner. The spinner knob requires good arm and hand function. (Fig. 8-2A).
2. The V-grip is shaped like the letter V (Fig. 8-2D). The palmar aspect of the fingers is slipped through the opening and then held in a vertical position by the uprights of the V. The V-grip is used when someone has weakness in the hand, such as occurs in quadriplegia, but has a reasonable amount of flexor muscle function in the fingers.
3. The flat spinner (Fig. 8-2C) permits the palm and fingers to be secure, palm facing downward. It is for those who have a functional wrist and a slightly functional grip.
4. The Tri Pin resembles the V-grip but has three adjustable pins arranged in a triangle. One pin contacts the palm, and the other two contact the volar and dorsal surface of the wrist and resist efforts of the hand to pull out of the Tri Pin. The hand is free, however, to life up and out at any time. This steering device is primarily used by people with quadriplegia who have no gripping muscle function.
5. The wrist splint type is a molded splint permitting a flaccid wrist and fingers to be retained securely by Velcro straps (Fig. 8-2F).
6. The quad grip with pin is similar to the flat spinner with a latch closure device on the extensor aspect of the fingers, which then holds the hand snugly in place.
7. The amputee ring is helpful for prosthetic wearers using a hook. The point of the hook is inserted into the hole, and the wheel can be maneuvered in any direction (Fig. 8-2C).
8. The upright quad spinner is used by quadriplegic persons with at least partial functional use of the wrist and some use of the extensor muscles of the

hand. The hand is held in a vertical position to the steering wheel (Fig. 8-2D).

New regulations under Federal Motor Vehicle Safety Standard 208 prevent anyone from installing anything that will disable an air bag. However, an exception may be granted for vehicles that are intended to be operated by disabled individuals. Manufacturers do have kits for disabling an air bag if the disabled person wants a steering aid installed. The choice is up to the vendor and the patient.

Gearshift

A gearshift extension bar is useful where motions are limited, as in the shoulder or elbow (Fig. 8-2B). Electronic gearshifts are now available and can be activated by pushing a button or touch pad.

Secondary Controls

Secondary controls are those devices necessary for driving other than the steering, acceleration, and braking systems. The placement and prescription of these control switches or extensions depend on individual needs.

1. The quad key holder is used by drivers who do not have a functional grip and cannot use a key. It provides pressure and leverage to turn the ignition key. (Fig. 8-2E)
2. Elbow switches are used for those operations that need to be performed while the vehicle is in motion. They are used when the driver cannot safely remove a hand from the brake/accelerator control and the steering device. These switches may be used for horn, turn signals, headlight dimmer switch, and/or cruise control.
3. Head control switches are used when an individual lacks enough upper limb function to operate the elbow switches. These switches may be used for horn, turn signals, headlight dimmer switch, and/or cruise control.
4. Driving consoles are used to relocate secondary control switches for easy access to the driver. They may be mounted on the steering column, driver side door, or in the center of the vehicle to the

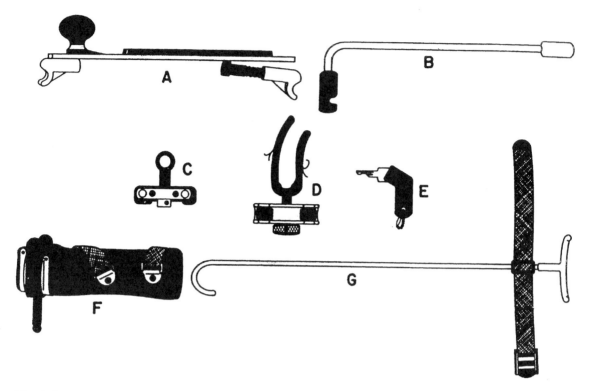

Fig. 8-2. Various steering aids and other devices. **(A)** Knob—spinner hand control. **(B)** Gear shift extension. **(C)** Spinner ring hand control. **(D)** Yoke hand control. **(E)** Quad-key ignition key holder. **(F)** Wrist splint. **(G)** Hook reacher.

driver's right. These switches formerly were in the form of toggles but now are primarily made as touch pads. The touch pads can be built up, depending on individual needs. The following switches and controls can be wired into the console:

Ignition
Wipers/washers
Heater/air conditioning
Power windows
Power door locks
Electric mirrors
Door/lift controls
Electric gear selector
Headlight dimmer
Electric parking brake
Emergency flashers
Electric wheelchair lockdown

Brakes

Power brakes are practically a necessity for most disabled drivers. Pedals can be elevated or locations changed. Standard parking brakes are manually controlled but, for the physically disabled, can be made electric so that they can be operated by a switch or other controls. A parking brake extension lever (Fig. 8-2G) allows for hand operation of a conventional foot-operated parking brake. In addition, sensitized or zero-effort brakes are now available.

Accelerator

Frequently, the accelerator pedal must be altered. When the deficit prevents the use of the right lower limb for acceleration and braking, a left foot accelerator can be installed. Two types of left foot accelerator pedals are available: one that is bolted to the floor and one that is attached to the right foot accelerator with a bar extending to the left. Hand-controlled accelerators are mounted on the steering column as described above in "Hand Controls." The level of the foot pedal can be raised by adding an extension for those who have short limbs.

Joystick Driving Systems

For those with severe physical disabilities who are unable to operate the steering wheel, accelerator, or brake, joystick driving systems are available. These systems typically use a joystick for the primary driving controls: acceleration, braking, and steering. Generally, moving the joystick forward causes acceleration; backward, braking; and side to side, steering. The joystick requires the use of only one upper limb to run this control and can be installed on either the right or left side.

VANS

Both full-size vans and minivans are used by those with more severe physical disabilities such as quadriplegia, multiple sclerosis, neuromuscular diseases, and postpolio syndrome. The vans can be modified to allow driving from a wheelchair if the person cannot transfer independently and safely into a power seat. For the individual who drives from a wheelchair, the floor of the van usually needs to be lowered. Special considerations include the following:

1. The amount of the floor that needs to be lowered varies with the size of the individual and the type of the van.
2. Instead of lowering the floor, a power pan or channels can be installed into the driver's position.
3. Wheelchair restraints or electric lock-downs to fasten the wheelchair to the floor are an absolute necessity. Sudden stops, acceleration, and so on can result in the driver becoming unstable and the chair moving about, imposing a safety hazard. Manually operated or electric tie-downs are available.
4. Vans modified for the disabled have regular car seats that can be quickly disconnected if desired, and a wheelchair used instead.

5. The seat can have a six- or eight-way power base to facilitate a transfer from wheelchair to the driver's seat.
6. Acceleration and braking can be operated by hand controls. If there is weakness of the upper extremities, the braking can be modified with reduced or zero effort.

Other Modifications

Obviously, all sorts of van modifications can be added and may be essential.

1. A raised roof may be required, because the elevated seat height of a person in a wheelchair makes the head come close to or in contact with the roof.
2. Mirrors of special design or placement are sometimes needed for rear or side vision.
3. Van rear or side entrance loading are options to be considered. Side entry needs wider parking space, but rear entry may need more road space.
4. Expanded doorway widths and heights are sometimes required, depending on the seated height of the individual and the size of the lift to be used.
5. Seat belts, together with some of the above modifications, must be altered as required. The patient's wheelchair should be properly secured in addition to a set of shoulder and lap belts. A chest strap may also be needed for those with weak trunk musculature to ensure stability in the wheelchair.
6. Steering wheel alterations—such as a wheel of smaller than usual diameter—steering column extensions, or horizontal steering can be made. The resistance of the power steering can also be reduced to low or zero effort.
7. Air conditioning is generally considered essential in hot climates, particularly for those with spinal cord injuries or multiple sclerosis. This includes rear air conditioning as well.
8. Two-way radio for communication is sometimes vital in rural areas, on freeways, or where vocational endeavors require it. Cellular telephones can also be used.

Figure 8-3 shows a minivan dashboard with various types of adaptive driving equipment.

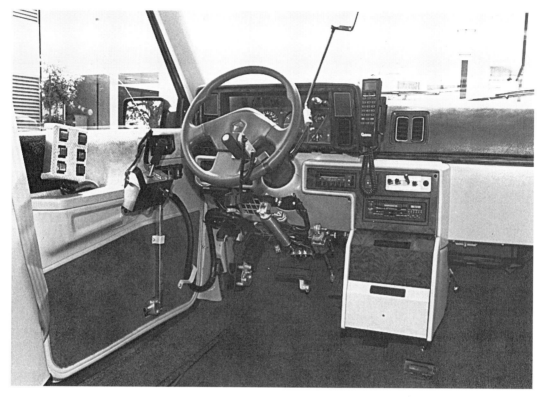

Fig. 8-3. Dashboard of a minivan with examples of adaptive driving equipment.

Equipment charts have been devised to make selections easier to recommend. Table 8-1 shows a modification guide for vehicles that might be considered essential, depending on the nature of the primary diagnosis. This table may be consulted for common neuromusculoskeletal diagnoses but is by no means inclusive. Of course, the modification will ultimately be determined by the functional disability, but it may include other related aspects, such as terrain, climate, and rural versus urban driving.

A list of suppliers of adaptive equipment for driving and sources of special vehicle modifications is given in Appendix 8-2.

Automobile Versus Van

Automobiles are used when the individual is able to independently transfer in and out of the vehicle. The most common disability category at this functional level is par-

aplegia. Persons with paraplegia are generally able to transfer into the driver's side by sliding from left to right. A transfer board is sometimes used. Alternatively, they may enter the passenger side of the vehicle and slide from right to left. Spastic conditions such as multiple sclerosis may require door or seat modifications. Diseases where muscle strength or lack of coordination are predominant necessitate many special adjustments to the controls and addition of other adaptive devices. Hand-control mounts should correspond to the opposite side of the disability. Consequently, interference by these mounts must be considered also. In addition, storage for the wheelchair must be arranged when automobile is in use. If the chair is placed behind the driver's seat, additional leg room to accommodate the medical condition must be anticipated. If the individual cannot independently load/unload the wheelchair, an automatic chair topper can be added. This device is a car-top carrier that can automatically load and unload the wheelchair.

A van (either full-size or minivan) is recommended

Table 8-1. Automotive Modifier Guide

Disability	Hand Controls	Steering Aids	Gear Shift	Switches	Brakes	Accelerator	Floor	Other
Spinal cord disease/ injury								
C5,6	+	+	+	+	+	+	+	+
T1,2	+	+			+	+	+	+
T10	+	+		+	+	+	+	+
L4,5	+	+			+	+	+	+
S1,2	+	+			+	+		
Brain disease/injury								
Left hemiplegia		+	+	+		+		
Right hemiplegia		+	+	+		+		
Cerebral palsy		+	+	+		+		
Amputee								
Upper right or left		+						
Lower right or left					+	+		
Bilateral upper	+	+			+		+	+
Bilateral lower	+	+			+	+		
Above knee					+	+		
Below knee	+	+			+	+		
Multiple sclerosis	+	+	+	+	+	+	+	+
Neuromuscular disorders	+	+	+	+	+	+	+	+
Poliomyelitis	+	+	+	+	+	+	+	+

when an individual uses a power wheelchair or cannot independently transfer in and out of the vehicle. In particular, the van has made transportation possible for persons with such disabilities as quadriplegia, muscular dystrophy, multiple sclerosis, and postpolio syndrome. In the van, the disabled person can function as either the driver or the passenger. As mentioned, if the individual drives from the wheelchair, then the floor of the van usually must be lowered for adequate visibility.

The greatest advantage of the van is the convenience of entry and exit without leaving the wheelchair. All that is required is an elevation system for either rear or side entry. The disabled person must decide which entry system is best for his or her vocational needs and life-style. With a rear entry conversion, all bench seats are removed. The rear bench seat can be retained in a side entry system.

In summary, it is necessary to ascertain the functional abilities of the individual to select the best vehicle for his needs.

Van Access Systems

Elevator and ramp methods for entry and exit depend on the type of vehicle. Some of these rely on the use of hoists, elevators, and ramps mounted on the side or rear. Cable winches, hydraulic systems, or other devices employed work electrically, with a mechanical backup for emergencies. Two basic types of elevator modifiers are now available, swing-away and fold-out.

Swing-Away Lift

In the swing-away lift, the wheelchair is rolled onto a platform, rotates 180 degrees as it swings out and then is gently lowered to the ground level. Safety ledges, switches, and other mechanical controls for emergencies are handily mounted.

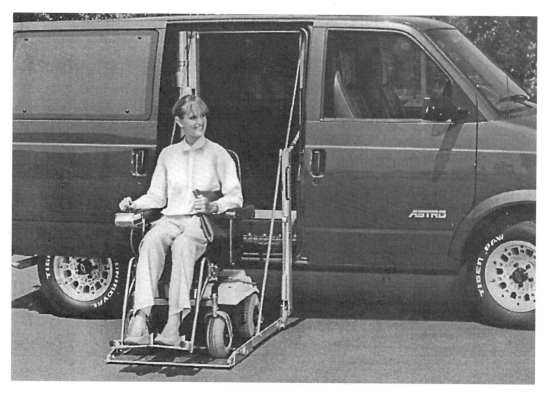

Fig. 8-4. Minivan with fold-out platform lift in lowered position.

Fold-Out Lift

In the fold-out platform lift, the platform folds out parallel to the ground and lowers like an elevator (Fig. 8-4). A safety guard is present to keep the wheelchair from rolling off. Switches and actuating devices are usually placed in accessible positions for the wheelchair user. When folded, the lift remains stationary and blocks the doorway. Platform lifts are now available that either split in the middle or fold in half and allow for ambulatory passengers to use this entrance/exit without deploying the lift.

Minivan Access System

Like vans, minivans are now being converted with a special system to allow people to drive from their wheelchairs. This includes an automatic door opener and fold-out ramp with a 10-inch lowered floor and "air kneel" suspension. When not in use, the folded ramp remains

positioned inside the doorway but can be disengaged and can swing away to allow for entry/exit of ambulatory passengers (Fig. 8-5).

INDICATIONS FOR VEHICLE MODIFICATIONS

Requirements for particular modifications in or on the vehicle are dictated by a thorough knowledge of the level of injury (if spinal cord damage has occurred), the extent of the disability (bone, joints, muscles, nerves, etc.), and whatever function remains. Consequently, three fundamental data bases must be derived: manual muscle tests, range of motion of joints, and activities of daily living (ADL) evaluations. Other considerations are related to the degree of brain damage and emotional stability, vocational requirements, and capability to satisfy the licensing laws of respective states. Social consequences to be considered relate to employment mobility, demands on family members, widening of recreational pursuits, and general encouragement of independence.

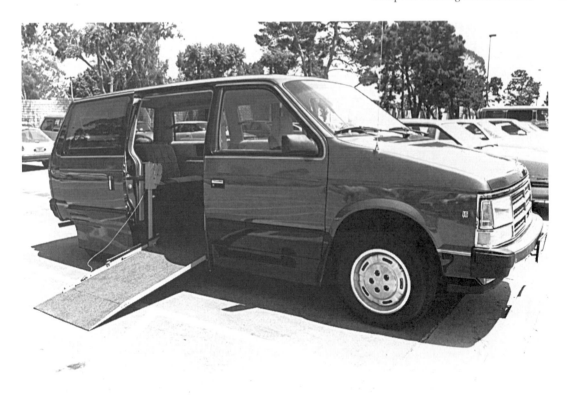

Fig. 8-5. Fold-out ramp in lowered position.

Upper Limb Impairment

When single or bilateral below-elbow amputees drive a vehicle, few adaptations are necessary. Using a prosthesis, the client may need certain dashboard functions modified with rings. An amputee ring steering device might also be needed. Automatic transmission is generally recommended.

An above-elbow amputee has a greater challenge when driving. The individual can use only one upper limb for steering and therefore would need a spinner knob for a steering device. For the right above-elbow amputee, tasks such as using the gearshift lever and turning on the ignition would be difficult. Devices such as a left-hand gearshift and a keyholder adapted for the left hand might be indicated. The person with a left above-elbow amputation may have difficulty using the turn signal lever or activating the left-hand parking brake. Devices such as a cross-over turn signal and a foot-operated or right-hand–operated parking brake lever may need to be added to the vehicle.

Bilateral above-elbow amputees cannot effectively operate the standard steering and dashboard functions and therefore require extensive vehicle modifications. The steering wheel and dash functions need to be relocated to the floor with special adaptations and must be operated by the feet.

In some cases, the person may have a disease or condition that limits the range of motion in the upper limbs. This can be caused by various types of arthritis or even quadriplegia. Adaptations made to the vehicle may include a steering column extension, smaller steering wheel, and relocation of dash controls to within the person's reach.

Lower Limb Impairment

The ability to operate the brake or accelerator pedals may depend on muscle strength in the leg or thigh muscles and also coordination of the lower limbs. Automatic transmission is needed in the case of a lower limb ampu-

Table 8-2. Recommended Match of Functional Disability to Adaptive Equipment

Functional Disability	Adaptive Driving Equipment
Right upper limb involvement	Steering device
	Left-hand gear shift
	Key adaptation
Left upper involvement	Steering device
	Cross-over turn signal
Bilateral upper limb involvement	Relocation of secondary control switches
	Foot-operated steering
	Electric gear shift
	Key adaptation or electric ignition
Right lower limb involvement	Left-foot accelerator pedal
Left lower limb involvement	Parking brake extension
Bilateral lower limb involvement	Hand controls for acceleration and braking
	Steering device
	Parking brake extension
Bilateral lower limb involvement and partial function of bilateral upper Limbs (i.e., quadriplegia)	Hand controls for acceleration and braking—possibly power-assisted controls
	Gear shift extension
	Steering device
	Reduced or zero-effort steering
	Relocation of secondary control switches
	Reduced or zero-effort brakes, if not power assisted
	Key adaptation
	Power ignition
	Electric gear shift
	Steering column extension
	Smaller diameter steering wheel

tation, and special consideration should be given to the individual's balance while driving a vehicle, depending on the level of the amputation. People with a left lower limb amputation may not experience any change in driving performance and usually do not need adaptations to their vehicles. Those with a right lower limb amputation, even prosthesis wearers, should not use their affected leg for acceleration and braking. A left-foot accelerator pedal should be used in those cases.

When both lower limbs are involved, such as with a high bilateral amputation, spina bifida, or paraplegia, acceleration and braking should be restricted to the upper limbs. Hand controls would be prescribed for these individuals. If the parking brake is foot operated, it will need an extension lever to allow for hand operation. The dimmer switch will also need to be hand operated.

Table 8-2 summarizes the adaptive driving equipment recommended for functional disabilities of the upper and lower limbs.

Spinal Impairments

The patient with arthrodesis of the spine poses a driving problem. The most common cause of total spine arthrodesis is rheumatoid spondylitis, and although patients with this disability can usually drive a car safely, they have difficulty checking vehicles to the right or left of them in their blind-spot range. By providing enough mirrors to give a 360-degree field of vision, this problem can be partly solved.

Patients with back pain may not require any special driving aids, but alteration of seating may be important. The average automobile seat is not well designed for the patient with low back pain, because the angle between the lower limbs and the spine is often such that it may well aggravate the back problem. Furthermore, automobile seats are often too soft for many patients. It may be necessary to install a firmer seat in the vehicle or, more simply, to use a spinal supporting device that can be placed on the seat. Usually, these devices are readily available and can be contoured to accommodate the lumbar spine in an optimal position.

Disabilities Associated With Incoordination

Persons with incoordination, rigidity, and other involuntary movements have difficulty controlling the steering wheel. Often, they cannot operate a vehicle safely. However, if involuntary motions are very mild, it may be possible for some such persons to drive a vehicle. If the involuntary movement or spasms are limited to the legs only, the individual may be able to drive with hand controls, while the legs are secured so that there is no interference with the "gas" and brake. With upper extremity involvement, a steering device, such as the V-grip or Tri-Pin may be used.

Disabilities With Impairment of Consciousness

Conditions in which there may be temporary loss of consciousness such as diabetes and epilepsy present a serious dilemma for licensing authorities and physicians who are asked to evaluate them. In giving permission to drive, the better the control of the condition that causes the disability and the more compliant the patient is with medical advice, the more liberal the advice should be. However, in many of these conditions, some patients exhibit genuine difficulty in remembering the hazards of failing to follow advice regarding their condition. Epileptics present a particularly complicated problem. Many authorities insist that no epileptic patient should be allowed to drive. This attitude has made it difficult to have an objective survey of the conditions of epileptics who drive automobiles; not only patients but also physicians, when asked for information, refuse to list the epileptic patients who drive a car. The general opinion seems to be that epileptic patients can be allowed to drive if they are under strict medical supervision, if it is proven that they take prescribed medication regularly, and if they have not had an episode of unconsciousness for at least 24 months.

DRIVER TRAINING

Automotive aids, by themselves, are not helpful without adequate training in their use. The disabled person, to operate the vehicle, must satisfy current and local driving regulations. Therefore, special driving instruction often is necessary, particularly when employment, social, and recreational goals are needed for independence. The ability to drive safely will determine whether the individual is an asset or burden to society.

Simulation of driving situations is widely employed in preliminary assessment of driving skills. Computerized devices are available to measure a person's ability to perform the basic control motions necessary in driving. Other tests consist of videotape presentations of driving situations to evaluate the driver's ability to perform visual-perceptual and decision-making tasks required to operate a vehicle safely in adverse conditions. Some driver training programs use especially adapted and equipped in-house vehicles that can simulate and actually measure road performance objectively. Because this equipment is very expensive, many driver trainers consider these systems a luxury, relying instead on their skill and experience in testing and training disabled drivers in real-life situations.

A conceptual outline of driver training for handicapped veterans was developed with much success at the Veterans Affairs Medical Center at Long Beach, California. It is an example of steps needed to examine and validate driving performance (Fig. 8-6).

Training programs are now widely available to help train driver teachers, examiners, and state official inspectors. These courses include didactic and practical instruction in testing, licensing, and evaluation to serve the special problems of the physically disabled. A list of adaptive driving resources, education programs, and associations is presented in Appendix 8-1.

RESEARCH IN AUTOMOTIVE MODIFICATIONS

Automotive modifications, practical and esthetic, are now used around the world, and significant research is being conducted in Sweden, Germany, Great Britain, and particularly, the United States. In particular, servo, or power-augmented, controls have been developed for easier operation of a van.

These assistive methods had been originally employed for braking and steering, but with increased demands, their use has widened with the physically impaired. One system has three degrees of freedom, providing backing, accelerating, and steering for the vehicle. The ignition and operation of all accessories, including doors, lift, and soon are accomplished by activating push buttons on a panel facing the driver. A small wheel on which the panel is attached actuates a direct linkage to the power brake servo valve, elimination foot-pedal push rods. When the wheel is pushed forward, acceleration occurs. Braking is accomplished by pulling backward. Steering is carried out by rotation.

As a result of servo mechanisms, it is possible to employ one ounce of energy to turn a wheel 90 degrees whereas previously six ounces were required. This is known by various terms: low-, minimal-, and "zero-effort" steering. Zero-effort systems are highly recommended for quadriplegic patients who have the required mobility but not the strength to operate conventional steering and braking controls.

Current information on adapted automobile research is available from a number of sources. Louisiana Tech

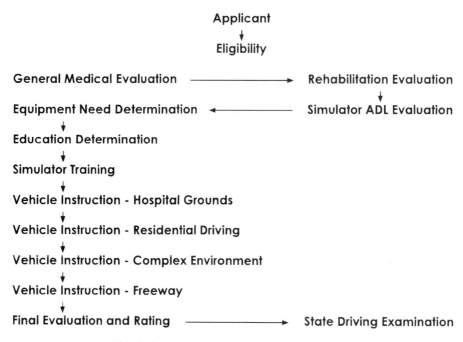

Fig. 8-6. Conceptual outline of driver training.

University Biomedical Engineering Center has been a site for research until recently. Currently, the University of Virginia Rehabilitation Engineering Center is a major site for research. Researchers there have a grant from the National Institute on Disability and Rehabilitation Research to study transportation needs of the disabled.

These centers are engaged in developing national standards in assessing performance; selecting and designing assistive devices and control systems; analysis of control devices for safety, reliability, and ergonomics; assessment of capability of disabled persons to match adaptive devices to their measured abilities; and driver training programs to rehabilitate disabled drivers for safe, reliable performance on streets and highways. For more information write to or telephone the following:

Louisiana Tech University Biomedical Engineering
P.O. Box 7923
Ruston, LA 71272
(318) 257-7562

Rehabilitation Engineering Center
Post Office Box 1885
Charlottesville, VA 22903
(804) 296-4216

Manufacturers of disabled driving equipment and suppliers of such equipment can also provide information concerning disabled driver education and adaptive driving resources. A selected group of these companies is listed in Appendix 8-2.

ACKNOWLEDGMENTS

For this chapter, assistance in updating information has been provided by James A. Guna, B.A., R.K.T., Charge Therapist, Driver Training Coordinator, Veterans Affairs Medical Center, Long Beach, California. We are also grateful to Mary M. Schwartz, O.T.R., who is in charge of driver evaluation and training program at the Rehabilitation Institute, Kansas City, Missouri, and Robert Newsome, Chief of Prosthetics Service, VA Medical Center, Kansas City, Missouri.

REFERENCE

1. Federal Register 40:15017, 1975

Adaptive Driving Resources and Associations

Adaptive Mobility Services
2201A E. Michigan St.
Orlando, FL 32856-0996
(407) 897-7074

American Automobile Association
1000 AAA Dr.
Heathrow, FL 32746-5063
(407) 444-7962

American Driver and Traffic Safety Education
  Association
IUP Highway Safety Center
Indiana, PA 15705-1092
(412) 357-4051

Association of Drivers Educators for the Disabled
P.O. Box 49
Edgerton, WI 53534
(608) 884-8833

The Chrysler Motors Physically Challenged Resource
  Center
P.O. Box 159
Detroit, MI 48288-0159
(800) 255-9877

The Department of Transportation
400 Seventh Street SW
Washington, DC 20591
(202) 366-4000 or (800) 424-9153
TDD (202) 755-8919 or (800) 424-9153

National Mobility Equipment Dealers Association
914 E. Skagway Ave.
Tampa, FL 33604
(813) 932-8566

RESNA
(An association for the advancement of assistive technology)
1700 N. Moor Street, Suite 1540
Arlington, VA 22209-1903

Society of Automotive Engineers
400 Commonwealth Dr.
Warrendale, PA 15096-0001

Transport Canada
Transportation Development Center
Complexe Guy Favreau
200 Dorchester St W. Suite 601
West Tower
Montreal, Quebec H27-1X4
Canada

Veteran's Administration
Prosthetic and Sensory Aids Service
810 Vermont Avenue NW
Washington, DC 20420
(202) 233-2011

Vendor/Manufacturer's Listing for Vehicle Adaptive Equipment

Bruce Ahnafield
President
Ahnafield Corporation
3219 W. Washington
Indianapolis, IN 46222
(317) 636-8061

Jeff Hermanson
1st Vice President
Braun Corporation
1014 W. Monticello
Winamac, IN 46996
(219) 946-6153

Jim Elliot
Sales Director
Collins Industry (Mobile Tech Corp.)
P.O. Box 2326
Hutchinson, KS 67504-2326
(316) 663-4441

Tom Stowers
President
Creative Controls Inc.
32450 Dequindre
Warren, MI 48092-5311
(810) 979-3500

Jerry Sirjord
Sales Manager
Crow River Industries, Inc.
14800 28th Ave., North
Minneapolis, MN 55447
(612) 559-1680

Sheldon Kronezk
President
Division Driving Systems, Inc.
9151 Hampton Overlook
Capital Heights, MD 20743
(301) 499-1000

Peter Ruprecht
Owner
Drive Master Corporation
9 Spielman Rd.
Fairfield, NJ 07004
(201) 808-9709

William E. Perry
President
Driving Aids Development Corporation
9417 Delancey Dr.
Vienna, VA 22182
(703) 938-6435

Bill Butt
Sales Representative
Driving Systems Inc.
16139 Runnymed St.
Van Nuys, CA 91406
(818) 782-6793
(Formerly MED VAN)

William Snyder
President
Electro Van Lift, Inc.
1915 W. County Road C
Roseyville, MN 55113
(612) 635-0655
(Complete Mobility)

Billy Ferguson
Vice President
Ferguson Auto Service
1112 N. Sheppard St.
Richmond, VA 23230
(804) 358-0006

Jan or Christine
Sales Representative
Gresham Driving Aids
P.O. Box 405
Wixom, MI 48393
(810) 624-1533
(800) 521-8930
FAX (810) 624-6358

Jerry Kittle
Owner
Handicaps, Inc.
4335 S. Santa Fe Dr.
Englewood, CO 80110
(303) 781-2062

William Hendrickson
President
Manufacturing & Product Service
7948 Ronson Rd.
San Diego, CA 92111
(619) 292-1423
(Has bought out Blatnik's Controls approved by VA
1982)

Curt Olson
General Manager
Mobility Products & Designs, Inc. (MPD)
148200 28th Ave. North

Minneapolis MN 55447-4834
(612) 559-1680
(Subsidiary of Crow River, Inc.)

Russ Gates
President
Originator Corporation
832 N West 1st St.
Fort Lauderdale, FL 33311
(305) 463-7231

Anthony Shamahs
President
Pick-a-Lift, Inc.
2051 E. Edgewood Dr.
Lakeland, FL 33803 (Company Address)
P.O. Box 1208 (Mailing Address)
Eaton Park, FL 33840
(813) 665-5355 or 666-5438

Linda Niederkohr
REB Manufacturing Company
P.O. Box 276
Carey, OH 43316-0276
(419) 396-7651

Terry Miller
Service Manager
Ricon Corporation
12450 Montague St.
Pacoima, CA 91331
(818) 899-7588
(800) 322-2884

Linda Galbraith
Sales Manager
Wells-Engberg Company
129 S. Phelps Ave., Suite 920
Rockford, IL 61108
P.O. Box 6388
Rockford, IL 61125
(815) 227-9765
(800) 642-3628

Thomas Wright
President/Owner
Wright-Way, Inc.
175 E. Interstate 30
P.O. Box 460907
Garland, TX 75046
(214) 240-8839

Adaptations in and to the Home Environment

Kirsten Kohlmeyer

9

Adaptive equipment is pervasive in our society. It is commercially available through stores, health-care facilities and catalogs (see Appendix 9-1). Health-care professionals also evaluate, train for, and make adaptive equipment. Many communities have exhibit areas for various pieces of adaptive equipment as a community service, not as a commercial venture.

It is very easy to get caught up in "gadget mania." Equipment can be costly and confusing to a client if not properly evaluated and presented. Third-party payers do not often cover smaller pieces of equipment. Commercial suppliers are helpful for replacing equipment and keeping abreast of new equipment on the market.

Specialized organizations and support groups can recommend diagnostic, specific equipment needs, and individuals who use them as personal contacts. Occupational therapists are specially trained in activity analysis and disability. They can train for adaptive techniques where specialized equipment may or may not be necessary. Occupational therapists also fabricate and issue adaptive equipment.

DEFINITIONS

The American Occupational Therapy Association[1] defines therapeutic adaptation as the design and restructuring of the physical environment to assist self-care, work, and play/leisure performance. This includes selecting, obtaining, fitting, and fabricating equipment, and instructing the client, family, and staff in proper use and care of equipment. Categories of therapeutic adaptation consist of orthotics, prosthetics, and assistive and adaptive equipment.[1]

By definition, a piece of assistive equipment gives support or aid, whereas adaptive equipment is made fit or suitable, often by modification.[2] Environmental adaptations are changes in physical space that facilitate access, mobility, and utility.

The goal of any piece of adaptive equipment, as well as environmental adaptation, is to maximize the person's desired participation in self-care, home, work, school, leisure, and community-based activities. Additional benefits may include health maintenance, energy conservation, and prevention of deformity.

This chapter examines commonly used assistive aids for a variety of disabilities. It addresses options for maximizing function, evaluation of fit, and interfacing adaptive equipment with the environment. Legislation affecting accessibility is outlined as well as a summary of recent home modification standards finalized by the American National Standards Institute (ANSI).

MAXIMIZING FUNCTION

Although a multitude of conditions that need orthoses and rehabilitation equipment exist (see Ch. 1, Table 1-1), several basic principles apply to a variety of disabilities:

1. Patients with range of motion limitations, such as those with amputation, burns, osteoarthritis or rheumatoid arthritis, and spinal cord injury, often need to compensate for lack of reach and joint excursion. Reachers, extended handles, and Velcro closures are several options.
2. For patients with decreased strength and endurance, such as those with cardiac disorders, chronic obstructive pulmonary disease, and multiple sclerosis, compensation principles include the use of lightweight or electrical devices and energy conservation techniques such as improving leverage in body mechanics.
3. Patients who have tremors, ataxia, and athetoid choreiform movements, sometimes seen in cerebral palsy, multiple sclerosis, or traumatic head injury may have significantly impaired coordination.

Stabilizing proximal limb segments, weighing distal segments, and provision of a safe environment help compensate for lack of balance and fine motor skill.

4. Those with decreased hand function, such as brachial plexus injury, burns, rheumatoid arthritis, and spinal cord injury, often use orthoses, universal cuffs, and/or straps to perform activities of daily living.
5. For patients with hemiplegic paralysis and those with upper extremity amputation(s), major compensation techniques include stabilization such as securing objects with Dycem or adaptive techniques to substitute for the role previously assumed by the affected side.[3]

Tables 9-1 to 9-3 list equipment options for personal care, communication, leisure, and home management activities. To use Tables 9-1 to 9-3, the reader should assess the patient's deficits in both a general and specific manner and then match this assessment with the suggested adaptive or assistive equipment under the appropriate headings of personal care, communication, or desired leisure or home management activities.

Table 9-1. Personal Care

Deficit Areas	Eating	Oral Facial Hygiene	Dressing	Toileting/Bathing
Range of motion	Universal cuff Elongated handles Built-up handles Cup holder Long straw/straw clip Plate guard Scoop dish	Sunbeam dental care system Electric toothbrush Water Pik Extended handles Extended comb/brush Hand-held shower Extended faucet handles Shampoo basin (for care giver)	Front-opening garments Large buttons Zipper pull Velcro fasteners Button hook Long shoe horn Reacher Sock aid/donner Dressing stick Elastic shoelaces	Reacher Spray deodorant Long-handled sponge/toilet aid Long-handled skin inspection mirror Hand-held shower Terry cloth robe (for drying) Raised toilet/tub seat Safety rails
Strength/arm placement	Balanced forearm orthosis Swedish sling/overhead suspension sling Lightweight utensils Serrated knife Water bottle Quad feeder Long straw/straw clip	Balanced forearm orthosis Swedish sling/overhead suspension sling Hand-held shower Extended faucet handles Lightweight comb/brush Razor holder Soap on a rope	Large buttons Velcro fasteners Dressing stick Leg lifters/loops Sock aid/donner Bed/dressing ladder	Hand-held shower Long-handled sponge Soap on a rope Lever soap dispenser

Continues

Table 9-1. (*Continued*)

Deficit Areas	Eating	Oral Facial Hygiene	Dressing	Toileting/Bathing
Coordination/ balance	Dycem Weighted utensils Weighted forearm cuffs Swivel utensils Long straw/straw guard Covered glass/sipping spout Rocker knife Scoop dish Friction mobile arm support	Wash mitt Soap stabilizer Soap on a rope Level faucets Suction brush for nail/ denture care Electric toothbrush Electric razor Shaving cream dispenser handle Shampoo dispenser Hair-dryer adapted with gooseneck	Front opening garments Large buttons Velcro closers Built-up button hook Elastic waists Zipper pull Elastic shoelaces	Roll-on deodorant Bath mitt Nonskid bath mat Bath seat/tub bench Hand-held shower Soap on a rope Safety rails Leg separator
Hand function	Dycem Adapted utensils (built-up handle, swivel, bent) Universal cuff Quad grip knife Sandwich holder Wrist–hand orthosis (WHO) Hand Orthosis (HO)	Built-up handles Universal cuff Denture brush Floss holder Shaving cream dispenser handle Shampoo dispenser Makeup basket Soap on a rope	Velcro closures Loops/rings Zipper pull cuff Thumb loop Button hook Elastic shoelaces W/c Gloves (for friction)	Terry cloth robe (for drying) Towel with loops Bath mitt Soap on a rope Skin inspection mirror Adapted catheter clamp Pneumatic/electric leg bag clamp Digital stimulator Suppository inserter
One-hand activities	Rocker knife Plate guard Dycem	Wash mitt Suction nail/denture brush Soap on a rope	Large, front-opening garments Velcro closures Button hook Reacher Dressing stick Long shoe horn	Wash mitt Long-handled sponge Soap on a rope Spray deodorant
Endurance	Flat-base utensils Lightweight utensils Balanced forearm orthosis	Electric toothbrush Lightweight comb/brush Balanced forearm orthosis	Reacher Dressing stick Long shoe horn Elastic shoelaces	Bath seat/tub bench Safety rail Hand-held shower

(Adapted from Kohlmeyer,[3] with permission.)

EVALUATION OF FIT

Before deciding to introduce, loan, or issue adaptive equipment, the health-care professional considers numerous factors. Do the patient, family, and/or care giver understand the purpose of the device to ensure proper use and carryover outside of the health-care setting? Is the equipment too difficult to obtain, don/doff, or use, although it ultimately may facilitate task performance? Does the patient want to use the equipment? Are there sociocultural issues to consider? What are the economic factors such as cost and reimbursement? Technologic sophistication not only affects cost and reimbursement but also future acquisition and repair needs.

(*Text continues on p. 240*)

Table 9-2. Communication and Leisure

Deficit Areas	Reading	Writing/Typing	Telephone Use	Games/Hobbies/Arts and Crafts/Sports
Range of motion	Electric page turner Mouthstick Book holder	Built-up pens/pencils Electric typewriter Word processor Typing sticks	Speaker phone Environmental control unit Push button Clip receiver holder	Mouthstick activities Bowling ball ramp Embroidery hoop Built-up handles
Strength/Arm placement	Electric page turner Mouthstick Book holder Balanced forearm orthosis Swedish sling Head wand	Inverted pencil in universal cuff Typing sticks Built-up pens/felt tip Stabilized clipboard Electric typewriter with self-correcting ribbon Mouthstick with interchangeable tips	Speaker phone Head set Mouthstick Gooseneck phone holder Environmental control unit	Mouthstick activities Pneumatic control camera W/c camera tripod holder Trigger release archery Built-up handles for pencil/brush grips Raised gardening Bowling ball ramp
Coordinator/ balance	Dycem Book holder	Typewriter holder Keyguard Weighted/enlarged pencil or pan Felt-tip Stabilized clipboard	Gooseneck phone holder Shoulder rest Large push buttons	Magnetic playing cards and board Enlarged/weighted game pieces Card holder Automatic card shuffler W/c bowling ball holder and ramp Chest strap/body harness Easy kneeler/seat
Hand function	Page turner Universal cuff with pencil inverted Pen holder with inverted pencil attached to orthosis Rubber "finger" Book holder	Wanchik Writer Writing frame The artwriter Figure-of-eight writing splint Universal cuff with pencil inverted Pen holder	Large push buttons Phone holder (shoulder or gooseneck) Speaker phone Universal cuff with pencil inverted Clip receiver holder	Spring-loaded cue stick Quad grip frisbee Universal cuff Velcro straps/grip Enlarged game pieces Spring-loaded bowling ball Orthosis with utensil slot and vertical holder with inverted pencil Clamp frames
One-hand activities	Book holder	Stabilized clipboard Paper weight	Receiver holder (stand or shoulder)	Embroidery hoop Knitting needle holder Card holder Recreation Belt Electric retrieve fishing reel W/c bowling ball holder Bowling ball ramp
Endurance	Book holder Electric page turner	Built-up pens/pencils	Portable cordless phone Phone holder	Built-up handles Camera holder Embroidery hoop Clamp frames Easy kneeler/seat Bowling ball ramp

(Adapted from Kohlmeyer,[3] with permission.)

Table 9-3. Home Management

Deficit Areas	Meal Prep/Clean-Up	Cleaning/Laundry	Environmental Control
Range of motion	Reacher Nonslip mats Lightweight utensils Sponge cloth mitt Countertop appliances	Extended handles for dustpans/mops Self-ringing mop lever Long-handled feather duster	Electric scissors Key holder Lever doorknob extension Reacher Environmental control unit
Strength/arm placement	Pan stabilizer Mirror over stove (if sitting) Push–pull oven rack piece Countertop appliances	Reacher Front-loading machines Extended handles for dustpans/mops Long-handled feather duster	Environmental control unit Automatic door opener Pad/rocker switch Light-touch controls
Coordination/ balance	Pots with bilateral handles Dycem/nonskid mat Cutting board with rails, suction cup feet and corner stabilizer Pot stabilizer Wall-mounted jar opener Heavy utensils/bowls Electrical appliances Countertop appliances Long oven mitts	Suction bottle brush Dust mitts Wheeled cart Heavy, upright vacuum	Lever door handle Friction tape/rubber-covered door handle Key holder Pad/rocker switch Environmental control unit
Hand function	Wrist loop/strap Modified handles with high-temperature plastic Rocker knife Electric can opener Box topper Carton holder	Wash mitt Liquid soap dispenser Automatic faucet Faucet-mounted spray attachment Built-up/cuff handles on duster	Loop scissors Quick clip scissors Key holder Pad/rocker switch Light-touch controls Lever handles Environmental control unit
One-hand activities	Dycem Suction devices Stabilized jar opener One-handed can opener One-handed rolling pin One-handed beater Cutting board with rails, suction cup feet, corner stabilizer	Standard equipment	Standard equipment Environmental control unit
Endurance	Pull-out shelves Lazy Susans Vertical storage Lightweight utensils Electrical appliances Wheeled utility cart	Self-propelled vacuum Wheeled service cart Permanent press clothing Dishwasher	Standard equipment Environmental control unit

(Adapted from Kohlmeyer,[3] with permission.)

Is the equipment clinically necessary? For example, various lower extremity handling/dressing techniques used by paraplegic or quadriplegic individuals may negate the need for dressing sticks, reachers, long-handled shoe horns, or leg lifters.

Often, adaptive techniques suffice for task performance rather than adaptive equipment. Ultimately, adaptive equipment should be reliable, facilitate performance, increase safety, and decrease time and/or energy expenditure. Temporary devices may be appropriate during the rehabilitation phase when a patient's functional abilities are changing.[4–9]

The most important basis for evaluating adaptive equipment is whether it satisfies the need(s) of the consumer from the consumer's viewpoint. Batavia and Hammer[10] identified four key evaluation and selection criteria for long-term users of assistive devices:

1. Effectiveness—the extent to which the function of the device improves one's living situation; functional capability or independence
2. Affordability—the extent to which the purchase, maintenance or repair of the device causes financial difficulty
3. Operability—the extent to which the device is easy to operate and responds adequately to demands
4. Dependability—the extent to which the device operates with repeatable and predictable levels of accuracy under conditions of reasonable use

These principles apply to all pieces of equipment regardless of cost and function. The relationship between the health professional and patient should be a partnership, with the pros and cons of equipment options presented candidly and discussed thoroughly. Sufficient time should be allocated for training before a definitive decision is made. Last, the provider should schedule follow-up services to meet the patient's changing needs.

INTERFACING ADAPTIVE EQUIPMENT WITH THE ENVIRONMENT

Patients need to be able to use their equipment in a variety of environments. What is functional in the rehabilitation treatment setting may not work at home or on the job. If equipment proves useless, money spent will be wasted. This financial loss might include cost of the equipment, time spent in training sessions, and indirectly, nonproductive time spent in the home, work, and/or community setting.

Categories

Adaptive equipment can be categorized in a number of ways:

1. Disposable medical products—medical, nursing, and urinary supplies
2. Daily living products—personal hygiene and self-help devices
3. Prosthetic/orthotic devices
4. Durable medical products—wheelchairs, crutches, and bathing equipment
5. Accessibility products—lifts, ramps, and hand controls

Because the home is the base of operations for daily living, the home environment is of utmost importance in the course of rehabilitation.

In reviewing the home setting, those providing adaptive equipment must consider the need for equipment changes, replacement, maneuverability, and storage.[11] An accessible environment may eliminate the need for some adaptive equipment.

Legislation

In attempting to define *accessible,* a review of legislation affecting environmental adaptation is in order. Legislation in the United States affecting accessibility includes the Architectural Barriers Act of 1968, Federal Rehabilitation Act of 1973, Comprehensive Rehabilitation Services Amendment of 1978, Fair Housing Amendment Act of 1988, and American With Disabilities Act (ADA) of 1990.

The Architectural Barriers Act of 1968 was the first federal legislation in the United States to require federally funded building projects to be accessible to people with physical disabilities.[12,13] The Federal Rehabilitation Act of 1973 further mandated that any institution receiving federal funds could not discriminate against people with disabilities because of existing architectural barriers.[14] The Architectural and Transportation Barriers Compliance Board was created to enforce provisions of the Rehabilitation Act. Federal legislatures passed the Comprehensive Rehabilitation Services Amendment in 1978 because of inadequate compliance with the Rehabilitation Act.

Uniform Federal Accessibility Standards were developed to be consistent with the Standards of the ANSI to establish accessibility guidelines.[12,15] The Fair Housing Amendment Act of 1988 extended the coverage of Title VIII of the Civil Rights Act of 1968 to prohibit discriminatory housing.[16]

The ADA, signed into Public Law 101-336 on July 26, 1990, is one of the most important pieces of legislation for people with disabilities in United States history. Based on the Civil Rights Act of 1964, the ADA significantly expands rights created by Title V of the Rehabilitation Act of 1973 in the areas of employment, public services and transportation, public accommodations, and telecommunication.[10,17–22]

Standards and Guidelines

Application of accessibility standards (considered as minimal guidelines in environmental planning) should be individualized, regardless of the environmental setting. In general, when adapting the home environment, four possibilities are (1) modifying the existing home to provide an accessible environment within a reasonable time and expense; (2) expanding the existing home to achieve desired results; (3) relocating to an existing home that may or may not need modification; and (4) designing and building a new home to suit the individual's needs. Factors to be considered when evaluating daily functions, space requirements, and modification or design of the home include general access, bathing/toileting, eating, general circulation and living space, and sleeping and transportation.[11] This chapter uses the revised ANSI Standards (1992)[15] as guidelines when making recommendations for environmental modifications.

GENERAL ACCESS

Dimensions

Tables 9-4 to 9-6 provide suggested dimensions for access to buildings, bathrooms, and kitchens.

Table 9-4. Considerations for General Access

Access	Specifications
Ramps	Slope/rise no steeper than 1:12 (new construction); maximum 1:30
	Width 36-inch minimum
	Landings 60 × 60 inches; at least as wide as widest ramp run leading to it
	Handrails 34–38 inches vertically required if rise 6 inches, >72 inches; circular cross section $1\frac{1}{4}$–2 inches; extended 12 inches beyond top and bottom of ramp runs
Stairs	Trends 11 inches deep, risers 4–7 inches
	Nosings 60-degree angle from horizontal; $1\frac{1}{2}$-inch maximal protrusion
	Handrails continuous full length; 34–38 inches above nosings; $1\frac{1}{2}$ inches from wall, extended 12 inches beyond, circular cross section $1\frac{1}{4}$–2 inches
Elevators	Call buttons centered at 42 inches above the floor, $\frac{3}{4}$-inch minimum in size
	Hall signals visible, audible, 72 inches above floor, $2\frac{1}{2}$-inches minimum in size
	Dimensions sufficient space to enter, maneuver to reach controls and exit
	Door protective/reopening device; open/close automatically (reopening device in effect minimum 20 s)
Wheelchair lift	Clear floor space 30 × 40 inches
	Forward approach 36 inches (when depth >10 inches)
	Parallel approach 60 inches (when depth >10 inches)
	Floor surface stable, firm, slip resistant
	Gratings less than $1\frac{1}{2}$ inches in one direction
	Operable parts within reach ranges
Doors/doorways	Clear width 32 inches with door open 90 degrees
	Thresholds $\frac{1}{2}$-inch maximum
	Door hardware easy to grasp; 3–4-feet height
	Door opening force 5.0 lb

Ramps

Ramps are essential for wheelchair users if elevators or lifts are not available to connect different levels. A wheelchair user's ability to manage an incline is related to both its slope and length. Ramps are recommended to be straight with the least possible slope. Level rest plat-

Table 9-5. Considerations for Bathrooms

Item	Specifications
Room	Clear floor space, unobstructed turning space, 60-inch diameter minimum
Toilet	Height 15–19 inches
	Mounted adjacent to side wall or partition with 18-inch minimum clearance to and from centerline of toilet to sink; 18-inch minimum from centerline of toilet to wall
	48-inch minimum clear space in front of the bowl and from side wall
Countertops and sink	Clear floor space 30 × 48-inch minimum in front; 19-inch maximum underneath
	Knee and toe clearances: Fixtures extend 17-inch minimum from wall between bottom & front edge of counter and floor; 29-inch minimum clear knee space
	Exposed pipes and surfaces covered
	Countertop mounted with rim 34-inch maximum above floor with clearance of 29-inch minimum from floor to bottom of front edge
	Sink mounted with counter or rim 34-inch maximum above floor; 6½-inch deep maximum
Shower	Transfer type with fixed bench
	Shower unit hose 60-inch minimum used as fixed shower head or hand-held shower
	Controls mounted on side wall opposite seat 38 to 48 inches above the floor
	Enclosures should not obstruct controls or transfers
	Grab bars should be across control wall and back wall to a point 18 inches from control wall
	Dimensions 36 × 36 inches with clear floor space of 36 × 48 inches
	Threshold maximum ½ inch
	Transfer type without fixed bench
	Same as above with exception: seat should be folding or nonfolding; L-shaped in transfer-type stalls mounted 17–19 inches above bathroom floor; extend full depth of floor
	Roll-in
	Same as above with exception
	30 × 60-inch inside dimensions
	Clear floor space 36 × 60 inches
	Grab bars on three walls of the shower
	Controls on back wall 38 × 48 inches above shower floor
Bathtub	Clear floor space in front 30 × 60-inch minimum for parallel approach; 48 × 60-inch minimum for forward approach; 30 × 93-inch minimum when seat is provided at head of tub
	Rim height 17–19 inches from floor to top of rim
	Shower unit provided with 60-inch hose minimum used as a fixed shower head or hand-held shower
	Seats and other structural attachments able to withstand 250 lb of vertical or horizontal force
	Grab bars with permanent seat 48 inches long along back wall, 15 inches on head end wall, 12 inches on foot end wall
	Grab bars without permanent seat 24 inches long along back wall, 24 inches on head end wall, 12 inches on foot end wall
Accessories	Mirror: bottom edge of reflecting surface 38 inches maximum above floor
	Cabinet: 44 inches maximum above floor inches
	Water controls
	33–36 inches above the floor located between rim of tub and grab bar at foot of tub
	Force required to activate 5 lb maximum
	Grab bars: 33–36 inches above the floor; able to withstand 250 lb of pressure
	Towel racks: 33–36 inches above the floor

Table 9-6. Considerations for Kitchens

Item	Specifications
Clearance	40-inch minimum between counters and opposing base cabinets, countertops, appliances, or walls
	60-inch minimum as above in U-shaped kitchens
Clear floor space	30 × 48-inch minimum for forward or parallel approach extend 19 inches maximum underneath counter
Work surface	At least one 30-inch wide minimum section of counter with 28–36-inch height from floor
	Base cabinets shall be removable under full 30-inch minimum frontage of the counter
	Knee space clear width of 30 inches minimum
Sink	28–36 inches in height from floor to top of counter surface
	6½-inch deep bowl maximum
	Faucets operable with one hand, no tight grasping, maximum force required 5 lb
Rangers and cooktops	Clear floor space as above; controls should not require reaching over burners
Ovens	Clear floor space as above
	30-inch clear knee space
	Controls on front panels
Refrigerator/ freezers	Clear floor space as above
	Side-by-side model should have 50% of freezer space and 50% of refrigerator space located 54 inches maximum above floor
	Other combination refrigerators and freezers should have at least 50% of freezer space and 100% of refrigerator space and controls 54 inches maximum above the floor
Dishwashers	Clear floor space same as above
	All rack space accessible
Storage	Cabinets, drawers, and shelf storage should have standard clear floor space; accessible storage spaces should be within reach ranges
	Forward unobstructed, 15–48 inches
	Forward obstructed, 0–26 (48) inches, 20–25 (44) inches
	Side unobstructed, 15–54 inches
	Side obstructed, 46 provided height of obstruction from floor is 34 inches and depth is 24 inches maximum

forms are necessary at 10-foot intervals for ascent/descent on a long or curved ramp. Continuous handrails should be installed with curbs on both sides so that the wheelchair does not run off the ramp. The ramp must have a nonskid surface and protection from the elements if possible (Fig. 9-1).

Stairs

Individuals using crutches or canes often prefer stairs. All steps on a flight of stairs should have uniform riser heights and tread depth. Undersides of nosings should not be abrupt and handrails should be provided.

Elevators

Some companies manufacture residential elevators to accommodate wheelchair users who need access between floors. Elevator doors should remain open for a sufficient duration, and their closing movement should stop when a person or object exerts sufficient force at any point on the door edge. Door and signal timing for all calls, inside dimensions of the elevator car, location of car controls, and an emergency communication system should meet individual needs.

Mechanical Lifts

The wheelchair user may require a mechanical lift where several stairs exist and space for ramps is not available. Vertical lifts are placed at the bottom of the stairs and

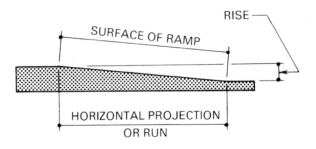

	Maximum Rise		Maximum Horizontal Projection	
Slope	in	mm	ft	m
1:12 to 1:15	30	760	30	9
1:16 to 1:19	30	760	40	12
1:20	30	760	50	15

Fig. 9-1. Components of a single ramp run and single ramp dimensions. (From Council of American Building Officials,[15] with permission.)

often require an upper landing to meet them. Inclined platform lifts are either post-mounted on tracks along the stairs or on the wall(s) or stairs themselves. For safety, both these lifts may have enclosing walls and interlocked gates. Chair lifts have built-in seats for individuals who are not wheelchair users but have difficulty climbing stairs.

Doorways and Doors

The minimum clear width opening for a doorway is 32 inches. Greater widths are needed if competing traffic is leaving, if sudden or frequent movements are needed, or if the wheelchair is to be turned at an opening. The provider should consider crutch extension and space for arms and hands, bulky clothing, and wheelchair accessories. Figure 9-2 shows typical dimensions of adult-sized wheelchairs. Thresholds should be minimal in height and hardware easy to grasp (i.e., lever-operated, push-type or U-shaped mechanisms). Side-hung doors may be suitable for individuals with limited arm placement and hand functions. Remote controls may be needed by others.

Types of doors to consider include hinged (regular or fold-back), pocket-sliding, sliding, folding (i.e., accordion-type), and automatic or pulley-operated openers and closers. Kickplates or doors reduce required maintenance by withstanding abuse from wheelchairs, walkers, or canes.

Bathroom

Generally, one can modify an existing bathroom with the adaptation of a shower chair, tub bench, grab bars, and hand-held shower for patients who can transfer themselves. If feasible, another bathroom style is that of a roll-in shower, which allows an individual or an attendant to wheel a shower wheelchair directly into the bathroom. Bathroom space should be safe and efficient. Table 9-5 shows suggested dimensions.

Toilet

Preferences for toilet seat heights vary considerably, ranging from 15 to 19 inches. Various designs of seats and filler rings are available in various designs to allow

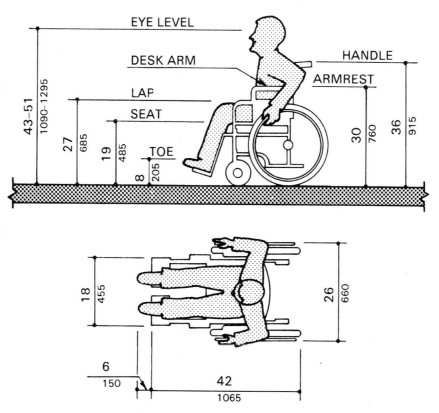

Fig. 9-2. Dimensions of adult-sized wheelchairs. Footrests may extend farther for very large people. (From Council of American Building Officials,[15] with permission.)

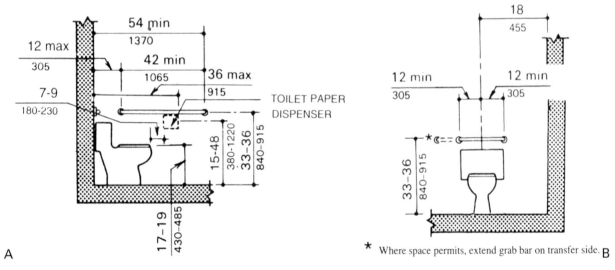

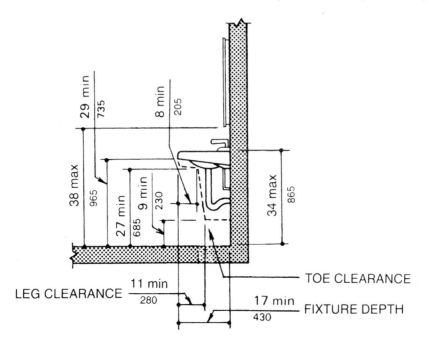

Fig. 9-3.   Toilet dimensions. **(A)** Side view; **(B)** front view. (From Council of American Building Officials,[15] with permission.)

for bowel/bladder programs and personal hygiene. Ample floor space should be available around the toilet for safe transfers whether assisted or unassisted. Grab bars should maximize a person's ability to move independently; flush controls should be operable and within reach (Fig. 9-3).

Countertops and Sinks
Built-in sinks should be placed close to the front edge of the countertop. Water supply and drain pipes should be insulated to prevent burns. If space allows, a work surface on the counter and storage for supplies often facilitates performance of personal hygiene (Fig. 9-4).

Fig. 9-4.   Leg clearances for countertops and sinks. Dashed line indicates dimensional clearance for optional under-fixture enclosure. (From Council of American Building Officials,[15] with permission.)

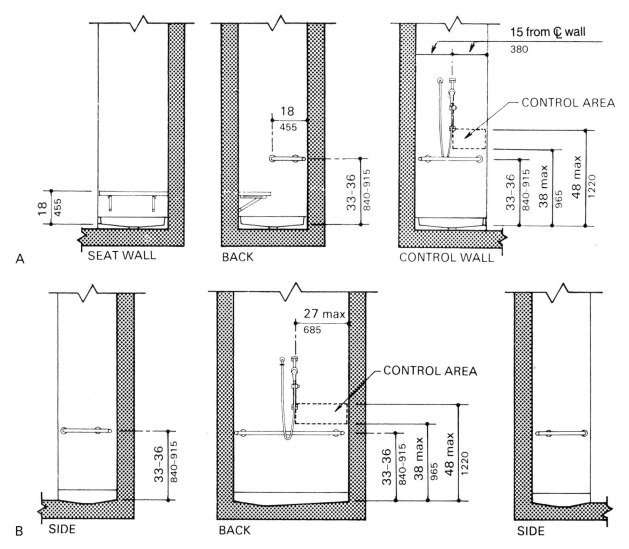

Fig. 9-5.   Grab bars at shower stalls. **(A)** A 36-inch by 36-inch stall; **(B)** a 30-inch by 60-inch stall. Shower head and control area may be on back wall (as shown) or on either side wall. (From Council of American Building Officials,[15] with permission.)

Showers

Three typical shower designs exist: transfer-type showers with a fixed bench and grab bars, roll-in with grab bars, and roll-in with a removable bench. A recessed shelf is helpful in all cases as is a hand-held shower with scald control. An angle-lever type handle should be used (Fig. 9-5).

Bathtub

Tub benches, bathtub seats, portable seats, built-in seats, and hydraulic seats can facilitate a transfer into the bathtub. Bathmats, friction strips, and grab bars also increase

safety. A hand-held shower with scald control and recessed shelving for supplies add to the individual's convenience (Fig. 9-6).

Accessories

If mirrors are to be used by ambulatory people as well as wheelchair users, their height at the topmost edge should be 74 inches. A single, full-length mirror accommodates all people. Medicine cabinets should also have easy access, generally with the bottom of the cabinet located 36 inches from the floor. The most convenient type of cabinets are mounted to the leading edge of the

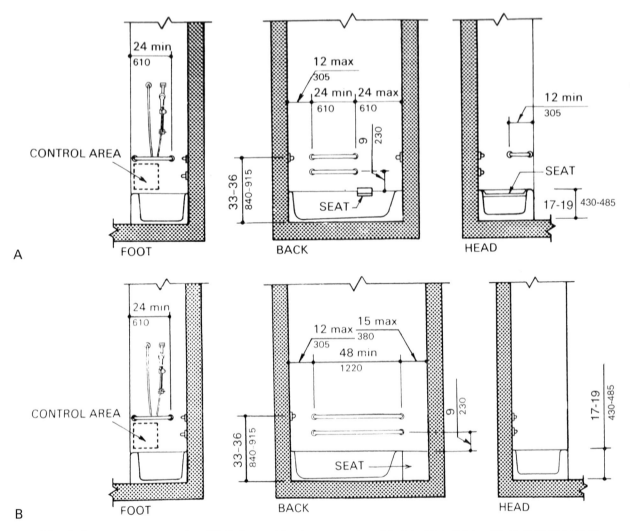

Fig. 9-6. Bathtub accessories. **(A)** Bathtub without permanent seat in tub; **(B)** bathtub with permanent seat at head of tub. (From Council of American Building Officials,[15] with permission.)

sink or vanity and recessed with single row storage. Valves with single-handle control and a lever blade shape that mixes the water to control temperature and adjust flow are recommended for water controls. Pressure balance and thermostatic control are essential safety features. One should mount grab bars 32 inches from the floor; however, the height may vary depending on an individual's transfer style, body mechanics, and equipment used. Grab bars, towel racks, and soap dishes should be positioned within easy reach and secured to withstand 250 pounds of pressure.

Kitchen

It is imperative to have unobstructed space around the refrigerator, sink, stove, and table. The floor should be smooth with nonskid surface. A U- or L-shaped design is often most efficient for a wheelchair user. Figures 9-7 to 9-10 and Table 9-6 show suggested reach dimensions.

Counters

Counter height is typically 30 to 33 inches with knee clearance underneath (Fig. 9-11).

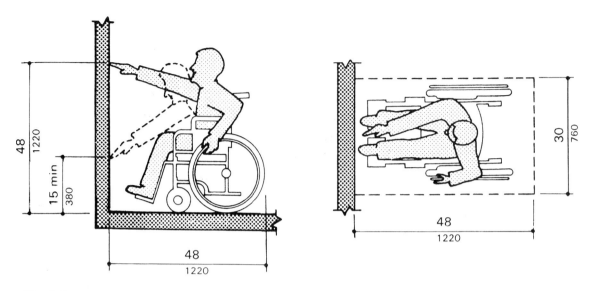

Fig. 9-7. Unobstructed forward reach limit. (From Council of American Building Officials,[15] with permission.)

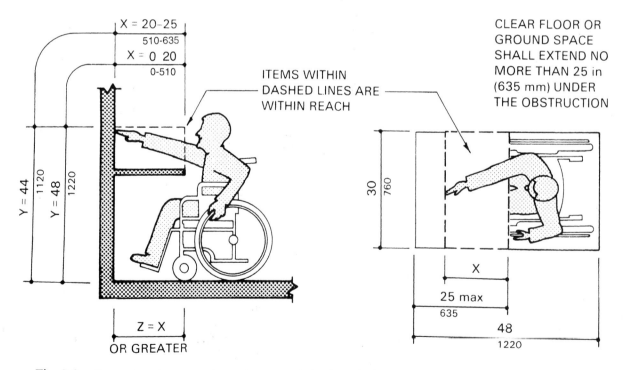

Fig. 9-8. Forward reach over an obstruction. x, reach depth; y, reach height; z, clear knee space (the clear space below the obstruction, which should be at least as deep as the reach distance, x). (From Council of American Building Officials,[15] with permission.)

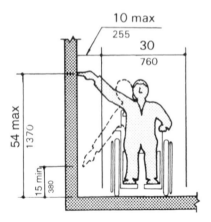

Fig. 9-9. Unobstructed side reach limit. (From Council of American Building Officials,[15] with permission.)

Sinks

Sinks should be no deeper than 6½ inches with a swivel arm lever faucet. A spray attachment and garbage disposal are helpful for cleanup. Knee space under the sink should be adequate, and all pipes should be insulated. Persons with impaired sensation benefit from a scald control. A work surface adjacent to the sink and/or a cutting board is helpful for efficiency and energy conservation.

Refrigerator

A two-door, side-by-side model allows for variations in reach for everyone. If a standard one-door refrigerator is the only option, it is helpful to have a bottom freezer. The most convenient refrigerators are self-defrosting models.

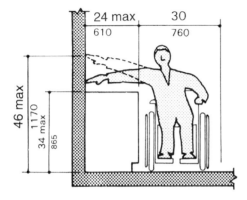

Fig. 9-10. Obstructed side reach limit. (From Council of American Building Officials,[15] with permission.)

Cooktop

Burners should be arranged in a single row and flush to adjacent surfaces to allow for sliding of pots and pans. No knee space should be allowed, because of the danger of spills, and controls should be located in front.

Oven

Controls should be located on the front panel of the oven. A built-in oven with a side-hung door is often more accessible than an oven with a drop door. A pullout board can be useful for both food preparation and transfer to prevent accidental removal. Oven shelves should have nontip stops.

Cabinets and Shelves

Hardware on doors, pullout boards, and drawers should be easily operated by those with impaired hand function. Pullout shelves with single-row storage can be installed. A kitchen tray cabinet on wheels is also helpful in transporting and storing objects. Cabinet base(s) should accommodate wheelchair footrests. Accessible lighting under cabinets as well as receptacles for hanging utensils are also convenient.

GENERAL CIRCULATION AND LIVING SPACE

Ground and Floor Surfaces

Surfaces of accessible routes and in accessible rooms should be stable, firm, and slip resistant. Although the static coefficient of friction is the basis of slip resistance, a generally accepted method to evaluate slip resistance of walking surfaces for all conditions does not exist. Feasible options for nonskid surfaces include wood, vinyl, and specifically treated tile. Carpeted surfaces should have a level loop or textured loop with level-cut pile or pile texture no greater than ½ inch. Gratings with long openings should be placed perpendicular to the dominant direction of travel and have openings no greater than ½ inch. A change in level of a walking surface greater than ¼ inch requires slope/edge treatment.

Hallways/Accessible Routes

To allow for easy access to and egress from adjoining rooms, hallways should be 4 feet wide (minimum is 3

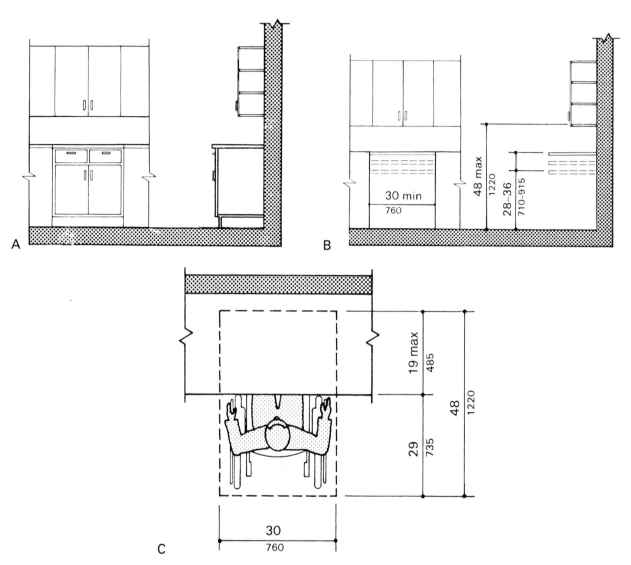

Fig. 9-11. Counter work surface. **(A)** Before removal of cabinets and base; **(B)** cabinets and base removed and height alternatives; **(C)** clear floor space under work surface. (From Council of American Building Officials,[15] with permission.)

feet) wherever possible. Where narrow hallways exist, door hardware, hinging mechanism, and/or size can be changed to facilitate easy movement. Adequate turning space at the beginning and end of each hallway is desirable. To make a 180-degree turn, a wheelchair requires the following minimum dimensions: a clear space of 60-inch diameter or a T-shaped space within a 60-inch square with arms 36 inches wide and 60 inches long. Turning space must also include knee and toe clearance.

Clients in different types of wheelchairs will have different space needs (Fig. 9-12).

For safety reasons, the living environment should have at least two accessible routes for entrances and exits. An emergency evacuation plan should exist in case of fire, with preparations made for detecting and dealing with the fire as well as contacting emergency personnel. Backup for electrical equipment such as a movable ramp may be necessary.

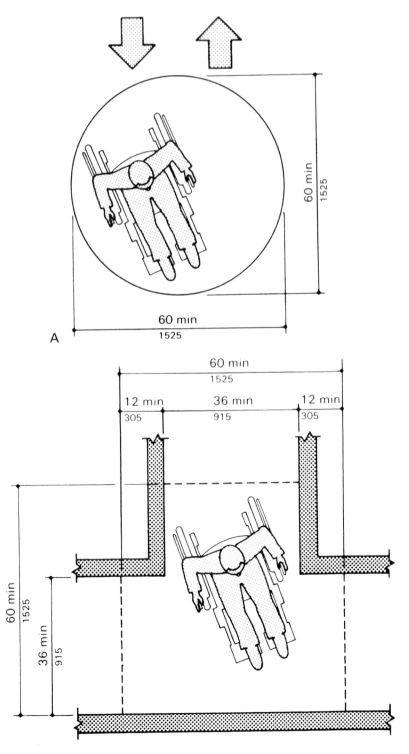

Fig. 9-12.   Wheelchair turning space. **(A)** A 60-inch-diameter space; **(B)** a T-shaped space for 180-degree turn. Dashed lines indicate minimum length of clear space required on each arm of the T-shaped space in order to complete the turn. (From Council of American Building Officials,[15] with permission.)

Walls should be made of easy-maintenance materials. Clear plastic corner edging and shields can be used in hard wear areas such as corners and where wheelchair footrests touch the walls.[11]

General Living Space

Windows should be easy to operate and open outward when possible. It is easier to operate double-hung and horizontal sliding windows than casement or awning windows that have cranks. Light switches should be placed within accessible reach at the point of entry to all rooms, staircases, and hallways. Rocker switches or light switch extenders can be used for individuals with impaired hand function. Remote control switches are available from hardware stores or could be used from an environmental control unit. Lighting needs to be safe and functional both inside the house and out. Table lamps should have a wide base of support; pull chains or pressure-sensitive switches may be helpful. Receptacles should be unobstructed and accessible. Fuses and circuit-breaker switches should be within easy reach. To control a variety of minor appliances, an electric tabletop strip console of switches and outlets can be used. Adequate and accessible heating and air conditioning should be available, especially for individuals who have difficulty with temperature regulation. A central vacuum cleaning system may eliminate the challenge of using a vacuum cleaner from a wheelchair as well as make the environment more tolerable for individuals with respiratory problems. Last, one should also consider the ease of providing recreation within the home, condominium, or apartment complex.[11]

Bedroom

The bedroom should have convenient access to the bathroom. There should be an easily accessible bedside light switch, telephone, and storage area for medical, urinary, or personal care equipment. The bed location, height, and surface should allow for easy transfer. Casters can give easy movability of furniture, such as a table or desk chair. Closets should be large, with rods hung at a maximum of 54 inches from the floor.

Transportation

All persons with disabilities must have their needs for transportation considered. Transportation provides access to employment, school, recreation, and medical care as well as feelings of overall independence and control in one's life. Persons requiring transportation can be divided into four categories: those requiring total assistance (i.e., a passenger van); those able to drive with adaptive equipment (i.e., full-size van, minivan or car); those who can use public transportation; and those who require no special equipment. Accessible parking spaces should measure a minimum of 96 inches wide with a minimum 60-inch adjacent access aisle. Accessible parking spaces, access aisles, and passenger loading zones should not have surface slopes steeper than 1:48 in all directions. Passenger loading zones should provide a minimal access aisle 60 inches wide by 20 feet long adjacent and parallel to the vehicle pull-up space. They should have a minimum vertical clearance of 114 inches. A van parking space should be at least 98 inches in height and have an access aisle 96 inches wide. The above dimensions are only minimal guidelines. One must consider whether the van has a raised roof and/or dropped floor, side entry, or rear entry, and the type/length of mechanical lift. A covered parking area with access to the home is ideal. Curb and entry ramps may provide access to home entry.

Strategies for Decision Making

In a similar manner to proposing choices of adaptive equipment, one must consider several factors when making recommendations for home modifications. Does the client live alone or with family members who might perceive changes as an intrusion or inconvenience? Does the client own or rent? This may dictate the level of modifications possible. What financial and physical resources are available to implement the modifications? Is the client's condition static or dynamic, is it likely to improve or worsen? In considering this matter, one should plan for the changes that may occur with aging. Does the environment need to be rearranged, structurally modified, or relocated? The client should try the suggested modification or simulated setup before the healthcare professional begins an intervention. The client's preference, desire, and ability to be independent should be the final determinant in the selection of intervention strategies. The home environment should provide a comfortable, stimulating, and convenient atmosphere from which people with disabilities can pursue happily their association with family and friends and their educational, vocational, and recreational aspirations.[23]

SUMMARY

Adaptions in and to the home environment promote independence on a multitude of levels. Adaptive techniques, alteration of standard equipment, commercially available rehabilitation equipment, and fabrication of custom equipment facilitate participation in self-care, work, school, and social activities for people with a variety of disabilities. Occupational therapists evaluate the need for, train in the use of, issue, and fabricate adaptive equipment. These and other rehabilitation professionals, in addition to third-party payers and case managers, help patients decide on equipment necessity, long-term use potential, repair and cost considerations. In general, the schematic approach of no-technology to low technology to high technology is most useful and cost-effective. The patients' active participation in all components of the decision-making and training process is key to successful outcomes and enjoyable, productive living.

REFERENCES

1. American Occupational Therapy Association: Standards of practice for occupational therapy. American Journal of Occupational Therapy 37:802, 1983
2. Webster's Tenth New Collegiate Dictionary. Merriam-Webster, Springfield, MA, 1990
3. Kohlmeyer KM: Assistive and adaptive equipment. p. 316. In Hopkins H, Smith H (eds): Willard and Spackman's Occupational Therapy. 8th Ed. JB Lippincott, Philadelphia, 1992
4. Malek M: Activities of daily living. p. 231. In Hopkins H, Smith H (eds): Willard and Spackman's Occupational Therapy. 7th Ed. JB Lippincott, Philadelphia, 1988
5. Pedretti LW: Occupational Therapy: Practice Skills for Physical Dysfunction. 2nd Ed. CV Mosby, St. Louis, 1985
6. Trombley CA, Scott AD: Occupational Therapy for Physical Dysfunction. Williams & Wilkins, Baltimore, 1983
7. Chiou L, Burnett C: Values of activities of daily living. Phys Ther 65:901, 1985
8. Garber SL, Gregorio TL: Upper extremity assistive devices: assessment of use by spinal cord injury patients with quadriplegia. Am J Occup Ther 442:126, 1990
9. Moy A: Which aid? p. 74. In Bumphrey E (ed): Occupational Therapy in the Community. Aspen Publishers, Maryland, 1987
10. Batavia DI, Hammer GS: Toward the development of consumer-based criteria for the evaluation of assistive devices. J Rehab Res Dev 27:419, 1990
11. Jackson RH: Home modifications for the physically-challenged. p. 183. In G. Yarkony (ed): Spinal Cord Injury Medical Management and Rehabilitation. Aspen, Rockville, MD, 1994
12. General Services Administration, Department of Defense, Department of Housing and Urban Development, U.S. Postal Service, and the Architectural and Transportation Barriers Compliance Board: Federal Register 49:153, 1984
13. US Department of Education Clearinghouse on the Handicapped: Pocket Guide to Federal Help for Individuals With Disabilities. US Department of Education, Washington, DC, 1987
14. Nugent T: The Problem of Accessibility to Building for the Physically Handicapped. The Stanley Works, Framington, CT, 1978
15. Council of American Building Officials/American National Standards Institute, Inc. Accessible and Usable Buildings and Facilities. Council of American Building Officials, Falls Church, VA, 1992
16. Department of Housing and Urban Development: Federal Register. 53:215, 1988
17. American With Disabilities Act of 1990. Public Law 101-336. 42 USC 12101
18. Antone TM, Falk RN: Physical access. Team Rehab Rep March/April:27, 1991
19. Baker & McKenzie US Employment Law Practice Group: Baker & McKenzie United States Employment Law Update Legislative Bulletin July 1991
20. Ellek D: The Americans With Disabilities Act of 1990. Am J Occup Ther, 45(2):177, 1991
21. Department of Housing and Urban Development: Federal Register 53:215, 1988
22. Verville R: The Americans With Disabilities Act: an analysis. Arch Phys Med Rehabil 71:1010, 1990
23. Barnes K: Modification of the physical environment. In Baum C, Christiansen C (eds): Occupational Therapy—Overcoming Human Performance Deficits. Slack, Thorofare, NJ, 1991

Sources for Adaptive Equipment and Accessibility Standards

ADAPTIVE EQUIPMENT SOURCES

Abrams A, Abrams M: The First Whole Rehab Catalog. Betterway, White Hall, 1990

North Coast Medical: ADL Catalog. North Coast Medical, San Jose, CA, 1991 (800) 821-9319

Hale G (ed): The source book for the disabled. Paddington Press, New York, 1979

McCluer S, Conroy EE, Gephardt SL, Rice W, Wilke R: Assistive devices and equipment for rehabilitation. Hot Springs Rehabilitation Center, Hot Springs, AK, 1971

Fred Sammons: Professional Healthcare Catalog. Fred Sammons, Burr Ridge, IL, 1994 (800) 821-9319

Vandengerg ADL Rehabilitation Supplies (800) 872-2347

ASSISTIVE TECHNOLOGY RESOURCES

See Chapter 10, Appendix 10-2.

ACCESSIBILITY STANDARDS

Accessible and Usable Buildings and Facilities (CABO/ANSI A117.1—1992)

American National Standards Institute
Sales Department
1430 Broadway
New York, NY 10018
(212) 642-4900

Accessibility Guidelines for Buildings and Facilities and Uniform Federal Accessibility Standards

U.S. Architectural and Transportation Barriers Compliance Board
1331 F Street N.W., Suite 1000
Washington, DC 20004-1111
(800) 872-2253

Environmental Control for Persons with Disabilities

10

Ruth Dickey
Arlette Loeser
Edward Specht

The presence and influence of technology in today's society are everywhere. Technology has in some ways changed the lives of all people in areas such as entertainment, medical diagnosis and treatment, communications, and computer applications. For persons with disabilities, the effective use of technology has frequently meant increased independence at home, at school, on the job, and in the community.

ASSISTIVE TECHNOLOGIES

Particularly in the last 35 years, the concept of independent living for persons with disabilities has increased the focus on the use of assistive technology. The greatest influence on this concept has been the consumer-based Independent Living Movement and the passage of equal opportunity legislation, such as the Technology-Related Assistance for Individuals With Disabilities Act of 1988[1] and the Americans With Disabilities Act in 1990.[2] Equal opportunity is the foundation of the concept that all persons with disabilities should be able to participate fully in all aspects of society. Both the goods and the services of technology support the creation of a level playing field for all participants including persons of all ages with physical, sensory, perceptual, and cognitive disabilities.

Parallel Components

Beginning with the creation of the first prosthetics research and development of centers formed after World War II to deal with the need for improved artificial limbs, the area of assistive technology has developed four parallel components. The successful delivery of assistive technology and related services requires a framework that includes all of these areas and addresses the needs of the person with a disability as a consumer and furthermore as an informed consumer.

Those parallel components include the following:

Products: the actual devices and aids
Services: evaluation/analysis, selection/prescription, product adaptation, environmental adaptation, technical consultation, design/customizing

257

Information: product listings, availability for demonstration, simulation, trials, training and technical support, networking and referral

Labor

Practitioners who are adequately trained to provide service delivery such as functional assessment, task/site analysis, using information and funding resources, integrating multiple technologies, providing effective long-term use information, identifying technical service providers, and customizing resources

Materials and management methods that are available to construct, adapt, and customize the personal and universal user environments

Categories and Products

Some current examples of assistive technology categories include computer applications (hardware and software); augmentative and alternative communication; personal care devices; seating and positioning; wheeled mobility; sensory aids; robotics; biofeedback; functional electrical stimulation; recreation devices; and environmental control. Support, research, and information services include funding sources for devices, quantitative functional assessment, technology transfer, legislation, advocacy programs, administration and management, networking, data bases, academic curriculums, and continuing education programs.

Assistive technology products can range from being simple single-function mechanical devices, such as a reacher or a ball-bearing forearm orthosis, to electronic and or computer systems, to complicated multifunction integrated systems. These services and systems can be used for direct therapeutic intervention for the following purposes:

1. Prevention (alarm systems, automatic sensors)
2. Remediation (biofeedback, functional electrical stimulation, cognitive retraining)
3. Functional tasks (work simplification, energy saving, substitution for loss or limitation of physical function)
4. Hands-on evaluation and equipment selection
5. User training
6. Identification of solutions for multiple needs requiring the integration of systems and devices

The process by which assistive technology is delivered is generic in nature. Although we look specifically at the area of environmental control in this chapter, the reader needs to be aware that the application of other areas of assistive technology, such as power mobility, augmentative communication, and computer access, is identical and interactive. The client may already have some of the information needed but may need assistance with some other aspects of the process. This is best achieved by making the client responsible for participation in the process to provide needed resources without reducing either consumer control of the outcomes or the client's responsibility in the process. The role of the professional and others in the service delivery process is that of a consultant and can be achieved by the process described in this chapter. Empowering consumers in the process provides them access to all the information and the people they need to make those informed decisions. The specific goals of this chapter are to provide the following:

A framework for and an understanding of the process of client needs assessment for assistive technology

Criteria for the selection of the equipment

A description of the current state of the art of environmental control units and systems and their applications

General assistive technology resources

CHARACTERISTICS OF DISABILITIES

Most individuals benefit somehow from technology that makes their daily living easier. Individuals who have lost function should be assessed for technology intervention, which not only can make their lives easier but more productive and independent as well. The evaluation of functional needs includes environmental, personal, and psychosocial aspects. In particular, the interaction with one's environment is a natural and constant occurrence. The lack of control over one's environment can create frustration, discomfort, and a compromise in the quality of one's life. Technology should be considered as an intervention strategy to regain the lost control by compensating for the disability.

Each disability offers a set of circumstances. Yet, we need to go beyond the general disability groups (e.g., spinal cord injury, amputation, and traumatic brain injury) and categorize them as they relate to function. Discussed below are six characteristics of disability that relate to all ages and follow a continuum of progress over time.

Motor Function

Motor impairment refers to a limitation of movement imposed on a body part. This movement is needed to perform purposeful motion in a consistent, predictable fashion to perform activities. The loss of strength can prevent one from gaining motion needed to perform activities, thus preventing one from pushing a button on a remote control for a TV or holding a telephone receiver for the duration of a conversation. Decreased range of motion can result from limited strength or other anatomic changes such as muscle contractures, fluctuating spasticity, or joint tightness. Functionally, this limits the body part's area of reach. This limitation often forces one's functional movement into a space with limitations or a window of function. Often, this window becomes overcrowded with various devices competing for the same area of available movement.

Motor Control

Uncontrolled and involuntary movements can interfere with the ability to initiate or complete a purposeful movement. Muscle weakness also reduces controlled, refined, and consistent movements. A client presenting with decreased motor control often leaves an evaluator with a limited number of control sites and movements to access a device. Further, a limited amount of durable switches and mountings can endure the multidirectional forces of varying degrees offered by uncontrolled movements.

Sensory Deficits

Individuals with compromised vision, visual perceptual skills, and hearing require extensive evaluation of their limitations to identify the extent of their deficits. The nature of the deficit will have an impact on equipment design and positioning such as display and monitor size. During the evaluation process, impaired vision, hearing, perceptual, and tactile sensibilities can influence the method of exchange of information and are therefore addressed early to establish a comfortable media for the evaluator to demonstrate and illustrate the equipment features. Equipment used by individuals with visual impairments needs to have clear auditory feedback, whereas individuals with auditory impairments require clear visual feedback. The selection of display size, design, and required positioning is affected by the extent and nature of the disability as well.

Cognition

The range of attentional, memory, and behavioral deficits dictates the learning curve for the functional use of an object. Ideally, the client should have the ability to understand cause and effect. This understanding enables clients to integrate the relationship between switch activation and the device it controls. Many individuals with impaired cognition require simple solutions that demand limited thought process. Cognitive deficits that interfere with learning and the carryover of information from one session to another can interfere with the level of complexity and variety of functions included in the equipment solutions explored.

Endurance

Clients with cardiac and degenerative conditions as well as those experiencing life's natural aging process have decreased endurance and are prone to fatigue. Usually, the loss of energy necessitates earmarking percentages of energy output for designated activities. The evaluator should gear these clients to thinking about their total daily energy output and how they want to use it. This process is often begun when conventional adaptive equipment is issued, introducing the concept that activities do not have to be chores when there are assistive devices to ease the performance. The integration of assistive technology (AT) can be done the same way. The introduction of electronic devices that conserve energy demonstrate to individuals that they can redirect their newfound energies elsewhere by effortlessly doing things they struggled to do before. Eliminating the need to stand up an additional time to adjust a light or shut off an appliance helps to free up residual energy for activities of the individual's choice.

Comfort

Medical conditions that are accompanied by pain and discomfort frequently necessitate the immediate change of the client's personal environment, body position, or need to call for assistance. Offering full control over changing the environment also helps to prevent anticipatory anxiety often accompanied by pain as well as preventing the onset of a pain cycle, which can take hours to stop. Altering room lighting, bed positioning, or noise levels or activating call buzzers are some of the functions that these clients use. Although many have never realized their options to control factors influencing their comfort, often these individuals accommodate and accept the discomfort. When exposed to these possibilities, most clients react with disbelief of the control they can have over their physical reactions and anger over past limited exposure to devices that could have prevented or enhanced the quality of their daily life.

In consideration of all these characteristics, useful strategies can facilitate a successful outcome. These strategies are most useful when categorizing the disabilities according to the continuum of time-related issues.

INTERVENTION STRATEGIES

Progressive Illnesses

Clients with progressive conditions require strategies to promote the most time-efficient outcome. Illnesses such as amyotropic lateral sclerosis (ALS), multiple sclerosis (MS), muscular dystrophy (MD), and Parkinson's disease vary in rate of progression, intensity, and life-threatening concerns. Because there is an acute awareness of limited life expectancy, the evaluator must be thorough in acquiring information that is affected by the condition's progressive nature. The following must be explored to outline a plan:

Client's level of acceptance and awareness of the disease process

Past and present rate of progression and estimated prognosis

Client and significant family member(s) expectations and goals

Physical activity as well as intense concentration can drain one's energy; therefore, providing solutions to be used in the most comfortable and supported positions as well as offering a resting position will maximize energy conservation. The client should be informed of the possibility of having good and bad days to allow for maximum flexibility and future modifications of the equipment solutions.

Lifelong Conditions

Diagnoses such as cerebral palsy, MD, and other chronic conditions require sensitivity to the client's history and how it has affected the client's function. Clients and their families find ways to function by using resources they are aware of. Options may have been rejected because of unsuccessful experiences. Clinicians therefore must demonstrate respect for the individual's *existing* life-style and focus on enhancing the client's existing life-style without passing judgment. A survey of the client's equipment history and current functional methods offer the evaluator an understanding of what is working for the client and what functions are difficult to perform. The practitioner should offer options using learned behaviors and familiar movement patterns. Familiarity can simplify the demands on the client and will encourage their cooperation in the process.

Traumatic Injuries

Patients with conditions such as spinal cord, brain, and back injuries or any other condition with a sudden onset can use assistive technology as early as during hospitalization for the acute injury. Environmental control is often introduced to in-patients offering control of the bed, TV, phone, and light. The early introduction of this equipment can help clients to recognize the role of technology as a strategy promoting early functional independence and equipment comfort. To implement the appropriately graded intervention, the practitioner should identify

The client's level of adjustment to the new circumstances (expectations and emotional acceptance)

The client's plans for change in environment and life-style

The client's changing physical status (it is better to halt the process until the client's function is stabilized)

If a temporary solution is required,

Explore flexible off-the-shelf equipment options that can be moved to various locations with little or no modification.
Implement lower cost solutions addressing the functions most important to the client.

PROCESS AND SUCCESSFUL OUTCOMES

Goals

The overall goal of intervention is the practical application of the technology. For a successful outcome, the process must be based on client-centered service delivery. Through practical application of this process, we have learned that a successful outcome is most likely achieved by including each of the following concepts:

Include each step of the process.
Complete each step in sequence as outlined so that the total process is accomplished in a framework from global to detailed analysis.
Overall case coordination should be provided by the team doing the actual technology service delivery to the client.
Use interdisciplinary team-oriented service delivery.
Use an analytical and detailed problem-solving process.
Implement early goal identification.
Encourage a high degree of consumer participation and responsibility in decision making.
Provide maximum client education to ensure informed consumer decision making.
Provide hands-on evaluation and training. Training is necessary in all aspects of equipment/technique selection and problem solving.
Offer comprehensive technical support to ensure access to current information and successful device/system integration.

Support all intervention with proper seating and positioning for functional activity, which provides comfort, deformity prevention, pressure relief, efficient respiration, positive body image, and maximum independence.[3]

Client Intervention

Screening/Intake

Initial phone contact with the referral source is done to confirm that the evaluation program is appropriate for the client's needs. This involves the request for demographic information, past medical and equipment history. The greater the amount of information available before the client's initial visit, the more prepared the evaluation team can be.

Initial Needs Assessment

The initial needs assessment session is the client's and the evaluator's opportunity to obtain and to share as much relevant information as possible. This lengthy information exchange enables the evaluator to ask a variety of questions pertaining to the client's needs. It should be clarified to the client that the object of the needs assessment session is to identify client expectations, goals, life-style requirements, daily routine, physical and functional status, past experiences, and future plans. Thirteen specific areas of inquiry are involved in this part of the process (Table 10-1).

On completion of the needs assessment, the evaluator should summarize and describe the services indicated for the client's specific needs. Reassure the client that all of the information will be applied toward the establishment of goals and a plan. An outline of the proposed goals and plan is crucial for the client. In addition, project an approximate overall length of time of the process and an approximate length to each session.

Be sure to request any additional information needed, which may include the following:

Confirmation of funding availability for service delivery and equipment
Referral for wheelchair positioning for function, comfort, and/or access
Examination of bed positioning for comfort and function and/or access

Table 10-1. Initial Needs Assessment—General Areas of Inquiry

Medical history	Social status	Activities of daily living
Past procedures	Supportive system	Dressing
Current intervention	Funding	Bathing
Future procedures	Limiting factors	Grooming
Physical function	Cognition	Toileting
Upper extremities	Orientation	Ambulation
Lower extremities	Memory	Other mobility
Neck	Problem solving	Bed mobility
Trunk	Sensory/perception	Transfers
Facial oral	Vision	Eating/food preparation
Characteristics	Auditory	Phone communication
Sensation	Tactile	Writing
Active movement	Psychological	Transportation
Strength	Motivation	Recreation
Endurance	Learning style	Call for assistance
Tone	Vocational pursuits	Equipment information
Discomfort/pain	History	Owned
Vital functions	Current status	Tolerance
Respiration	Environments	Considerations
Swallowing	Home	Past experiences
Sitting tolerance	School/work	Future plans
Speech	Other	Life-style requirements
Weight shifting		Personal goals
Posture		

Identification of pending environmental changes
Identification of desired functions
Generation of a floor plan
Arrangement of a site visit
Outline of the daily routine and schedule

Access Evaluation and Control Movement and Site Selection

Information gathered at the initial needs assessment regarding general physical function is a springboard for the access evaluation. The evaluator should explain what access is and why a comprehensive evaluation is necessary to operate environmental control units (ECU). The client must understand that in order to determine how they will operate the equipment, specific functional movements, control sites, and input devices must be evaluated, selected, and then integrated.

The access evaluation identifies the available functional control movements, their anatomic locations, and the quality of the available movements. Consistent, func-

tional, and comfortable positioning should be established before access evaluation to ensure maximized body function and consistency of movements. Multiple body positions may need to be considered (e.g., sitting, reclining, or lying down) as well as a variety of positions of the individual control sites (e.g., the head stabilized by a headrest, the arm positioned in a gravity-eliminated plane).

One specific case is gaining access when the person is in bed. It may be advantageous for the client to operate a call signal, a telephone, or a TV from bed. A complicating factor is that a person's functional movements may be significantly compromised in a reclined position versus an upright seated position. It is advisable to perform a second control movement evaluation based on the bed position if a device is to be accessed from the bed.

Control movements can be used to operate an input device, a switch, standard or alternate keyboard, or a pointing device. The control site is the anatomic location and specific spot at the location that interface with the input device. Once the movements are identified, the degree of controllability (resolution) is determined to select consistent and predictable responses with regard to input. This is done by monitoring the strength, range of motion, endurance, and muscle control (as noted earlier in "Characteristics of Disabilities"). The identification of multiple usable movements and control site options is useful to give the client choices. Individuals with fatiguing conditions in particular require more than one movement for alternating control movements and/or locations. The greater the number of reliable control motions and sites available, the greater the number of individual input devices that can be controlled. As the availability of control motions decrease in number, the greater the need to integrate the tasks to be controlled (Fig. 10-1).

With an understanding of how to identify the available control movements and sites, options for input devices must be explored and analyzed.

Input Devices Selection

The input device is the object that is operated by the user to activate a device or system. Input devices can include switches, keyboards, joysticks, microphones, or sensors. Specific input devices are chosen because of the specific characteristics that match the output characteristics of the control motion and site. Input device characteristics include the following:

Excursion which is the distance or range required to move the part of the input device for activation

Force which is the amount of momentary and/or sustained pressure required to activate the output device

Size and shape which are considered when interfacing with the control site location and mounting requirements

Auditory and tactile feedback which confirms successful activation of the input device in isolation of the functional device

Durability which is necessary when movements have varied motor control and in case of multidirectional and/or heavy forces

With the maximum control motions and sites identified, the evaluator can now identify input devices to match the available control motions and sites based on the required characteristics (Fig. 10-2).

Once the potential input devices have been selected for evaluation, the evaluator should connect the input device being evaluated in a switch tester. A switch test is usually a battery-operated device with a variety of connector options that is used to obtain objective visual and auditory feedback when a switch is activated. The switch tester provides feedback independent of any connected system, thereby preventing the client's switch evaluation to affect later equipment selection. Once the process is explained, the client should be positioned properly and instructed in specific objective tasks, which will reflect the potential success of the interface between the motion and the input device. Specific tasks may include the following:

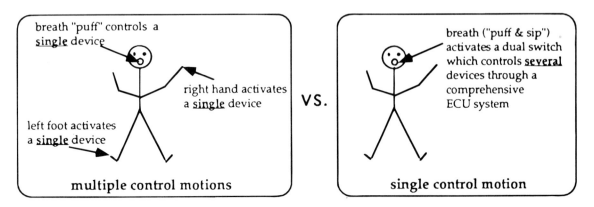

Fig. 10-1. Comparison of the impact of control motion availability.

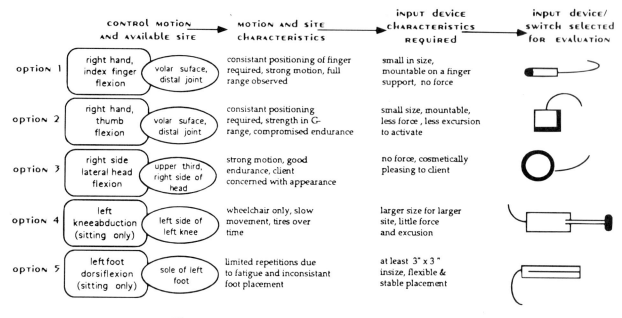

Fig. 10-2.   Matching control motion with input device.

Activate the input device 10 times to obtain short beeps.

Activate the input device 25 times and count to 5 with each input.

The evaluator then quantifies and numbers the successful actuations and documents accompanying responses by the client. This process is repeated with various input devices until the client and evaluator can construct a hierarchy of motions to be used based on the successes (Fig. 10-3).

After access options have been identified, the preferred motion and input device are used in conjunction with the environmental control options.

Equipment–Client Matching

Equipment Trials

Client education and the opportunity to get hands-on equipment experience is a necessary investment for the most successful end result. This opportunity is used to obtain feedback from the client and for the evaluator to assess the appropriateness of each solution option chosen for the client. This includes a three-step process: (1) client education, (2) identifying the number of systems for evaluation, and (3) client training.

    Step 1: Client education
        Introduction to ECU operation
        Identification of functions
        Explanation and demonstration of various generic ECU components

Almost all ECU functions are accessed through electronic devices. In some cases, these functions substitute for mechanical functions such as opening a door or turning the pages of a book, but in most cases, the ECU substitutes for the standard controls of an electronic device, such as a telephone, a TV, or a lamp, which are difficult to operate with a given physical disability. An understanding of environmental control operation is helpful in evaluating ECU requirements for a specific individual.

Environmental control operation uses the process by which machines operate. A machine can be conceptualized as a system that accepts external inputs, processes them, and then generates outputs that affect the environ-

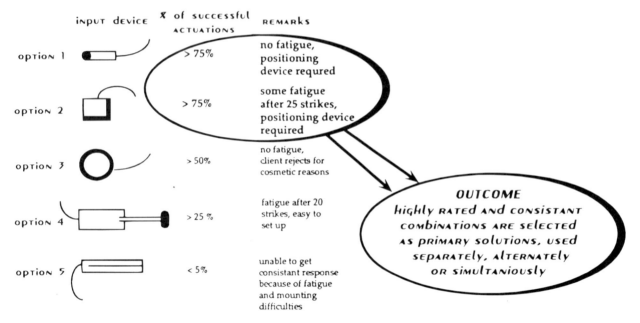

Fig. 10-3. Access evaluation outcome.

ment. Most such systems also include a feedback mechanism so that the inputs can be adjusted to those inputs so that the desired outcome is achieved. A simple example is a lamp: The switch is the input; the light produced, the output. The feedback system in this example is the light, which is equivalent to the output. When the switch is activated, the operator recognizes the desired result when the light is produced. The feedback system (Is the light on?) is equal to the output (the light is on).

Other devices provide separate feedback systems. Consider choosing which channel to watch on TV. Suppose it is 11:00 PM, and we wish to watch the news on Channel 2. If the TV did not have a channel indicator (feedback system), we would have to wait for the news to start in order to know if we were indeed watching Channel 2 (Fig. 10-4).

Step 2: Number of systems
Identification of projected number of systems to be evaluated by the client

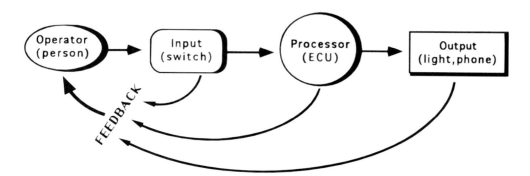

Fig. 10-4. Environmental control feedback loop.

Step 3: Training (repeated with each system evaluated):

Explanation and demonstration of components of each system being evaluated

Client training and use of ECU system with setup based on information obtained from prior sessions

Implementation of solution changes (positioning, input device) as feedback is obtained

Cumulative comparison of each system evaluated (Table 10-2).

Equipment Selection and Generation of Specifications

On completion of the equipment trials, the next session is dedicated to the identification of the equipment most appropriate for the client's needs. This begins with the following procedures:

A summary of findings from evaluation process

Identification of preferred input device and ECU processor

Examination and problem-solving of the equipment's integration with client's

Daily routine

Various environments (bedroom, living room)

Positions (manual wheelchair, motorized wheelchair, bed)

Available funding

Generation of detailed equipment report in narrative or chart form (Table 10-2) and a letter of medical necessity when required

Equipment Installation

Once funding is obtained and the equipment is ordered and delivered, the equipment is ready to be installed. Installation should be done by a party designated by the evaluation team and the client. Depending on the complexity of the system setup and mounting requirements, this party can include a client's friend or family member, the rehabilitation technology equipment supplier (RTS), ECU evaluation team (if service is available), or the manufacturer's representative. Instructions for installation found in the equipment report should be followed, and any questions should be directed to the evaluation team. If any component requires substitution or a significant amount of time has lapsed since the evaluation was performed, the evaluation team should be consulted.

User Training

Because a client must understand basic system operation during the evaluation stage, informal user training begins with the client's initial hands-on experience. Once the client's equipment is installed, the training is performed either in the client's home or in the setting where the evaluation was performed. The client should be taken through various practical situations using the system to perform each of the functions available. Training should be performed by someone who has a complete understanding of the system's operation as it pertains to the individual's specific physical disability and home situation. Failure to obtain adequate training can result in client frustration, ranging from an inability to operate the device with reliability to a total abstention from its use.

Table 10-2. Sample Client-Evaluation Chart, ECU Comparison

System Name	Description	Input Device Used	Likes (Strengths)	Dislikes (Weaknesses)	Possible Changes
Brand XXX	Integrated, dual-switch entry, scan/select	Puff and sip breath switch	Can move to another location if necessary, compact design	Takes too long to get to function, does not need all functions included	Increase speed of scan, look at another system with fewer functions
Brand YYY	Speaker phone with single switch, phone operator assistance only	Toggle switch	Easy to understand	No phone number memory	Explore other phone options with memories

Follow-Up

The evaluation team is encouraged to track the client's status for the purpose of monitoring successes and failures. Follow-up is often difficult because of time constraints and a lack of client response. Most often, follow-up is initiated by the client who either has had a change in physical function, life-style, or environment. When indicated, a client will return to the evaluation team for a reevaluation of his equipment needs, modification, reconfiguration, or replacement of his current system.

GUIDELINES FOR THE SELECTION OF REHABILITATION TECHNOLOGY

The value of assistive technology devices lies in their practical application. Clients prefer devices that are reliable and moderately priced. The selection of appropriate assistive technology not only involves the needs assessment and the client evaluation process but also must include information about the devices themselves. Currently, no consumer reports contain comprehensive product information that can assist in equipment selection. For anyone involved in the device selection, the guidelines discussed below should be considered in developing criteria for this part of the process.

Functional Operation

What does the device do or not do? Is the device easily learned and operated (including the clarity of operational manuals)? Is the operation accurate and not time-consuming? Is it noninterfering with concurrent activities? Can it be operated by others in the environment, such as the nondisabled or by other persons with disabilities? Are desired user functions available, and are they safely and reliably performed? Are the displays and feedback adequate?

Technical Complexity

These devices range a gamut of technical sophistication. Some are very simple, single-function devices that can be purchased off the shelf, while others are electronically sophisticated with a variety of adjustments or can be customized for individual users. Both the clinician and the user need to have information on this degree of complexity, because it may affect a variety of issues from operation to training, maintenance, repair, service, and installation.

Competition

What other devices currently perform similar or identical functions? Many devices and systems do similar functions but may have different access methods or may be more or less difficult to operate or install. The service provider must know what systems are currently on the market and be able to secure appropriate ones for hands-on evaluation and training.

Compatibility/Flexibility

Can the devices/systems be interfaced with others? Do they need to be interfaced, or can they be operated as stand-alone devices? Does the compatibility represent current and future device interfacing?

Consumer Evaluation/Perceived Value

The purchase of most of the devices in a given category (e.g., environmental controls) is based on their nationwide availability and cost. Clinical testing facilities can provide some information if they have done any comparative clinical evaluation. Clinical evaluation facilities generally have the devices available, and their methods of service delivery allow the client to become an informed consumer based on hands-on evaluation. Clients who have been involved in this process can make suggestions to device manufacturers and designers for changes. This kind of information, along with feedback from clinicians and care givers can help formulate some general advantages and disadvantages regarding current device use.

Engineering Evaluation

Does any formal evaluation address consumer concerns about system construction, which includes how easily the devices can be installed both mechanically and electrically and whether they can be easily transported and customized?

Availability

Are the devices commercially available? Who is the supplier, and how long will it take for delivery? It is important, especially with the more sophisticated devices, for the client to know with whom he will be dealing, for example, the local vendor, the manufacturer, a clinician, an engineer, or a combination of these sources.

Maintenance/Repair

All of the devices in general will need maintenance and eventually repair and/or service. Who is available to do this, the local vendor or manufacturer, and what is the process for this? What is the reliability of these suppliers? Are rentals or loaners available during the period when a device would be away from the client? Can the repairs/servicing be accomplished within a reasonable time?

Training

Is training necessary? If use training is necessary, who will do this, and how long will it take, what will the costs be, and where will it be provided? It is necessary to provide proper evaluation of consumer training for device selection, as well as operational training and follow-up. Technical support is a kind of training that refers more frequently to assistance provided for computer applications. It is necessary to provide technical support to the user after the equipment has been delivered to ensure successful functional use. Technical support may also come from the vendor from whom the equipment was purchased. Equipment should be warranted, and the client should be aware of the support due them from this source. Other technical support can come from companies that are in business for this specific purpose, for example, user and special interest groups as well as user manuals and built-in programs that may come with software programs.

Cost Issues

Everyone involved with the equipment needs to be aware of the individual costs and the comparative cost data. What funding sources are available (e.g., insurance, vocational services, workers compensation, etc.)? Are any hidden costs involved, (e.g., installation, maintenance, repair, training, engineering support, customizing, extra charges due to a warranty)? It is also necessary for prescribers to be able to provide adequate justification for both the equipment and the services surrounding them.[4,5]

ENVIRONMENTAL CONTROL SYSTEMS

Environmental control units and systems (ECSs) are electronic scanners or a series of components that allow persons with severe physical disability to control their environments by controlling electrical appliances with limited physical output.[6] A system consists of four parts (Fig. 10-5):

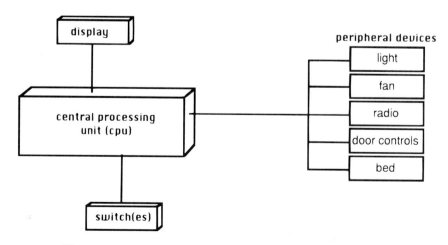

Fig. 10-5. Configuration of a typical environmental control unit.

1. A central processing unit (CPU) or control box containing the electrical switches and the receiving and transmitting components necessary to receive, process, and send signals, which activate, deactivate, or otherwise control the appliances.
2. Input devices or control switches connect the user with the appliances. Either hardwired directly or remotely connected to the central processing unit, they replace standard hand-operated switches found on individual appliances.
3. A display or monitor, either integral or remote from the unit, provides visual and/or auditory feedback that allows the user to identify available functions and the status of those functions.
4. Peripheral devices are the actual appliances operated via the ECS. Table 10-3 provides a listing of typical peripheral devices and the operation that an ECS can provide. The majority of device operations require either latching or momentary control. Latching control devices are those devices that turn on with a single input from a switch and remain in the "on" position until a second input returns it to the "off" position (e.g., a light, radio or TV). Momentary control refers to functions or subfunctions of device operation that require the operator to maintain switch closure continuously for the function to operate (e.g., raising the head of a motorized bed, intercom talk/listen, and TV channel change and volume control).

Remote operation of the ECS is achieved by three means of transmission: (1) radio waves, (2) infrared signals, and (3) ultrasonic control, or sound, frequencies:

Radio frequency waves are used to control equipment located at a distance from the control site. The signals pass through walls, with a range (dependent on the design and battery strength) of 15 to 200 feet.

Infrared signals pertain to radiation lying outside the visible spectrum at its red end. An infrared light beam is pulsed in the direction of a sensor to provide wireless control frequently associated with entertainment devices such as TV or VCR operation. The control is direct line of sight, requiring the user to be able to line up the input accurately for transmission. The range is 15 to 40 feet.

Ultrasonic control, or sound-control frequencies are above the range of human hearing. The transmission of

Table 10-3. Typical ECU Functions

Radio[a]
Fan
Air conditioners
Stereo[a]
Television
    (On/off; channel change; volume control
Motorized bed:
    Bed up/down; head up/down; foot up/down
Telephone controls
    Answer/hang-up
    Dialing (operator assisted/total digit dialing)
    Memory capability
    Redial (busy or unanswered numbers)
    Battery backup
    Listening/speaking (speaker phone; handset)
Lights (on/off or dim)
Assistance call/alarm/security systems
Room heaters/thermostat controls
VCR (on/off, play, rewind, fast forward)
Intercom
Electric blinds/curtains
Electric door locks/door openers and operators

[a] Volume and tuning capability for some systems.

the signal is nondirectional and does not pass through walls. The range is 15 to 25 feet. These signals sometimes are good if the user cannot direct a signal accurately enough at the receiver (e.g., as a result of coordination problems).

A fourth means of transmission, though not "remote" in the usual sense, is the sending of signals over existing house wiring. This concept is seen in the X-10 system and is used in virtually all of the current environmental systems in some manner. It is one of the simplest and inexpensive kinds of environmental control using existing house wiring. The X-10 consists of a series of off-the-shelf modular components. By sending signals from the CPU to a series of numbered lamps, appliances, and wall modules into which individual devices have been plugged, the user can turn the devices on and off (Fig. 10-6).

The system uses latching control only. There is no momentary control, except for an ability to dim and brighten lights, and no telephone function is available. Each system can control up to 16 appliances on one

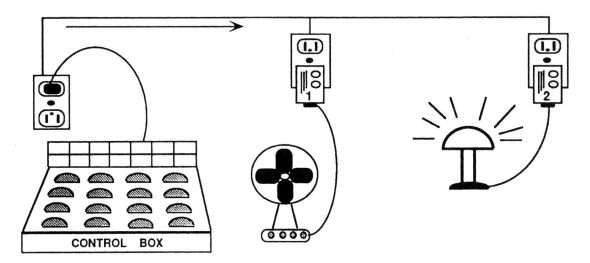

Fig. 10-6.   Signals sent over existing house wiring from the control box to numbered modules.

house code that can be plugged in all over the house. There are 16 house codes available and 16 functional options per house code, which equals a maximum total of 256 access options. Most systems use only a portion of these options. A variety of control boxes are available with various input sizes of input keys.

The RC 5000 (Fig. 10-7) is a remote control version of this system that consists of a portable transmitter that sends radio frequency signals to a transceiver, which in turn transmits signals via the house wiring to the modules installed at various locations. A variety of other functions have been added to this system, but it remains easy to install and operate and can save energy and provide some simple work simplification on the low-cost end of environmental control.

Disadvantages include the fact that it has latching-only control, has no telephone component, and inadvertent operation of devices (if there is a great deal of electrical activity on the house lines) can accidentally turn devices on or off. This modular ECS has been adapted by a number of manufacturers, which allows the modules to be accessed by alternate switch input and scanning selection methods for users who cannot operate any of the commercially available switches.

The Prentke Romich company and TASH both have scanning systems that have alternate switch access. Most all of the other commercially available ECSs today in some way incorporate the X-10 into their systems to

expand the function of the systems. Also, interfaces allow this control to be used from personal computers. In this instance, the computer becomes the control box from which the signals are transmitted to the individual modules.

ENVIRONMENTAL CONTROL OPERATION

The control or operation of the peripheral devices through these systems is accomplished via three methods: direct selection, encoding, and scanning selection.

Direct selection provides the user immediate selection or operation of a function or key by devices such as a mouthstick, optical viewpoint indicator, voice input, or touch screen.

Encoding uses a series of character sequences, which are converted to electrical signals that control switch operations This method can be used to transmit coded signals (e.g., morse code) by single or dual switch input for appliance control. Coding is commonly used in accessing augmentative communication systems (e.g., using semantic compaction or abbreviation expansion) or computers (e.g., using chordic keyboards in which multiple keys are simultaneously activated in different combinations to produce alphanumeric inputs or functions).

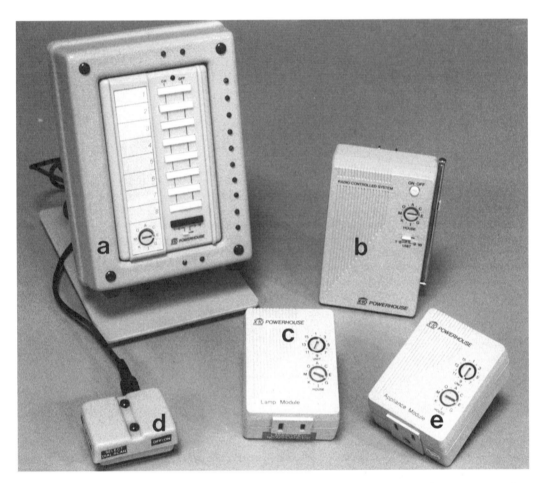

Fig. 10-7.   Prentke Romich Scanning X-10 Powerhouse uses the RC 5000 remote, radio-frequency control system and includes **(A)** table-mounted transmitter, **(B)** transceiver, **(C)** lamp and appliance modules, and **(D)** a dual-input switch (minirocking lever).

Scanning selection is typically the slowest input method involving moving a signal light or indicator across an array of selections from function to function by the operation of an input switch. The desired selection is activated by a second input selection or automatically by release of the initial input. Usual access is by two switch input (e.g., pneumatic "puff and sip"), where the user puffs from function to function and then sips to operate the selected device. A variety of switches are available for users who have differing physical capabilities. These switches can be interchanged on the units or can be operated in parallel when the user needs more than one kind of switch because of varying input locations (e.g., from a wheelchair or from bed).

Categories

Currently there are hundreds of devices available for people with disabilities that can be classified as environmental controls. Some of these perform a single function such as signaling for assistance, others allow the user to operate many devices from a single switch. Some can be controlled by voice, whereas others are simply variations of standard equipment, such as large-button telephones. To better understand the many devices available and to organize the search when trying to identify a device to assist an individual, it helps to identify categories of devices.

The method of categorization that we have chosen is based on the type of environment in which the device is to be used. This method discriminates between portable and stationary devices. It identifies systems that are to be used in a hospital setting and those based on home automation. In some cases, it defines unique categories based on technology that creates its own set of characteristics or requirements, such as voice-recognition–based ECUs. These are considered in greater detail below. This method reduces, but does not eliminate, the problem of devices falling into overlapping categories. It assists in beginning the search for a device that addresses a specific persons' needs.

Using this categorization method, we sometimes can quickly limit the search to only those devices that are portable or those that are based on a computer system. Other times, we find we can eliminate those devices that only address a single function or that are integrated with another controlled system such as a wheelchair or a communication device. By categorizing according to environment, we are encouraged to consider very carefully the environment in which the device or devices are to be applied. This careful examination will often make apparent requirements for the device that otherwise may not have been recognized.

Whatever the method we use to categorize devices, we end up using all available information about a device to further distinguish between equipment options. This includes the information identified above, such as what functions are controlled and what movements or senses are required for operation as well as information about cost, available local support, training and maintenance requirements, and much more.

Category Descriptions

This section describes eight current categories of environmental control.

Single-Function/Stand-Alone Devices
Individual devices are available for nearly every function described above including telephones, intercoms, bed controls, fans, and lamps. Sometimes these devices are simply an unusual model of a standard appliance that has characteristics that make them more accessible for persons with disabilities. These may include a lamp with large switches, or a TV remote that has extra-large buttons in the shape of the functions to be operated, or a telephone with large, easily read, and easily depressed

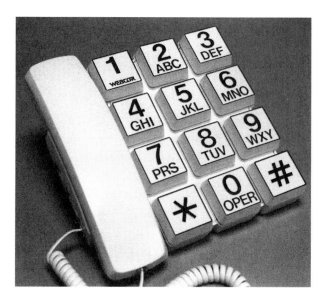

Fig. 10-8.   The Webcor large-button telephone.

keys (Fig. 10-8). Other devices have been specifically modified for persons with disabilities but are intended to meet a single and specific need. A telephone designed to operate by a single switch or an electric door opener with a remote control are examples.

This category is by far the largest and includes many items that are readily available from local merchants. Because they include many commercially available devices, they are often less expensive. They are often items designed for general applications and do not have an appearance that characterizes the user as a person with a disability. Their wide availability, low cost, and positive appearance are key advantages. Another advantage is that when necessary, they can often be used as a component of a more complex system. Most single-function appliances that can be operated by a single switch or by electric power can be incorporated as part of a more complete ECS (see "Comprehensive ECUs," below).

The main limitation is encountered when trying to incorporate several single-function devices for use by a person with more limited physical movements. When each device requires its own control switch and its own display or feedback system, each takes up space, and it may not be possible to position them so that a person with severe impairment can reach all of the necessary input devices. When this problem is encountered, it is necessary to consider a more comprehensive solution.

Comprehensive ECUs

Comprehensive ECUs are the classic system that originally defined what an ECU is. It typically consists of a box that sits in a central location and has a display—often a series of light-emitting diode (LED) lights, which indicate the status of various controlled devices. Attached to the box are the assorted devices to be controlled, such as a telephone, alternate current (AC) outlets, switch contacts, and probably an infrared or X-10 transmitter. The system may be controlled by one or two switches or by voice (see "Voice-Activated ECUs" below). If it is necessary to control devices when out of view of the display, it may be possible to obtain a second display for a remote location in the home. One specific example of this category is the Imperium 200H from Teledyne Brown Engineering.

The Imperium 200H (Fig. 10-9) has a CPU with a built-in telephone, which has either speaker phone or head phone capability and user microphone; a remote back-lit display with visual and voice feedback; an infrared remote control (One for All) for entertainment device control, and an X-10 power line interface for light and appliance control. The control box receives signals from a single input switch. Other functions such as bed controls, tape recorder, and call systems come through control box connections. A battery backup is available in case of power failure. Figure 10-9 depicts the setup of this system, which is similar to most comprehensive systems.

Ten to fifteen of these types of devices are currently available. The cost of a complete and installed system may be several thousand dollars and would typically be installed in a combined bedroom/living area. These systems are especially appropriate for those persons who spend extended periods of time in bed or in a single living space. One advantage of this type of system is that all devices are accessed in the same manner. Learning the intricacies of a particular unit may require some training, but once it is mastered, the same procedure is used to access all devices. Another benefit is that these systems are usually flexible in accommodating a wide assortment of controlled devices, including many of the single-function devices described above, which can be used as controlled accessories by a comprehensive ECU.

The major disadvantage of these systems is that they are centrally located. For the person who moves around the house and may need to control several different devices in any one of several locations, they are very limit-

ing. Another limitation is location requirements. For a person who may already have a motorized and a manual wheelchair and assorted other devices in his living space, the ability to find space for this box where it can be seen and accessed can be problematic.

The miniaturization of equipment design is reducing this second concern, with several of the newest devices being much smaller. As miniaturization continues, we will most likely see this category subsumed into the next one, that of multifunction ECUs that are also portable.

Portable ECUs

Portable ECUs are smaller, battery powered, and generally less full featured than a comprehensive ECS. They are usually designed to be mounted on a wheelchair and in some cases are an integral part of the powered wheelchair control system. As a result, they can be used to control different devices in different rooms and move about with the user. Fewer of these types of devices are currently available, and they are often significantly less expensive than a comprehensive ECS. For this lower cost, fewer functions are available on a portable ECU. Most often, this lower cost is evidenced by a single output, which can be adapted to provide several different functions. The output might be a radio frequency signal, which is converted at a transceiver to an X-10 signal, or an infrared or ultrasonic signal.

The Prentke-Romich Scanning Director is one example of a portable ECU (Fig. 10-10). Its base unit can be stationary or portable and operated by either a single or dual switch. The face of the unit contains a two-line, 16-character, backlit display. The side of the device has a jack for the input switch, an on/off switch, display contrast control, a jack for the AC charger, and a serial port. The scanning director allows control of infrared devices and X-10 beeper relay appliance control. Once programmed, the base unit receives infrared LED transmission from other devices. A memory transfer interface allows the user to store the information on a computer disc.

When the ECU is configured for two-switch operation, the user operates one switch to advance from menu item to menu item and the other switch to select the currently displayed menu item. In single-switch mode, the user may either operate and release the switch to begin an automatic scanning process or tap the switch to scan to the next item. In both cases, a long switch operation selects the current menu item.

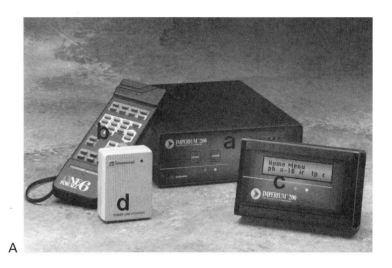

A

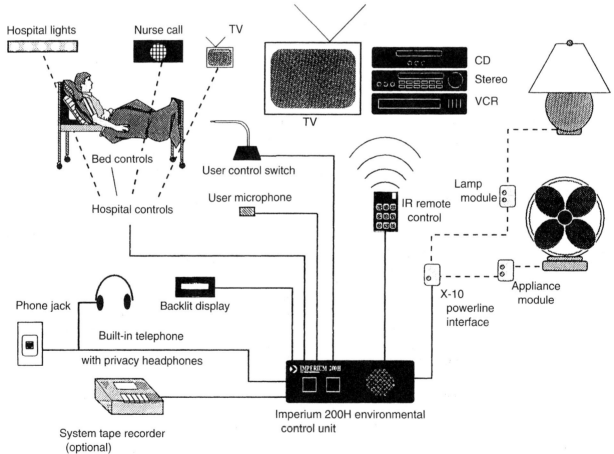

B

Fig. 10-9. **(A)** Imperium 200H infrared environmental control configuration with *(A)* control box, *(B)* infrared remote controller, *(C)* remote display, and *(D)* X-10 module. **(B)** Schematic diagram of a possible configuration of the Imperium 200H in the home. (Fig. A courtesy of Teledyne Brown Engineering, Huntsville, AL.)

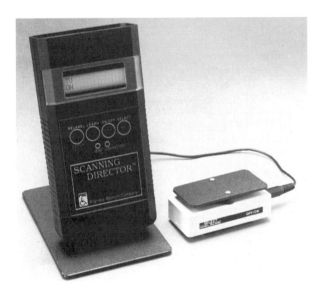

Fig. 10-10.   Prentke Romich Scanning Director and dual input switch.

Another similar unit, called the Director (not shown), also manufactured by Prentke-Romich, attaches to their augmentative communication devices. Signals are transmitted from the communication device by key or switch activation, which is programmed for device control.

As electronic miniaturization continues, more of these of devices with more output capabilities will be developed. They will most likely be integrated into other devices such as wheelchairs or communication devices that are already being used and moved around the home or other environment. This move toward integration presents both opportunities and pitfalls, which we examine in the section that follows.

Integrated ECUs

An integrated ECU is a device that is designed for some purpose other than environmental control but that includes some ECU functions as part of its operation. In some cases, the ECU functions are a well-developed component of the overall system, whereas in other cases, the ECU features are more of an after-thought and may be quite limited in their true functionality. Typical systems that integrate ECU features include powered wheelchair control systems, augmentative communication devices, and computer access systems. The trend is to incorporate ECU functions or the capability to add ECU functions

in many of these high-end electronic devices, which are targeted toward persons with severe disabilities. As this feature becomes standard on many of these devices, the availability of more comprehensive and well-designed systems is likely to increase.

Careful thought must be given to all potential circumstances when choosing an integrated ECU, and the following questions must be addressed:

> Will the combined system be available from all locations where it is needed, as in the case of a wheelchair-based system for someone who also wants to control some devices when in bed?
> If one part of the system must be removed or replaced for maintenance or repair or upgrading, will the loss of or change to the rest of the system create an untenable situation?

A balance to these limitations is the fact that inclusion of ECU functions as part of another device is usually less costly than purchasing a separate ECU. Also, the integrated ECU will sometimes be covered by a third-party payer who is purchasing the host device and would not pay for the stand-alone ECU. The integrated ECU is a most effective solution in those cases where the ECU requirements are minimal, primarily for the purpose of convenience, or only necessary at specific locations where the combined device will be available.

One example of the integrated concept is UCS1000 Tongue Touch Keypad (TTK) System from newAbilities, which uses a computer-based system with its components interacting to allow environmental control, wheelchair operation, and computer access via the Keypad. The TTK is a battery-operated, radio-frequency–transmitting device resembling an orthodontic retainer. Nine pressure-sensitive keys embedded in the retainer and operated by tongue touch send signals to a keypad receiver, which in turn sends signals to a universal controller, where they are interpreted and send outputs to appropriate devices (Fig. 10-11). These nine switches are operated in a variety of sequences to access the main function and then narrow it down (e.g., to the room) and then to the device and finally to the operation.

Computer-Based ECUs

Computer-based ECUs offer easy attachment of an assortment of peripherals to a personal computer to provide ECU functions. X-10 offers software and a box that

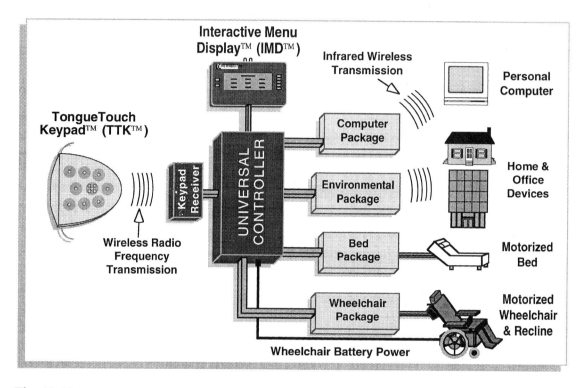

Fig. 10-11. The new Abilities UCS 1000 Tongue Touch Keypad System. (Courtesy of New Abilities Systems, Inc.)

attaches to almost any personal computers' serial port and allows control of up to 256 different X-10 modules. Several companies offer infrared controllers that can be attached to a serial port and control any infrared device through software. A standard modem with common communication software can be used as an automatic telephone dialer, and several devices permit the phone line to be turned on and off via software control. By combining these devices, integrating the software, and adding a computer access system, a particular type of ECU is customized.

One example of this category is the SenSei System from Safko International, which combines the Safko Server and Navigational Software. The Server augments a standard computer by extending control from the computer via the Solution Series. This allows the user to choose from functions displayed on the monitor in an easily recognizable picture format (Fig. 10-12). The functions include control of up to 256 modules (lights, appliances, security, heating, etc.); a telephone; emergency call; infrared remote control for entertainment de-

vices (TV, CD, stereo, cable, VCR); bed control and auxillary outputs. Alternate-input devices include pneumatic control, joystick, trackball, penmouse, and voice.

Voice-Activated ECUs

Although voice-based ECUs are not a category of their own and may be configured as any of the categories above, we isolate them here as a separate category because they present certain unique characteristics. Speaking to a device and having it respond to commands is so intriguing that persons who would otherwise not consider an electronic assistive device are willing to consider this as a solution.

The input device is the microphone, and its selection and placement can be an important part of the process. Some systems depend on its being within as little as a quarter of an inch of the speaker's mouth, presenting problems for persons who do not have consistent positioning or who have uncontrolled head movements caused by severe spasms. The speaker's voice quality and consistency are important considerations. Many systems

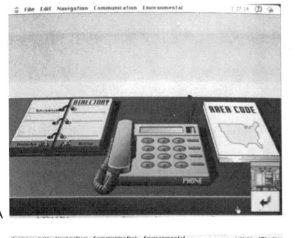

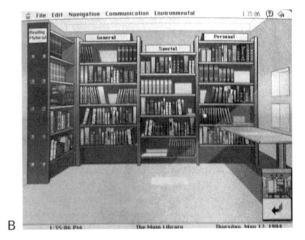

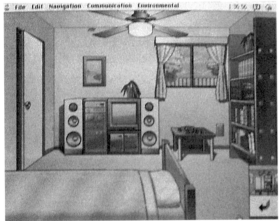

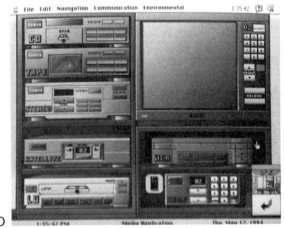

Fig. 10-12. SenSei's pictorial format on the monitor allows easy selection of control functions. Examples include **(A)** telephone, **(B)** a library of books, **(C)** room functions, and **(D)** entertainment devices. (Courtesy of Safko International.)

rely on the user's training with the system. Consistency is important; often, the voice entry system trains the user as much as the user trains the system.

In essence, the user must learn to speak with the same intonation and emphasis as when the system was first trained. This is becoming less of a problem as advances are made in the algorithms that interpret the voice sounds and in the speed of the microprocessors used.

It is very difficult to perform an objective evaluation of voice-operated devices because the characteristics of the input, the voice, cannot be evaluated independently of operation of the device and the sound environment into which a voice-operated device will be placed. The potential for the proposed environment to generate sounds that can cause unintended operation and the ability of the environment to tolerate the voice commands required to operate the device must be examined by the evaluator.

A current example of a voice-operated ECU is the Simplicity System Series Four in One (Fig. 10-13). It is both a voice- and switch-activated system with voice output. The control requires the user to program his or her voice into the system (speaker-dependent speech recognition). The functions provided are those outlined for previously discussed systems. A special computer interface is available for any IBM PC/XT/AT or PS/2 personal computer or IBM-compatible PC. A remote microphone can be mounted on a wheelchair.

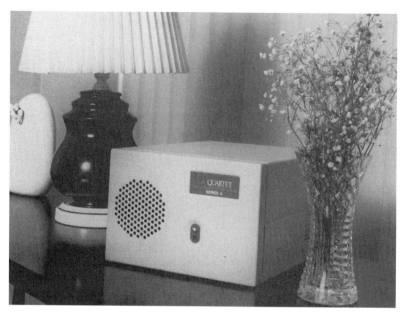

Fig. 10-13.   The Simplicity System Series Four in One voice-activated system. (Courtesy of Quartet Technology.)

As this technology develops, dedicated microprocessors that easily and inexpensively incorporate voice recognition into the control system of almost any device—from the TV to the washing machine—probably will be developed. If such control systems can be made practical and functional, rather than mere oddities, they could prove to be one more step toward achieving universal access for persons with severe disabilities.

Hospital-Based ECUs

The requirements for hospital room ECUs are both more limited and more demanding. Functions desired include control of the TV, phone, nurse call, bed, room lighting, and perhaps a radio or fan, with very little variation from this list. For the devices to pass in-house electronic regulations, be adaptable to the many different hospital phone and TV systems, and survive subjection to installation and manipulation by assorted personnel, they must be more adaptable, durable, and simple to operate than typical residential devices. They must also be protected from theft, vandalism, and inadvertent damage. While the output requirements are relatively stable, they should be flexible in accepting a variety of inputs and providing several feedback methods—the simpler the better.

Although several comprehensive systems have been incorporated into hospital rooms in the past, a few devices have been developed specifically for this purpose. The previously described Imperium 200H can also be included in this category of systems. Among the units designed specifically as a hospital system is the Hill-Rom Enhancemate Voice Activated Control System (Fig. 10-14). This system allows for voice activation and is a speaker-dependent system requiring user programming before use. This system allows operation of the typically needed functions at bedside (e.g., nurse call, bed adjustments, room/reading lights, TV control, and telephone access).

The specialized nature and requirements of these devices and the fact that they are primarily sold to large hospitals make them quite expensive as compared with other ECU systems. In spite of this, demand for these systems most likely will increase, as will the types of systems. This is the result of the Americans With Disabilities Act requirements that businesses, including hospitals, make the services they provide accessible to all people with disabilities.[2]

Home Automation Systems

The electronic age we live in continually presents us with devices that simplify and automate everyday tasks. Only a few years ago, the only way to turn on your patio light when returning home was after you were inside the house

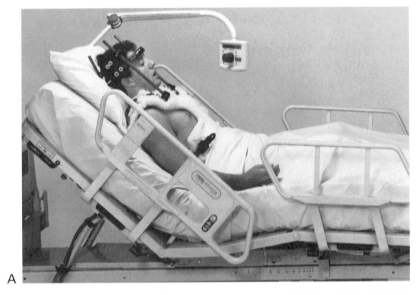

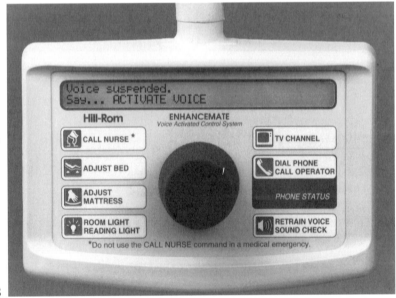

Fig. 10-14. **(A & B)** The Hill-Rom Enhancemate Voice Activated Hospital Control System shown with the typical functions of these systems. (Courtesy of Hill-Rom.)

and no longer needed its use. Now many homes have an automatic detector that turns on the outside lights whenever anyone enters the yard. This trend toward home automation creates many opportunities for persons with disabilities. Not only does it create beneficial devices, but it also lowers their cost and availability as they are mass marketed.

There has always been cross pollination between the ECU market and the home automation market, starting with the first introduction of X-10-type devices. As house-wide automation systems become more economical and widely distributed, we will see even more crossover. These systems will likely include integration of more sophisticated communication systems including in-

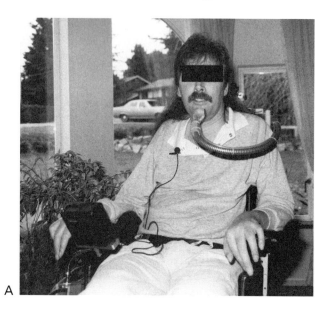

A

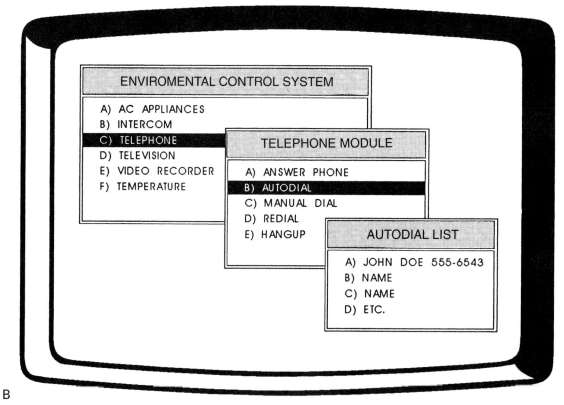

B

Fig. 10-15. The remote terminal of the Remote Gateway system **(A)** (mounted on the wheelchair) displays currently accessed functions, a sequence of which is depicted **(B)**.

tercoms or video intercoms and cellular phone tie-ins. The future 500-channel cable network will include a plethora of interactive services. Heating, cooling, and air-quality systems that allow individual control by room may also become more common. Another necessary fact of modern life, the home security system, will certainly be integrated into the whole fabric of the typical family home, as well as numerous conveniences and contraptions that we cannot yet imagine.

Only a few developers are working out ECU systems based on home automation designs. One of these designs is the Remote Gateway from the Neil Squire Foundation in Vancouver, Canada. The Remote Gateway is a communications link that will enable people with disabilities to access home automation systems. The system consists of three parts:

Base controller: This interfaces with and integrates the home automation components. In communication with the wireless link, it supports the user interface and the voice recognition.
Communications link: This wireless audio and data link uses a digital transmission format based on telephone technology.
Remote terminal: This small, portable, LCD display screen displays menu-based home control information (phone, entertainment, lights and appliances, doors and windows, intercom; security, temperature, timed events and setup).

The user has access to the device either through a keypad on the remote unit or through alternate single- or dual-switch operation or voice input. The remote terminal has been modified to allow the display of video information on the screen. The base controller communicates with the remote terminal by putting the commands and display information into an output buffer. With the remote screen initialized and cursor position established, characters are sent through the link and displayed on the screen. Some characters have been reserved for commands and with their activation, the devices or functions are completed (Fig. 10-15).

Summary
As all of our environments become more automated, integrated, and computerized, we will see a tremendous increase in availability and application of devices that make people with disabilities more independent. Ten years ago, there were only a handful of ECU devices, now there are hundreds. This has created a need for a well-educated consumer who can effectively evaluate all the choices and match the correct device to his requirements. Clinicians, especially in the area of occupational therapy, are learning how to assist in this process by using many of the techniques described above. The end result is selection of the appropriate device to enable greater independence.

COMPUTERS AND ECUs

Comparison and Contrast

As with nearly any other topic or subject today, no discussion is complete without examining the impact of computers. In many ways ECUs, especially integrated ECUs, are simply one more application of computer technology. The application of computers as ECUs imposes its own constraints and concerns on the design of the computer system, but the issues to be resolved are often computer issues. In fact, people with disabilities are gaining access to ECU-type functions much more quickly as a result of increased access to computers. Does this mean that the two subjects can be successfully merged into one area of study? Not quite. The requirements for successful operation of a computer are significantly more extensive than those necessary for ECU implementation. In this section, we briefly consider how the process of a computer access evaluation is similar to and different from an ECU evaluation.

Evaluation
The professional evaluation process will be the same in its generic elements (needs assessment, access evaluation, device identification, equipment trial, and solution recommendation) as that described above. When an evaluation for computer access produces a successful result, a subsequent ECU evaluation can draw from the computer experience. The goals have been identified, an access evaluation has been completed, and the required ECU outputs often can be added as extensions to the computer system. The computer can provide the ECU outputs as well as the more standard computer functions.

Functional Differences

Although the process will be similar, certain considerations are specific to a computer access evaluation.

A computer system has many more possible inputs than a typical ECU. A typical computer keyboard has 101 keys whereas the typical ECU can control about 50 different functions, and many people can be accommodated with only a dozen or two individual functions.

The speed of input required to be effective on a computer is much faster than that to operate an ECU device. Ten seconds to change TV channels is not an unreasonable requirement, but 10 seconds to enter a key stroke resulting in a typing speed of one word per minute is not reasonable.

To make computers more user friendly, manufacturers have incorporated a graphical user interface. These require the use of a proportional pointing device such as a mouse or trackball. This imposes an additional control movement requirement of being able to control a proportional input device. Alternatives for the mouse exist in the form of various mouth- and head-controlled pointing devices as well as solutions that allow the user to control the mouse with a single switch, scanning in different directions. For the person with a mobility impairment, this task can be significantly more difficult than operating a key or set of keys on the keyboard, especially in those cases where the accuracy of available movements is affected.

ECU requirements may exist at locations different from where computer access is provided. Typically, a computer can be located at a specific workstation, and the user can move to that location when it is necessary or desirable to perform typical computer tasks such as word processing. The workstation location may not be the only location where ECU access is functioning. Often, a client will use an ECU from different rooms and in various positions.

Input Characteristics

How do the operational input characteristics used to operate a computer system compare with those for operating a set of appliances through an ECU system? Operating a computer usually involves many more input operations in a given period of time than operating an ECU. Creating even a short letter can require several hundred inputs, whereas even the most aggressive cable clicker is unlikely to change TV channels more than a few dozen times in a half hour. This must be taken into consideration during the evaluation process. The potential user may be at risk for cumulative trauma disorders at the control site, both because of overuse of fewer available sites and because those sites may not be typical high-use areas that can accommodate repeated movements. These complications would also be more devastating to the client because of the already compromised function.

Strategies to Decrease Input Volume

Because computer access requires so many more input operations, various strategies have been developed over time to attempt to reduce the number of inputs required. The most common include word prediction and abbreviation expansion.

Word prediction consists of displaying on the screen a word or list of words that have the same beginning letters as those already entered by the user. If the word being entered is the same as one of the predicted words, the user can complete the word with only one additional entry, usually a number that corresponds to the entry. This can decrease the overall number of entries by about one half. Although word prediction reduces the number of entries required, it will not generally speed up the time required to enter text except for the person who enters characters very slowly. This is because the time required to visually scan the predicted words significantly reduces the speed of entry.

Abbreviation expansion consists of using a set of entries, the abbreviation, which consistently represent a common word or phrase or block of text. This is essentially the same process as using text macros or glossary entries from common word processing programs. The effectiveness of this technique depends on the ability of the user to recall the various abbreviations and the repeat rate of the abbreviated text within the text to be generated.

Feedback Systems

Just as the inputs required to operate a computer are more complex than those required to operate an ECU system, so are the feedback systems. Computers present the user with lots of information in a visual screen-based format as well as some audible information and some in a printed format. For candidates who have sensory impairments in addition to their mobility impairments, these methods of feedback must also be considered. Other users may find it difficult to remain in a standard seated position for the amount of time required to complete necessary computer operations. In these cases, the ability to view the screen from different positions may require specialized support furniture or mounting systems. Whenever possible, these position changes should be achievable without outside assistance.

Output

One great strength of computer systems is the ability to generate an incredible variety of outputs. These may take such diverse forms as electronic signals that are interpreted by other computers, physical operations performed by motors, hydraulic systems or other mechanical actuators, and visual or auditory displays including film clips, sound effects, and other sensual phenomena.

Typical ECU functions are only a small part of this menagerie. One reason the two areas overlap is primarily because they address the needs of individuals with disabilities. Someone who has difficulty answering a ringing telephone is likely to also have a hard time operating a computer keyboard or a pointing device.

A computer system's output capabilities include all of the functions of a typical ECU system as well as many others.

Information

The primary output generated by a computer system is often information. It may include information about personal finances, social communication, study notes and resources, or work-related reports and proposals. For much of this information, only screen viewing is necessary. Other information requires the generation of a printed copy, which can range from the simplest typed output to four-color printing equal to any printshop.

Audible Communication

Computer outputs may be organized to generate speech for those unable to communicate verbally. The ability of computers to act as communication devices is undergoing a dramatic increase, as computers are being linked through wired and wireless connections to transmit and receive faxes, electronic mail, pager messages, and telephone calls.

Manufacturing Equipment

Computers can be connected so that the products designed on the computer screen (computer-aided design, CAD) are directly produced by the factory (computer-aided manufacturing, CAM). As this trend toward increased computerization of everything from the office copier to the construction crane continues, along with the increased ability of all types of computers to communicate and exchange information, the possibilities for a person with a physical disability, no matter how severe, are limitless.

Future Trends

The trend toward computerization is gradually reaching people with disabilities. Whether at school, work, home, or in the community, more people with disabilities have access to computers, which are being applied in all of the ways described above and many more. This presents a wonderful opportunity for those with severe physical disabilities to take advantage of the ability of computers to control the electronic environment around them, whether that includes the TV across the room, the lamp next to them on the desk, or the apartment door buzzer 10 floors below.

Some of the ways these systems can increase independence are readily apparent, such as the ability of a modem and software to dial the telephone. Others, such as the ability to turn on the TV and change the channel, are less apparent and may require some research by the consumer to identify and implement. The integration of these multifaceted machines into every aspect of daily life brings with it many opportunities for greater independence and control for persons with severe physical impairments.

REFERENCES

1. Technology-Related Assistance for Individuals With Disabilities Act, Public Law 100-407
2. Americans With Disabilities Act of 1990, Public Law 101-336
3. Dickey RE: Workstation simulation laboratory for persons with severe physical disabilities. p. 11. Grant H128A91022. Rehabilitation Services Administration, Washington, DC, 1992
4. Shaver MS: Retrospective study of electronic technical aid use among high-level quadriplegic males. In Dickey RE (ed): Electronic Technical Aids for Persons With Severe Physical Disabilities. Rusk Institute of Rehabilitation Medicine, New York, 1985
5. Batavia DI, Hammer GS: Toward the development of consumer-based criteria for the evaluation of assistive devices. J Rehabil Res Dev 27:4, 1990
6. Dickey RE: High technology at home. p. 415. In Portnow J (ed): Physical Medicine and Rehabilitation, Home Health Care and Rehabilitation. 2:3. Hanley & Belfus, Philadelphia, 1988

Current Manufacturers of Commercially Available Environmental Control Systems

ACS Technologies Inc.
1400 Lee Dr., Suite 3
Corapolis, PA 15108
(800) 227-2922
(412) 269-6656

APT Technology, Inc.
8765 Township Rd., Suite 513
Shreve, OH 44676
(216) 567-2906/2001

Arroyo & Associates, Inc.
2549 Rockville Center Parkway
Oceanside, NY 11572
(516) 763-1407

Automated Voice Systems, Inc.
17059 El Cajon Ave.
Yorba Linda, CA 92686
(714) 524-4488

Baylor Biomedical Service
2625 Elm Street, Suite 102
Dallas, TX 75225
(216) 365-1890

Bloorview Children's Hospital
25 Buchan Court
Willowdale, Ontario, Canada
M2J 4S9
(416) 494-2222

CyberLYNX Computer Products, Inc.
2885 E. Aurora, Suite 13
Boulder, CO 80303
(303) 444-7733

High Tech Intelligence, Inc.
1602 S. Parker Rd., Suite 312
Denver, CO 80231
(303) 695-0609

Hill-Rom Company, Inc. A Hillenbrand Industry
1069 State Route 46E
Batesville, IN 47006
(800) 445-3730
(802) 934-7777

KY Enterprises Custom Computer Solutions
3039 E. 2nd St.
Long Beach, CA 90720
(213) 433-5244

LC Technologies, Inc.
4415 Glenn Rose St.
Fairfax, VA 22032
(703) 425-7509

Med Labs, Inc.
28 Vereda Cordillera
Goleta, CA 93117
(800) 968-2486
(805) 968-2486

285

NanoPac, Inc.
4833 S. Sheridan Rd., Suite 402
Tulsa, OK 74145-5718
(918) 665-0329

Neil Squire Foundation
1046 Deep Cove Rd.
North Vancouver, BC
V7G 1S3
Canada
(604) 929-2414

New Abilities Systems, Inc.
470 San Antonio Rd., Suite G
Palo Alto, CA 94306
(415) 856-6999

Prentke-Romich Co.
1022 Heyl Rd.
Wooster, OH 44691
(800) 262-1984
(216) 262-1984

Quartet Technology, Inc.
52 Davis Rd.
Tyngsboro, MA 01879
(508) 692-9313

Safko International
1438 West Broadway Road
Suite B240
Tempe, Arizona 85282
(602) 731-9470

TASH, Inc.
91 Station St., Unit 1
Ajax, ON L1S 3H2
CANADA
(219) 462-8086
(416) 686-4129

Teledyne Brown Engineering Imperium Products
300 Sparkman Drive, NW
P.O. Box 070007
Huntsville, AL 35807-7007
(800) 944-8002

Toys for Special Children Enabling Devices
385 Warburton Avenue
Hastings-On-Hudson, NY 10706
(800) TEC-TOYS
(914) 478-0960

Words +, Inc.
44421 10th Street, W., Suite L
P.O. Box 1229
Lancaster, CA 93535
(800) 869-8521
(805) 949-8331

X-10 (USA), Inc.
91 Ruchman Rd.
P.O. Box 420
Closter, NJ 07624-0420
(201) 784-9700
(800) 526-0027

Zygo Industries, Inc.
P.O. Box 1008
Portland, OR 97207-1008
(800) 234-6006
(503) 684-6006

Assistive Technology Resources

The following lists provide some guidelines to professionals looking for technology-related resources; they are not intended as a complete directory of those resources. Each interdisciplinary resource has multiple, comprehensive lists of technology resources. Disability/disease-specific organizations have national organizations, some of which have technology-assistance services and/or information special interest groups.

DISCIPLINE-SPECIFIC ORGANIZATIONS

American Occupational Therapy Assoc. TSIS
1383 Piccard Dr.
Rockville, MD 20850
(301) 948-9626

American Rehabilitation Assoc.
1910 Association Dr., Suite 200
Reston, VA 22091
(703) 648-9300
(800) 368-3513

American Speech-Language-Hearing Assoc.
10801 Rockville Pike
Rockville, MD 20852
(301) 897-5700
(ASHA publishes "Augmentative Communication")

The Institute of Electrical and Electronics Engineers, Inc. (IEEE)
345 East 47th St.
New York, NY 10017
(212) 705-7900

Orthotic and Prosthetic Assoc.
717 Pendleton St.
Alexandria, VA 22314
(703) 836-7116

INTERDISCIPLINARY ORGANIZATIONS

Closing the Gap
P.O. Box 68
Henderson, MN 56044
(612) 248-3294

International Society for Augmentative and Alternative Communication (ISAAC)
428 East Preston St.
Baltimore, MD 21202-3993

287

National Institute on Disability and Rehabilitation Research (NIDRR)
U.S. Department of Education
400 Maryland Ave. S.W.
Washington, DC 20202
(202) 732-1134
(Program Directory)

National Rehabilitation Information Center (NARIC)
8455 Colesville Road, Suite 935
Silver Spring, MD 20910-3319
(301) 588-9284
Directory of National Information
Sources on Disabilities (800) 346-2742)

RESNA (Society for the Advancement of Rehabilitation & Assistive Technology)
1700 North Moore St. Suite 1540
Arlington, VA 22209-1903
(703) 524-6630
(RESNA Technology Related Assistance
Project—list of Technology-Related Assistance States)

Trace R & D Center
S-151 Waisman Center
1500 Highland Ave.
Madison, WI 53705
(608) 262-6966

DISABILITY-RELATED ORGANIZATIONS

Alexander Graham Bell Assoc. for the Deaf
3417 Volta Pl. NW
Washington, DC 20007
(202) 337-5220

American Academy of Physical Medicine and Rehabilitation
122 S. Michigan Ave., Suite 1300
Chicago, IL 60603
(312) 922-9366

American Amputee Foundation, Inc.
P.O. Box 250218
Little Rock, AR 72272
(501) 666-2523
(800) 553-4483

American Assoc. of Retired Persons (AARP)
601 E St. N.W.
Washington, DC 20049
(202) 434-2277

American Congress of Rehabilitation Medicine Assoc. Management Center
5700 Old Orchard Rd.
Skokie, IL 60077
(708) 965-2776

American Deafness and Rehabilitation Assoc.
P.O. Box 251554
Little Rock, AR 72225
(501) 663-7074

American Foundation for the Blind
15 W. 16th St.
New York, NY 10011
(212) 620-2000
(800) 232-5463

American Geriatrics Society
770 Lexington Ave., Suite 300
New York, NY 10021
(212) 308-1414

American Lateral Sclerosis (SLS) Assoc.
21021 Ventura Blvd., Suite 321
Woodland Hills, CA 91364
(818) 340-7500

American Parkinson Disease Assoc.
60 Bay St.
New York, NY 10301
(718) 981-8001

American Printing House for the Blind
1835 Frankfort Ave.
P.O. Box 6085
Frankfort, KY 40206
(502) 895-2405

American Spinal Injury Association
250 E. Superior St., Room 619
Chicago, IL 60611
(312) 908-3425

Arthritis Foundation
1314 Spring St. N.W.
Atlanta, GA 30309
(404) 872-7100
(800) 283-7800

Associated Services for the Blind
919 Walnut St.
Philadelphia, PA 19107
(215) 627-0600

The Association for Persons With Severe Handicaps (TASH)
7010 Roosevelt Way N.E.
Seattle, WA 98115
(206) 523-8446 (Voice)
(206) 524-6198 (TDD)

Association for the Retarded Citizens of the United States (ARC)
2501 Ave. J
P.O. Box 6109
Arlington, TX 76005-6109
(817) 640-0204

AT&T National Special Needs Center
2001 Route 46, Suite 310
Parsippany, NJ 07054
(800) 233-1222 (Voice)
(800) 833-3232 (TDD)

Courage Center
3910 Golden Valley Rd.
Golden Valley, MN 55422
(612) 588-0811

Job Accommodation Network (JAN)
809 Allen Hall
West Virginia University
Morgantown, WV 26506
(800) 526-7234
(800) 526-4698 (in WV)

Muscular Dystrophy Assoc.
3561 E. Sunrise Dr.
Tuscan, AZ 85718
(602) 529-2000

National Arthritis and Musculoskeletal and Skin Diseases Information Clearinghouse
9000 Rockville Pike
Box AMS
Bethesda, MD 20892
(301) 495-4484

National Association for the Visually Impaired
22 W. 21st St.
New York, NY 10010
(212) 889-3141

National Association of the Deaf
814 Thayer Ave.
Silver Spring, MD 20910
(310) 587-1788 (Voice)
(310) 587-1789 (TDD)

National Clearinghouse on Technology and Aging
University Center on Aging
University of Massachusetts
Medical Center
55 Lake Ave. N.
Worcester, MA 01655
(508) 856-3662

National Easter Seal Society
70 E. Lake St.
Chicago, IL 60601
(312) 726-6200 (Voice)
(312) 726-4258 (TDD)
(800) 221-6827

National Multiple Sclerosis Society
205 E. 42nd St., 3rd Fl.
New York, NY 10017
(212) 986-3240
(800) 624-8236 (Information Resource Center)

National Parkinson's Foundation
1501 N.W. 9th Ave.
Miami, FL 33136
(800) 327-4545
(800) 433-7022 (in FL)
(305) 547-6666

National Spinal Cord Injury Assoc.
600 W. Cummings Park, Suite 2000
Woburn, MA 01801
(800) 962-9629

National Spinal Cord Injury Hotline
American Paralysis Assoc.
2201 Argonne Dr.
Baltimore, MD 21218
(800) 526-3456 (Outside MD)
(800) 638-1733 (MD only)

Paralyzed Veterans of America
801 18th St. N.W.
Washington, DC 20006
(202) 872-1300

Sensory Aids Foundation
385 Sherman Ave., Suite 2
Palo Alto, CA 94306
(415) 329-0430

Spinal Network
P.O. Box 4162
Boulder, CO 80306
(303) 449-5412

Technical Aids and Assistance for the Disabled
1950 W. Roosevelt Rd.
Chicago, IL 60608
(313) 421-3373
(800) 346-2959

United Cerebral Palsy Assoc.
1522 K St. NW, Suite 1112
Washington, DC 20005
(202) 842-1266
(800) 872-5827

ELECTRONIC RESOURCES/BULLETIN BOARDS

AppleLink
Apple Computer, Inc.
Office of Special Education and Rehabilitation
20525 Mariani Avenue, MS 43S
Cupertino, CA 95014
(408) 974-7910

CompuServe
Compuserve Information Service
500 Arlinton Centre Blvd.
Columbus, OH 43220
(800) 848-8199

Deafteck, USA
International Communications Limited
P.O. Box 81
Fayville, MA 01745
(508) 620-1777

4-Sights Network
Greater Detroit Society for the Blind
16625 Grand River
Detroit, MI 48227
(313) 272-3900

HyperABLEDATA
TRACE Research & Development Center
1500 Highland Ave.
Waisman Center
Madison, WI 53705-2280
(608) 262-6966

Project Enable
Rehabilitation Technology Associates
West Virginia Research & Training Center
One Dunbar Plaza, Suite E
Dunbar, WV 25064-3098

Rehabdata and Abledata
National Rehabilitation Information Center (NARIC)
8455 Colesville Road, Suite 935
Silver Springs, MD 20910
(301) 588-9284

Scan-GTE Education Services
GTE Place
West Airfield Dr.
P.O. Box 619810
DFW Airport, TX 75261-9810
(800) 927-3000

TECHNOLOGY-RELATED ASSISTANCE–FUNDED STATES (NIDRR)

Alabama Statewide Technology Access and Response Project (STAR)
2125 East South Blvd
P.O. Box 20752
Birmingham, AL 36120-0752
(205) 288-0240

American Samoa Assistive Technology Project
Division of Vocational Rehab.
Dept. of Human Resources
Pago Pago, American Samoa 96799
(684) 633-2336/1806

Arizona Technology Access Program (AZTAP)
2600 N. Wyatt, 2nd floor
Tucson, AZ 85712
(602) 324-3170

Arkansas Increasing Capabilities Access Network
2201 Brookwood, Suite 117
Little Rock, AR 72202
(501) 666-8868

Assistive Technologies of Alaska
400 D Street, Suite 230
Anchorage, AK 99503-7445
(800) 770-0138
(907) 562-5609

California Assistive Technology System
CA Department of Rehabilitation
830 K St., Room 307
Sacramento, CA 95814
(916) 327-3967

Colorado Assistive Technology Project
Rocky Mountain Resource & Training Institute
6355 Ward Rd, Suite 310
Arvada, CO 80004
(303) 420-2942

Commonwealth of the Northern Mariana Islands Assistive Technology Project
Developmental Disabilities Planning Office
Office of the Governor
P.O. Box 2565
Salpan, MP 96950
(670) 322-3014

Connecticut Assistive Technology Project
Bureau of Rehabilitation Services
10 Griffin Road N.
Windsor, CT 06095
(203) 296-2042

Dakota Link
1925 Plaza Blvd.
Rapid City, SD 57702
(800) 645-0673
(605) 394-1876

Delaware Assistive Technology Initiative
U of DE/A.I. duPont Inst.
1600 Rockland Rd. Rm 154
Wilmington, DE 19899
(302) 651-6790

D.C. Partnership for Assistive Technology
801 Pennsylvania Avenue, S.E., Suite 210
Washington, DC 20003
(202) 546-9164

Florida Alliance for Assistive Service and Technology
2002 Old St. Augustine Rd.
Building A
Tallahassee, FL 32399-0696
(904) 487-3278

Georgia Tools for Life
Division of Rehabilitation Services
2 Peachtree Street N.W., Suite 23-411
Atlanta, GA 30303
(800) 726-9119
(404) 894-4960

Guam System for Assistive Technology
University Affiliated Program
Developmental Disabilities
House #12, Dean's Circle
University of Guam
UCG Station
Mangilao, Guam 96923
(671) 734-9309

Hawaii Assistive Technology Training and Service Project
677 Ala Moana Boulevard, Suite 403
Honolulu, HI 96813
(800) 532-7110

Idaho Assistive Technology Project
129 W. 3rd Street
Moscow, ID 83843
(208) 885-3630/3621

Illinois Assistive Technology Project
110 Iles Park Place
Springfield, IL 62718
(800) 852-5110
(217) 522-7985

Indiana Attain (Accessing Technology Through Awareness in Indiana) Project
P.O. Box 7083
402 W. Washington Street
Room W453
Indianapolis, IN 46207-7083
(317) 232-1410

Iowa Program for Assistive Technology
Iowa University Affiliated Program
University Hospital School
Iowa City, IA 52242
(800) 331-3027

Assistive Technology for Kansas Project
2501 Gabriel
P.O. Box 738
Parons, KS 67357
(316) 421-8367

Kentucky Assistive Technology Services Network
Coordinating Center
427 Versailles Rd.
Frankfort, KY 40601
(502) 573-4665

Louisiana Assistive Access Technology Network
P.O. Box 14115
Baton Rouge, LA 70898
(800) 922-9152

Maine Consumer Information and Technology Training Exchange (Main CITE)
Maine CITE Coordinating Center
University of Maine at Augusta
46 University Dr.
Augusta, ME 04330
(207) 621-3195

Maryland Technology Assistive Program
Governor's Office for Individuals With Disabilities
300 W. Lexington St., Box 10
Baltimore, MD 21201
(800) 832-4827

Massachusetts Assistive Technology Partnership Center
Children's Hospital
1295 Boylston Street, Suite 310
Boston, MA 02115
(617) 355-7153

MonTECH
The University of Montana,
MUARID, MonTECH
634 Eddy Ave.
Missoula, MT 59812
(406) 243-5676

Nebraska Assistive Technology Project
301 Centennial Mall South
P.O. Box 94987
Lincoln, NE 68509-4987
(402) 671-3647/0735

Michigan Tech 2000
Michigan Department of Education
Rehabilitation Services
P.O. Box 30010
Lansing, MI 48909-7510
(517) 373-9233

Minnesota Star Program
300 Centennial Building
658 Cedar St.
St. Paul, MN 55155
(800) 331-3027
(612) 297-1554

Mississippi Project Start
P.O. Box 1000
Jackson, MS 39205-1000
(601) 987-4872

Missouri Assistive Technology Project
4731 South Cochise, Suite 114
Independence, MO 64055-6975
(800) 647-8558
(816) 373-5193

Nevada Assistive Technology Collaborative
Rehabilitation Division
Community-Based Services Development
711 South Stewart St.
Carson City, NV 89710
(702) 687-4452

New Hampshire Technology Partnership Project
Institute on Disability/UAP
#14, Ten Ferry St.
The Concord Center
Concord, NH 03301
(603) 224-0630

New Jersey Technology Assistive Resource Program
135 East State St.
CN 398
Trenton, NJ 08625
(609) 292-7498
(609) 633-6959

New Mexico Technology Assistance Program
435 St. Michael's Dr., Building D
Santa Fe, NM 87503
(800) 866-2253

New York State Triad Project
Office of Advocate for the Disabled
One Empire State Plaza, Tenth Floor
Albany, NY 12223-1150
(518) 474-2825

North Carolina Assistive Technology Project
Department of Human Resources
Division of Vocational Rehabilitation Services
1110 Navaho Dr., Suite 101
Raleigh, NC 27609
(800) 852-0042

North Dakota Interagency Program for Assistive Technology (IPAT)
P.O. Box 743
Cavalier, ND 58220
(701) 265-4807

Ohio Train
Ohio Super Computer Center
1224 Kinmear Road
Columbus, OH 43212
(614) 292-2426

Oregon Technology Access for Life Needs Project (TALN)
Chemeketa Community College
P.O. Box 14007
Salem, OR 97309-7070
(503) 399-4950

Pennsylvania's Initiative on Assistive Technology
Institute on Disability/UAP
Ritter Hall Annex 433 (004-00)
Philadelphia, PA 19122
(215) 204-1356

Puerto Rico Assistive Technology Project
University of Puerto Rico
Medical Sciences Campus
College of Related Health Professions
Dept. of Communication Disorders
Box 365067
San Juan, PR 00936
(800) 496-6035

Rhode Island Assistive Technology Access Project
Office of Rehabilitation Services
40 Fountain St.
Province, RI 02903-1898
(401) 421-7005

South Carolina Assistive Technology Program
Vocational Rehabilitation Department
P.O. Box 15, 1410-C Boston Ave.
West Columbia, SC 29171-0015
(803) 822-5404

Washington Assistive Technology Alliance
DSHS/DVR
P.O. Box 45340
Olympia, WA 98504-5340
(206) 438-8051

West Virginia Assistive Technology System
Division of Rehabilitation Services
P.O. Box 50890, State Capital
Charleston, WV 25305-0890
(800) 841-8436
(304) 766-4698

WISTECH
Division of Vocational Rehabilitation
P.O. Box 7852
1 W. Wilson St., Room 950
Madison, WI 53707-7852
(608) 266-5395

Wyoming's New Options in Technology (WYNOT)
Division of Vocational Rehabilitation
1100 Herschler Building
Cheyenne, WY 82002
(307) 777-6947/4386/7450

Virginia Assistive Technology System
8004 Franklin Farms Drive
P.O. Box K300
Richmond, VA 23288-0300
(804) 662-9993

Tennessee Technology Access Project
710 James Robertson Parkway
Gateway Plaza, 11th Floor
Nashville, TN 37243
(615) 532-6530

Texas Assistive Technology Project
University of Texas at Austin
UAP of Texas
Department of Special Education
EDB 306
Austin, TX 78712
(512) 471-7621

Utah Assistive Technology Program
Center for Persons With Disabilities
UMC 6855
Logan, UT 84322-6855
(800) 333-UTAH
(801) 797-1982

Vermont Assistive Technology Project
103 South Main Street, Weeks 1
Waterbury, VT 05671-2305
(802) 241-2620

CONFERENCES

Abilities Expo
> Durable medical equipment

American Occupational Therapy Association Annual Conference
> Professional, product demonstrations, papers, workshops

American Physical Therapy Association Annual Conference
> Professional, seminars, product data

American Speech-Language-Hearing Association (ASHA) Annual Conference
> Professional, some product data, seminars

The Association for Persons With Severe Handicaps (TASH) Annual Conference
> Product demonstrations, seminars

California State University at Northridge (CSUN) Technology and Persons With Disabilities Annual Conference on Contemporary Applications of Technology
> Extensive product demonstration, seminars

Closing the Gap Conference
> Microcomputer technology, educational emphasis

International Society for Augmentative and Alternative Communication (ISAAC) Conference
> International conference, communication based, seminars, demonstrations

National Home Health Care Exposition
> Home health-care products, durable medical equipment, showcase for new products

National Symposium on Information Technology (NSIT)
> Information access to assistive technology

President's Committee on Employment of People With Disabilities (PCEPD) Annual Meeting
> Vocational rehabilitation, law, legislation regarding employment

RESNA Conference
> Extensive rehabilitation engineering services, applications, product demonstrations, seminars, workshops, multidisciplinary

ADA RESOURCES

Employment

Equal Opportunity Commission
1801 L St., N.W.
Washington, DC 20507
(202) 663-4900
(800) 800-3302 (TTD)

Public Accommodation and State and Local Government Services

Department of Justice
Office on the American With Disabilities Act
Civil Rights Division
P.O. Box 66118
Washington, DC 20035-6118
(202) 514-0301
(202) 514-0318

Accessible Design in New Construction and Alterations

Architectural and Transportation Barriers Compliance Board
1111 18th Street, N.W., Suite 501
Washington, DC 20036
(800) USA-ABLE

Transportation

Department of Transportation
400 Seventh St., S.W.
Washington, DC 20590
(202) 366-9305
(202) 755-7687 (TDD)

Telecommunications

Federal Communications Commission
1919 M St., N.W.
Washington, DC 20554
(202) 632-7260
(202) 632-6999 (TDD)

Tax Credits and Deductions for Business

Internal Revenue Service
Department of the Treasury
1111 Constitution Ave., N.W.
Washington, DC 20044
(202) 566-2000

NEWSLETTERS/JOURNALS

Augmentative Communication News (Bimonthly)
One Surf Way, Suite 215
Monteray, CA 93940

Assistive Technology (Biannually)
RESNA Publication

Careers and the Disabled (Published 3 times a year)
Independent Living (Published 3 times a year)
Equal Opportunity Publications, Inc.
150 Motor Parkway, Suite 420
Hauppauge, NY 11788

CRT News Update
Center for Rehabilitation Technology
Georgia Institute of Technology
Atlanta, GA 30332-0156

Durable Medical Equipment Review (Bi-monthly)
Benkei Publishing Company, Inc.
Queen Executive Center
167 Washington Street
Norwell, MA 02061-9911

Journal of Rehabilitation Research and Development (VA Quarterly)
Rehabilitation Research and Development Services
Department of Veterans Affairs
103 South Gay Street
Baltimore, MD 21202-4051

Journal of American Occupational Therapy Association (Monthly)
Occupational Therapy Newsletter for Special Interest Sections (Quarterly)
Published by American Occupational Therapy Association

Occupational Therapy Journal of Research (Quarterly)
Slack Inc.
6900 Grove Road
Thorofare, New Jersey 08086-9447

Proceedings of RESNA Conferences (Annually)
Assistive Technology (Biannually)
Published by RESNA

Rehabilitation Robotics Newsletter
Alfred I. DuPont Institute
P.O. Box 269
Wilmington, DE 19899

Team Rehab Report (Monthly)
Miramar Communications Inc.
23815 Stuart Ranch Road
P.O. Box 1987
6133 Bristol Parkway
Malibu, CA 90265-8987

Technology and Disabilities (Quarterly)
Butterworth and Heinemann
225 Wildwood Avenue, Unit B
Editors Mann and Lane
Center for Assistive Technology
University of Buffalo
Buffalo, New York

Orthotic and Rehabilitation Terminology

Mark Agro

11

The effectiveness of orthotic practice depends on the clarity, accuracy, and efficiency with which the language is used or understood. This chapter on terminology used in the field of orthotics provides a reference for the technical terms used by orthotists, physiatrists, orthopedic surgeons, therapists, and other specialists. Compiling an orthotic and orthopedic lexicon is never complete since word usage continually changes. Language is never static; new terminology appears every day, while old terms fall out of use. This evolution is necessary to ensure effective communication among allied health professionals.

Over the last 20 years, a significant effort has been made to clarify and systematize terms used in orthotics. The confusing convention of naming orthoses by their designer fortunately has been replaced by a more pragmatic approach. In 1989, the International Standards Organization (ISO) in Geneva published recommended orthotic and prosthetic terms in an attempt to standardize words used in orthotics. The ISO advocates that orthoses be named by the anatomic joint(s) incorporated within the brace's structure. Ankle–foot orthosis, knee–ankle–foot orthosis, and hip–knee–ankle–foot orthosis are some common examples of the ISO nomenclature. Practitioners use acronyms such as AFO, KAFO, and HKAFO. This system is repeated for all areas of the body that are braced. Although orthoses are named for the joints they cross, their biomechanical effects often

extend more proximally. Particularly with ankle–foot orthoses (AFOs), they frequently control the knee, even though they do not traverse it.

The eponymic tendency in naming an orthosis is rare today; however, the names of cities such as Boston, Milwaukee, Philadelphia, Toronto, and Charleston continue to live on in the names of our orthoses. In addition, many old eponyms have been included because occasionally an older practitioner will inquire about an orthosis. No other book in print describes these terms, which were first compiled in *Orthotics Etcetera* in 1966.[1]

This chapter is designed as a resource for information regarding usage, etymology, acronyms, and eponyms used in the orthotic and rehabilitative field. The list of terms represents common terminology found in today's clinical environment. Every attempt has been made to use ISO conventions for vocabulary to prevent misunderstandings among allied health professionals and thus ultimately benefit the patient.

A-frame orthosis Bilateral hip abduction knee–ankle–foot orthosis (KAFO) applied to abduct the hip joints to maintain a stable position of the head of the femur in the acetabulum. Used for the treatment of disorders of the hip joint, notably Legg-Perthes disease.

Abouna splint Distal interphalangeal orthosis. Made of one piece of steel wire enclosed in a tube of latex rubber, it is shaped to fit over the two distal phalanges. Used in treatment of mallet finger.[2,3]

Accommodative foot orthosis Foot orthoses that conform to the abnormal foot shape or position to equalize pressure distribution on the foot. cf. *Functional foot orthosis.*

ADL Activities of daily living.

AFO Ankle–foot orthosis. An orthosis that encompasses the foot and lower leg. Biomechanically, it exerts control over the foot–ankle complex in the sagittal plane. Nearly all AFOs offer some mediolateral stability to control inversion or eversion. However, by altering the direction of the ground reaction force, an AFO can exert a more proximal controlling force on the knee, even though it does not cross the joint. See *Floor reaction AFO.*

Air splint Immobilizing orthosis for temporary use consisting of air cells that are inflated to encircle the limb and joints where desired.

Airplane splint Shoulder–elbow–wrist–hand orthosis (SEWHO) used to position the shoulder joint in an abducted position. Often prefabricated, it consists of adjustable segments with support for the arm and hand, while connected by a frame to a foundation on the patient's trunk and pelvis. Adjustable bars allow various abduction positions to be selected by the orthotist.

AMBRL or USAMBRL U.S. Army Medical Bioengineering Research and Development Laboratory, where several orthoses and prostheses were developed.

Ankle–foot–orthosis, flexible Plastic ankle–foot orthosis (AFO) that through the plastic architecture about the ankle allows desired motion in one plane. Generally, there is a restriction of plantarflexion while dorsiflexion is permitted.

Ankle–foot–orthosis, rigid Ankle–foot orthosis (AFO), which by design restricts both sagittal and frontal motion about the ankle joint. Biomechanically a rigid ankle can have a proximal effect on the knee during midstance to toe-off by inducing knee extension or flexion. See *Floor reaction AFO.*

APL Applied Physics Laboratory of John Hopkins University, Baltimore, where electromechanical devices were developed to be used in conjunction with orthoses.

Aplix French company manufacturing hook and loop fasteners (Velcro) used for numerous applications in orthotics such as belts and straps. In 1977, Velcro-France changed its name to APLIX S.A.

Arch support Colloquialism for foot orthosis (FO). Orthosis used to control abnormal foot positions or relieve pressure by redistributing weight-bearing forces on the foot.

ARGO Steeper advanced reciprocating gait orthosis, a TLSHKAFO using a modular version of the reciprocating gait orthosis (RGO) principle to assist paraplegics to attain bipedal gait. The ARGO has cables and assistive gas struts on the lateral uprights to stabilize the knees. See also *Reciprocating gait orthosis.*

Arnold back brace Thoracolumbosacral support consisting of a large pelvic belt, two paraspinal and two lateral uprights, and a transverse steel band at below scapular level, which drops under the axilla and terminates in a padded knob under the clavicle.[4]

Ashley heel A shoe with particularly large base of support built for greater stability in walking.

Assist Descriptor of orthotic joint motion control. A joint with assist includes springs or elastics to enhance joint motion.

Axial rotation The pivoting of a body part around its central longitudinal axis in the transverse plane.

Baeyer dropfoot brace   An ankle–foot orthosis (AFO) with posterior upright and a pair of elastic or leather straps from the calf band to the lace stays of the shoe.

Bail lock   An addition to mechanical knee joints consisting of a ring of metal linking medial and lateral knee joints passing posteriorly to the knee joint. This addition automatically locks the knee in extension. The "bail" description is taken from the handle of a metal pail that aptly depicts the appearance of the lever that controls the locking mechanism. When the patient is standing, the joints are locked in extension. For flexed knee sitting, the patient pulls up on the bail, and the knee becomes unlocked. Also known as a French or Swiss lock.

Baker spinal brace   A hyperextension back brace with pubic and manubrial pads and elastic straps.

Balanced forearm orthosis (BFO)   Elbow orthosis attached to a wheelchair frame to assist arm positioning for individuals with spinal cord injuries, shoulder muscle, or upper arm paresis. Some limited arm motion is required to manipulate this device, which balances so that gravity provides or assists the motions that are missing or weak. The BFO has an adjustable fulcrum-trough in which the forearm rests. The orthosis is articulated and swivels to assist hand positioning.

Balmoral shoe   A front-laced ankle-high shoe in which the lace stays meet in front, being stitched along their anterior borders to the vamp, and forming a V-pattern. It was introduced in 1853 and named after Balmoral Castle in Scotland. Also known as a Bal.

Barlow splint   X-shaped metal splint applied to the back of an infant with congenital dislocation of the hip. The four ends of the splint are molded over the shoulders and thighs to keep the latter abducted and flexed.

Barton wedge   A wedge inserted inside the shoe at its medial border.

Becker brace, joint, lock   Refer to various orthotic components made by the Becker Orthopedic Appliance Company in Troy, Michigan. The company was founded by Otto Karl Becker.

Bell-Grice splint   A bilateral shoe clamp spreader bar.

Bender splint   Fifth-finger adduction splint with spring wire.

Bennett finger splints   Simple orthoses for the digits of the hand to control instabilities and deformities commonly encountered in rheumatoid arthritis. These are mostly metal devices to be slipped on a digit ("slip-on splints"), occasionally also with a strap of metal or textile material.

Bisgrove hand or splint   Tenodesis wrist–hand orthosis (WHO) developed by John G. Bisgrove. A functional dynamic wrist–extension–finger–flexion hand splint.

Blucher   A front-laced shoe pattern with the tongue as part of the forepart and in which the quarters lap over the vamp or forepart.

Bluhm clubfoot splint   A modification of footplates to provide a corrective force in adduction deformity of the forefoot.

Bobath sling   A soft support for the upper limb, designed to counteract the tendency to glenohumeral subluxation in hemiplegia. A figure-eight bandage around the shoulder girdle with a small foam-rubber cushion or roll in the axilla (to provide some abduction of the humerus) or a cuff around the proximal segment of the arm (to hold the humeral head in place).

Body jacket   Generic term used to describe various spinal orthoses (TLSOs) used to immobilize and provide support to the spine.

Boldrey brace An orthosis for immobilization of the cervical spine without a chin piece. It reaches from the forehead and occiput to the lower ribs. From each side of the occiput, a prong advances below the ear and is molded individually to the contour of the maxillary and infrazygomatic region. Developed in 1945 by neurosurgeon Edwin B. Boldrey (San Francisco). It provides supportive immobilization of the cervical spine.

Boston brace or jacket A prefabricated thermoplastic thoracolumbosacral orthosis (TLSO with interface) used for the conservative treatment of scoliosis. Prefabricated modules are ordered by the orthotist based on measurements taken from the patient. Manufactured by Boston Brace International, Avon, Massachusetts.

Boutonnière splint Proximal interphalangeal finger orthosis (FO) used for the treatment of Boutonnière deformity. This is a disorder of the finger(s) exhibiting flexion deformity of the proximal interphalangeal joint and hyperextension of the distal joint. The splint reduces the flexion of the proximal interphalangeal joint and hyperextension of the distal joint.

Bowden cable A special cable and housing, resembling the cables used for bicycle brakes, to transmit forces from one area to another. Consists of a central wire inside a housing to reduce friction and binding. The cable links the hip joints in a reciprocating gait orthoses and is also found in some upper extremity orthoses.

Brace Vernacular for *orthosis* used interchangeably throughout this text.

Break The wrinkle or crease formed in the vamp of a shoe when the shoe is flexed at the ball.

Buckling Failure of a long thin object or sudden giving way of a joint through instability in compression, for example, uncontrolled knee.

Bunnell splints Prefabricated hand orthoses of padded metal straps joined by wires. Operates as a dynamic orthoses through elastic bands. Named for Sterling Bunnell, a hand surgeon.

CAD-CAM Computer-aided-design, computer-aided-manufacture. Computer technology sometimes used to construct orthoses and prostheses for the disabled.

Calcaneus The largest bone of the foot, the heel bone. Also used as an adjective to describe a position of deformity involving fixed or tight dorsiflexion of the foot, which makes the calcaneus more prominent.

California crutch See *Canadian crutch.*

Caliper Medial and lateral metal uprights (usually round) used in lower extremity bracing to transmit forces from the shoe to the calf portion of an orthosis. The caliper fits into an attachment plate on the heel and allows easier interchangeability of shoes.

Camp brace, corset, collar A variety of upper and lower extremity orthoses manufactured and distributed by Camp International, Jackson, Michigan.

Canadian crutch A wooden crutch, resembling an axillary crutch, but slightly shorter and ending with a leather cuff at or slightly above midarm level. It prevents flexion (buckling) of the elbow and assists triceps weakness. Also called California crutch. Suggested term: wooden triceps crutch.

Canty long leg brace Knee–ankle–foot orthosis (KAFO) with ischial seat and a knee joint with axis posterior to weight-bearing line, used in flaccid paralysis and fractures of lower limb.[5]

Carpal tunnel splint Static wrist–hand orthosis (WHO) used to restrict flexion and extension about the wrist to reduce motion and pain caused by carpal tunnel syndrome.

CARS-UBC knee orthosis   Named after the Canadian Arthritis and Rheumatism Society–University of British Columbia, it consists of two plastic cuffs, one for the thigh, one for the leg, connected by a telescoping rod. It is designed to correct a valgus or varus deformity of the knee, providing freedom to the flexed knee and a force to straighten it on extension, as in the stance phase of gait.[6]

Case hardening   The process of increasing the hardness of a metal by heating and then quickly cooling the part. Many orthotic components are case hardened to increase their durability.

CASH brace   The acronym CASH refers to a prefabricated spinal orthosis called a cruciform anterior spinal hyperextension. A lightweight modular thoracolumbosacral orthosis (TLSO) to help maintain extension of the spine. Manufactured and distributed by Ralph Storrs, Inc., Kankakee Illinois. See also *Hyperextension brace.*

Caudad   A position in the direction of the feet.

Cavus   Common term used to characterize a higher than average medial longitudinal arch in the foot.

CCO   Craniocervical orthosis. Orthosis encompassing the head and cervical spine, which controls motion in the cervical spine.

Center of gravity   The point at which the gravitational force is assumed to act on a body. It is often identical to center of mass.

Center of mass   The point about which the mass of an object is assumed to be concentrated.

Cephalad   Refers to a position in the direction of the head.

Certified orthotist (CO)   A health professional engaged in the practice of orthotics. To obtain certification, an orthotist must successfully pass a national set of examinations. Certified orthotists have demonstrated capabilities to design, manufacture, and fit orthoses and may use the initials CO.

Chairback brace   See *Knight spinal brace.*

Chandler felt collar   A felt collar, usually covered with stockinet, a machine-knitted, washable cloth. Illustrated in *Dorland's Illustrated Medical Dictionary*[7] under splint.

Charleston bending brace   A thoracolumbosacral orthosis (TLSO) used for conservative treatment of idiopathic scoliosis and designed in 1978 by R. Hooper, CPO, in cooperation with Dr. F. Reed of Charleston, South Carolina. The application purposely bends the abnormal spinal curvature into an overcorrected condition. This orthosis is considered for nocturnal use, because the axial loading on the spine is eliminated when the patient is horizontal.

Charnley caliper   A short-term adjustable splint with a padded ring for the groin, to be used immediately after the removal of the cast for a lower-limb fracture. Designed by British orthopedic surgeon J. Charnley.[8]

Cloran mouthstick   Motor-operated telescoping stick held in the mouth by means of a custom-fitted mouthpiece. Developed by Ohio dentist Arthur J. Cloran.[9]

Closure   Method of fastening together, closing, binding, or confining. Usually refers to straps on orthoses or shoes.

Clubfoot splint   Ankle–foot orthoses (AFO) used to apply a three-point pressure system to correct a talipes equinovarus foot.

CO   Cervical orthosis. Often called a cervical collar. This orthosis is used to treat conditions of the cervical spine, and it may be soft or rigid with a variety of names, such as Thomas, Mayo, Philadelphia, or Queen Anne.

Cockup splint   Wrist–hand orthoses (WHO) to maintain the wrist in a desired position.

Coleyne   Also known as *copolymer*. A common hybrid plastic used in orthotics and prosthetics consisting of a mixture of approximately 80 to 90 percent polypropylene and 10 to 20 percent polyethylene. The addition of polyethylene makes it a less brittle plastic.

Collins spring splint   A spring splint for paralysis of the long extensors or the fingers, leaving the finger pads and the palm of the hand free. Developed by D.W. Collins and R.D. Muckart.[10]

Compression garments   Elastic garments used to prevent hypertrophic scar formation and contractures or to control edema.

Continuous passive motion (CPM) machine
Uses an external energy source to provide occasional, interrupted, or continuous motion to affected joints. It consists of an orthosis encompassing one or more joints that is driven by an electric motor. It has been widely used after joint surgery to maintain range of motion and reduce edema and pain. A common example is its use after a total knee joint prostheses.

Contracture   An abnormal condition caused by tight or shortened soft tissues around a joint that prevents the full extension or flexion of a joint. A fixed flexion deformity is the most common type, but there can also be a contracture in extension.

Cook anterior heel   Metatarsal bar placed between the inner and outer soles.[11]

Cook shingle   Pressure pad used as an accessory to a flexible orthosis (corset). It is of rectangular shape, about 8 cm high and between 25 and 35 cm long and is most often applied to the lumbosacral area.

Cook walking caliper   An ischial weight-bearing brace with or without knee joint manufactured by the Zimmer Manufacturing Company.

Cookie   A wafer-shaped piece of material placed in a shoe as a pad under the medial longitudinal arch of the foot.

Copolymer   A common hybrid plastic used in orthotics and prosthetics consisting of a mixture of at least two types of plastic. The resultant plastic has many of the desirable features of each of the component plastics. See also *Coleyne.*

Coronal plane   A plane that divides the body into anterior and posterior sections (same as frontal plane).

Corset   Cloth or similar fabric spinal orthoses, or the fabric front of various spinal orthoses. Used to increase intra-abdominal pressure. The term also is used to describe the reinforcement of firm leather or stays incorporated in the upper of a shoe to support or restrict ankle motion.

Cotrel cast   Body cast made with slow-setting plaster during cephalopelvic traction while the patient is suspended by derotation slings applied to the outside of the cast.[12,13] Developed for the treatment of scoliosis by Yves Cotrel et al. at Berck-Plage, France.[12] It is also called elongation, derotation and [lateral] flexion (EDF) cast.

Coughlin shoulder splint   A body harness with outrigger arranged so that the patient receives assisted abduction by actively extending the shoulder.[14,15]

Cowhorn brace   A metal thoracolumbrosacral orthosis to control thoracic kyphosis similar to the Arnold brace. Flat curved metal extensions arise from the lateral ends of the thoracic band to end in small discs in the subclavicular area. The extensions resemble the horns of a cow.

Craig bar or (hip) splint   Spreader bar to which shoes are attached. Used in the treatment of Legg-Calvé-Perthes disease while allowing weight bearing. Similar to Illfeld abduction splint.

Cranial halo orthosis A cervicothoracic orthosis (CTO) used for maximum immobilization of the cervical spine. Fixation pins secure the halo into the skull. Adjustable distraction rods link the halo to a padded vest or spinal jacket to restrict spinal motion.

CTLSO Cervicothoracolumbosacral orthosis, often used in treatment of scoliosis.

CTO Cervicothoracic orthosis.

Cuban heel A heel that is higher than the heel of an Oxford shoe, approximately 3 to 5 cm. Usually only found in women's shoes, the heel is still large and low enough to secure a conventional ankle–foot orthosis structure.

Cushioned heel(s) Heel added to shoe made from soft cushioned material to provide a shock absorbing effect during gait. See *SACH.*

Custom-fitted orthosis Orthosis that requires customizing or assembling a prefabricated orthosis to fit a patient.

Custom orthosis An orthosis fabricated to fit a single patient. A cast, tracing, or a computer digital impression of the involved body part is taken and used as a model to make the orthosis. The orthosis cannot be worn by others. Custom orthoses can also be made by forming a low-temperature thermoplastic directly on the patient.

D Ring D-shaped loop of wire or plastic used to anchor the closing of webbing or other fastening material when it is folded back on itself.

De Puy splint Term used to describe various orthoses from the De Puy Manufacturing Company, Warsaw, Indiana.

DeLorme brace Knee–ankle–foot orthosis with adjustable uprights and shoe clamp by which it is attached to the heel of the shoe.[16]

Denis Browne splint Orthosis consisting of a bar clamped or riveted to Oxford-type shoes to abduct and externally or internally rotate the leg. This puts a torque on the lower extremities to counter torsional deformities. Primarily for pediatric treatment of club foot (talipes equinovarus). Named for its designer, Dr. Denis John Browne, a London Orthopedic surgeon (1892–1967).

Denison arm sling, brace, collar, etc. Any of various orthoses manufactured by C.D. Denison Orthopaedic Appliance Corporation, Baltimore, founded by orthotist Cedric D. Denison (1900–1980).

Denison cervical brace A two-poster occipitalcervicothoracic orthosis designed to immobilize the cervical spine. One poster connects a mandibular support with a breast plate; the other connects an occipital support with a plate over the scapulae. The two plates are connected by shoulder straps. Developed around 1960 by Cedric D. Denison.[17]

Denver bar, Denver heel A variant of the metatarsal bar, it is attached to the outsole of the shoe but is usually thinner and extends farther posteriorly, to about the level of the tarsometatarsal joints. Used to relieve pressure on the metatarsal heads. An internal Denver bar is inserted between outsole and insole.[18,19] According to Milgram and Jacobson,[20] the name originated with H. Sonnenschein, a New York orthopedist who referred to this orthoses as the *Denver bar,* since he had seen it used, in the late 1930s, by Dr. Lyle Pacard in Denver.

DIP joint Distal interphalangeal joint.

Direct formed See *Molded to patient.*

Dorsal The back or upward-facing segment of the body. cf. *Volar*

Dorsiflexion Flexion of a joint in the direction of the dorsum of the body part. Often used with reference to the foot or hand.

Double-action ankle joint Mechanical ankle joint that allows assistance or resistance of dorsiflexion or plantar flexion range of motion.

Double-bar AFO An ankle–foot orthoses (AFO) consisting of metal medial and lateral uprights attached to the shoe distally and connected proximally to a padded calf band. It will control sagittal and frontal plane mobility at the ankle.

Dropfoot Also known as *footdrop*. During gait, the foot plantarflexes and the toes drag on the floor because of loss of antigravitational effect from weak or absent dorsiflexors.

Dropfoot brace Any number of ankle–foot orthoses (AFOs) used for treatment of weakened ankle dorsiflexors during ambulation.

Durr-Fillauer Durr-Fillauer Orthopedic, Chattanooga, Tennessee. Manufacturer and supplier of components used by orthotists and prosthetists to fabricate orthopedic appliances for the disabled. A Fillauer bar is a type of Denis Browne splint for hip abduction. The company is now Fillauer, Inc., in Chattanooga, Tennessee.

Dutchman Traditional term applied to wedges added to shoes. A wedged piece of leather inserted between layers of heel or sole. Usually, it is a lateral sole wedge under the fifth metatarsal bone.

Dynamic orthosis An orthosis, usually with articulations, that generally provides assistive movement with springs or elastic bands.

Engen extension orthosis Based on the three-point pressure principle to correct joint deformities such as knee, elbow, or wrist flexion contractures.[21]

Engen reciprocal finger prehension unit A flexor tenodesis splint.[22]

Equilibrium In biomechanics, equilibrium is the state in which forces and moments on an object are balanced—an important concept in applying corrective forces about a joint with an orthosis.

Equinus A plantar flexion deformity of the foot, often associated with a tight Achilles tendon.

European lock Mostly used for the knee joint of a knee–ankle–foot orthosis (KAFO) its sturdiness allows the use of a unilateral lock on the lateral side of the joint. It is opened (for bending the knee) by a small lever at the lateral thigh upright. Its use is similar to that of a Swiss lock. Developed by Otto Bock Orthopädische Industrie, Duderstadt, West Germany, hence also called O.I. lock.[23]

Eversion A movement in the frontal plane only whereby the plantar surface of the foot is moved to face away from the midline of the body. This motion is caused by a combination of pronation, dorsiflexion, and abduction.

EWHFO Elbow–wrist–hand–finger orthosis.

EWHO Elbow–wrist–hand orthosis.

Ewing long leg brace A knee–ankle–foot orthosis (KAFO) incorporating a modification of the upper portion of the medial thigh upright, aimed at decreasing the bulkiness in the crotch, particularly in bilateral orthoses. The upright is bent posteriorly and slightly spiraled to conform to the contour of the thigh.[24]

Exeter splint One of several splints, typically a "lively" coiled-spring wrist or hand splint, developed in Exeter, England, notably by orthopaedic surgeon Norman Capener.[8,25]

Extrinsic posting A distinctive wedge modification added to the external part of a foot orthosis. The wedge accommodates a specific foot deformity. On weight bearing, the wedge prevents unwanted motion. It can be added to the forefoot in the case of forefoot varus leading to excessive pronation or to the rear foot, for example, calcaneal valgus. cf. *Intrinsic posting.*

Ferrari orthosis Various static or dynamic pediatric orthoses (AFO, KAFO, HKAFO) used in the management of myelomeningocele. The concept was developed by Italian Neurologist Dr. Adriano Ferrari of Bologna, Italy. Depending on the lesion level, the orthosis allows limited range of motion at selected joints. Patients with high lesions wearing HKAFOs are allowed a three-dimensional range of motion at the hip joint.

Fillauer bar of splint See *Durr-Fillauer.*

Filler Various materials, such as cork, felt, rubber, placed between the innersole and outersole to provide leveling and cushioning in shoes.

Flaccidity Absence or great reduction in muscle tone. Often associated with lower motor neuron lesions.

Flexible orthosis Refers to the ability of the material used in an orthosis to bend.

Floor reaction AFO Various forms of ankle–foot orthoses that provide knee stability during mid-to-late stance phase, usually by keeping the knee in extension. The orthoses require a dorsiflexion stop or rigid ankle to prevent the tibia from flexing over the foot. The orthotic alignment of the tibia–foot angle is critical to achieving the desired anteriorly directed force on the tibia. A modification can be incorporated to keep the knee in flexion.

Florida brace See *Jewett hyperextension orthosis.*

FO Foot orthosis. Orthosis below the ankle that encompasses all or part of the foot. Used to reposition an abnormal foot or relieve pressure by redistributing weight bearing on the plantar aspect.

Force A measurable influence causing or preventing motion or causing deformation. In biomecha-

nics, force is measured in Newtons and is always accompanied by a vector designating its direction.

Force couple Two equal and opposite parallel forces with different lines of action. An orthosis may provide such an action to achieve a desired effect on a limb.

Forrester collar A cervical orthosis with four uprights. See *Four poster.*

Four poster Cervical orthosis to restrict range of motion of cervical vertebrae. Consisting of a mandibular support connected to an anterior sternal pad and an occipital support connected to posterior suprascapular pads. Each of the anterior and posterior connections is made up of two supports, for a total of four, hence the term *four poster.*

Fracture orthosis Used primarily for fractures with nonunion after conventional treatment. Fracture orthoses used for lower extremity fractures commonly allow some axial loading through the bone. Most of the forces of walking are redirected from the bone to the external structure of the orthosis.

Free Descriptor of orthotic joint motion control. A free motion joint most commonly allows unrestricted motion in one plane.

Free motion joint Orthotic joint that allows full range of motion in one plane. A free motion ankle joint will allow full dorsiflexion and plantarflexion of the ankle joint but will restrict subtalar mediolateral motion.

Frejka pillow Pediatric hip abduction orthosis used for the treatment of congenital dysplastic hips or hip dislocation. Constructed of a fabric-covered foam, the pillow is worn between the legs and shoulder straps keep it in place. The bulk of the pillow causes abduction of the femora to keep the hips in a more stable position. Devised by orthopedic surgeon Dr. Bedrich Frejka, of Brno, in the Czech Republic.

French lock   See *Bail lock.*

Frontal plane   A plane drawn through the body at right angles to the sagittal plane. The frontal plane divides the body into anterior and posterior segments. Sometimes referred to as the *coronal plane.*

Functional electrical stimulation (FES)   Use of electrodes on the skin or implanted in orthoses to stimulate muscles and recruit stronger contractions or train patients to activate certain muscle groups. Essentially, the power source is a compact battery-operator stimulation unit and useful only when the nerve supply is intact.

Functional foot orthosis   Foot orthosis that alters the foot position to allow the foot to function more closely to normal. cf. *Accommodative foot orthosis.*

Gaffney ankle joint   Low-profile metal single-axis ankle joint. Formed into an ankle–foot orthosis by vacuum forming plastic on top of the joint, the mechanical joint is then integrated into the orthosis to provide articulation at the ankle. The joint allows free motion in one plane. Control of range of motion of dorsiflexion and plantar flexion through stops is achieved by the final trim lines of the moulded plastic around the ankle. The joints were developed by Philip D. Gaffney, Orthotic Technician, Hillsboro, Oregon.

Gait cycle   The repeated reciprocal movement of the upper and lower limbs in a recurring manner during walking. It is usually described from heel strike of a given foot until the next heel strike of the same foot. The cycle is divided into a swing and stance phases for a single limb.

Generation II knee brace   A knee orthosis (KO) commonly called the *G2,* consists of thermoplastic thigh and calf shells connected by a unilateral polycentric knee joint. Custom-made knee orthoses are made from casts sent to Generation II Orthotics Ltd., Richmond, British Columbia, Canada.

Gillette joint   Commercially available injection-moulded polyurethane ankle joints. These plastic joints are without a customary hinge and rely on a narrowing in the polyurethane that allows repeated bending without material fatigue. Dorsiflexion and plantar flexion occur as a result of the flexibility of the polyurethane. Gillette joints are vacuum moulded into the thermoplastic shell of ankle–foot orthoses (AFOs). Dorsiflection and plantar flexion range are controlled by the final trim lines of the plastic shells where the joints are imbedded. Developed at the Gillette Children's Hospital, St. Paul, Minnesota, and manufactured by Becker Orthopedic Appliance Co.

Gillette sitting support orthosis   Custom-molded plastic shell conforming to the sitting body posteriorly and laterally from the knees to the upper thorax. It is mounted on a base to be put on a wheelchair or any other seat. Developed for nonambulatory children with severe cerebral palsy or muscular dystrophy at Gillette Children's Hospital, St. Paul, Minnesota.[26]

Glimcher orthosis   Orthosis relieving weight bearing of a hip affected by Legg-Calvé-Perthes disease. Allowing walking, it consists of a steel bar for the lower limb, ending in a small stilt under the shoe. Its upper end is attached to an ischial ring, which is held in place by a strap over the opposite shoulder. A shoe lift is used on the uninvolved side. Developed by Melvin J. Glimcher (Boston orthopedic surgeon), E.L. Radin, and M.M. Amrich.[27]

Goniometer   Tool consisting of two bars articulated by a central pivot point. Designed to measure relative angle changes or range of motion of an anatomic joint.

Gordon-Barach belt   Emphysema belt. Suprapubic pad on which are placed two elastic metal bands connected to a canvas belt. It compresses the abdomen and thus pushes the diaphragm slightly higher. Both abdomen and diaphragm assume positions closer to expiration, which is thus facilitated, notable in pulmonary emphysema. Devised by American physician Burgess L. Gordon (1892–1984).[28]

Goring   A woven elastic fabric inserted in the front or sides of a shoe upper, the expansion of which allows a larger opening to insert the foot.

Greenville spinal orthosis   Vacuum-formed polypropylene body jacket incorporating the neck and pelvis for immobilization after spinal fusion. Developed at the Shriners Hospital for Crippled Children and manufactured by Greenville Orthopaedic Appliance Company, both in Greenville, South Carolina.[29]

Ground reaction force   The ground reaction force (GRF), usually expressed in Newtons, refers to the force that the ground exerts back on the foot during gait. It can be resolved in two components including the vertical, as result of body weight (and weight carried), and a horizontal, the result of the body's inertial force. The line of action of the ground reaction force is always from a point of contact with the ground through the body's center of gravity (C of G). Often referred to as the *weightbearing line.*

Guilford cervical orthosis   A two-poster cervical orthosis (CO) with one anterior and one posterior poster, shoulder straps, and axillary straps attached to a sternal plate. Named after its designer, a Cleveland, Ohio, orthotist, G.A. Guilford & Sons.[30]

Hallux valgus splint   A foot orthosis used to adduct the great toe in cases of hallux valgus. Usually worn at night or at rest.

Halo   See *Cranial halo orthosis.*

Harris brace   A lumbosacral orthosis (LSO) devised by Dr. R.I. Harris, orthopedic surgeon at the Hospital for Sick Children, Toronto, Ontario, Canada. Comprises a rigid aluminum frame posterior section and a corset front. The brace had its beginnings as an alternative to the cumbersome plaster casts frequently used after spinal surgery.

HdO   Hand orthosis. Sometimes HO is used. HdO designation is recommended by the ISO to allow greater accuracy in the description of the orthosis. HO is commonly used, which could mean hand orthosis or hip orthosis.

Heel breast   The forward face of the heel, often concaved toward the shank.

Heel elevation   An orthopedic modification, measured in a vertical line at the back of the heel from the plantar surface to the heel point at the heel seat.

Heel pitch   Inclination of the heel from the vertical at the posterior surface.

Heel seat   Either a place to which the heel is attached to the shoe or the area on which the anatomic heel rests within the shoe.

Heel stabilizer   A thermoplastic cup to position the calcaneus and contain the shock-absorbing calcaneal fat pad under the heel. See *UCBL heel cup.*

Heel wedge   Alteration to the heel on a shoe to provide corrective forces to the foot at heel strike and mid stance of gait. A medial wedge will cause a varus force to the heel. A lateral wedge will cause a valgus force.

Heel wedge SACH   Wedge of soft cushioning material added to the heel on a shoe to provide a shock-absorbing effect. It also provides a minor rockering component to the foot at heel strike by mimicking ankle plantar flexion.

HKAFO   Hip–knee–ankle–foot orthosis. Describes an orthosis that encompasses the hip, knee, and ankle joints.

HKO   Hip–knee orthosis. An orthosis that encompasses the hip and knee joints.

Hoke corset High-fitting thoracolumbosacral (TLSO) corset, (although occasionally an LSO) of cotton or similar material with multiple stays, front opening, and perineal straps. Hoke corsets have friction buckles that have alternating pull from left to right then right to left. It was widely used in poliomyelitis involving lower trunk muscles. Introduced by Michael Hoke (1874–1944), chief surgeon at the Georgia Warm Springs Foundation, in about 1930.

Hook hemiharness A soft support for the upper limb in hemiplegia, designed to counteract its tendency to glenohumeral subluxation. It consists of two cuffs, one around each arm, and a connecting strap that crosses the shoulder girdle posteriorly. Developed at the August F. Hook Physical Rehabilitation Center of the Community Hospital, Indianapolis, Indiana.

Hoover cane Long light aluminum cane used by a blind person when walking and probing for his way. Developed during World War II by Richard E. Hoover, a medical student who later became an ophthalmologist.

Horizontal plane See *Transverse plane*.

Hosmer-Dorrance Corp. Manufacturer of various prefabricated orthoses and prosthetic components used by orthotists and prosthetists. Located in Campbell, California.

HpO Hip orthosis. An orthosis that encompasses and controls the hip joint. Sometimes HO is used. HpO designation is recommended by the ISO to allow greater accuracy in the description of the orthosis. HO is commonly used, which could mean either hand orthosis or hip orthosis.

Hyperextension Extension of a joint beyond its normal range. An abnormal condition caused by lax or overstretched soft tissues about the joint.

Hyperextension brace Spinal orthosis used to maintain an extended position of the spine by the application of a three-point pressure system. Various prefabricated hyperextension braces are available that are used to stabilize compression fractures. See *Jewett hyperextension orthosis* for further description.

Ilfeld abduction splint Abduction splint consisting of an adjustable spreader bar and two thigh cuffs, used for infants with dislocation of the hips. It gives the child much freedom to move.[31]

Inflare shoe Shoe with inward swing of shoe forepart to apply pressure and position the metatarsals in optimal adduction.

Instep The arched dorsum middle portion of the human foot or that part of the shoe over the anatomic instep.

Interface material Padding or lining material added to the inside of an orthosis to provide cushioning or protection to the skin.

IP extension stop Interphalangeal extension stop. Addition to a wrist–hand orthosis that limits the extension range of the interphalangeal joint, while allowing flexion.

Intrinsic posting A modification to the positive cast of the patient's foot before the plastic orthosis is molded. This modification causes the resultant orthosis, on weight bearing, to maintain the foot into the desired position. This type of posting results in a low-profile orthosis. Intrinsic posting can be used in the rear foot or forefoot section of the orthosis, for example, forefoot varus leading to excessive pronation or calcaneal valgus. cf. *Extrinsic posting*.

Inversion A movement where the plantar surface of the foot is moved to face in the direction of the midline of the body in the frontal plane. A combination of supination, plantar flexion, and adduction motions.

IPMR, IRM Institute of Physical Medicine and Rehabilitation, now Institute of Rehabilitation Medicine, of New York University Medical Center, New York City. Several orthoses and orthotic parts were developed there.

Ischial brim Proximal portion of a knee–ankle–foot orthosis (KAFO) made from plastic, leather, or metal fabricated to contain the upper thigh in a cylindric or quadrilateral shape. The function redirects weight-bearing forces from the bones of the leg to the pelvis through the ischial tuberosity and surrounding upper thigh tissues.

Ischial ring Proximal portion of a knee–ankle–foot orthosis (KAFO). The frame is a metal oval-shaped frame (skeleton), contoured to the shape of the upper thigh and padded. Used as the proximal portion of KAFOs and fracture frames for stabilizing the lower limb by applying upward force on the pelvis to counteract the distal force of traction.

Isocentric RGO Reciprocating gait orthoses (RGOs) developed by Wallace Motloch, C.O., Redwood City, California. The unique feature of this RGO is the connecting link between the hip joints. It pivots on a bearing in the center of the pelvic band. See *Reciprocating gait orthosis.*

Jewett hyperextension orthosis Prefabricated thoracolumbosacral orthosis (TLSO) designed to maintain extension of the spine. The frame applies a three-point pressure system, two anterior (sternal and suprapubic) and a counter-pressure pad between in the thoracolumbar area. Frequently used during the acute stage for patients with spinal compression fractures. Devised by orthopedic surgeon Dr. E.L. Jewett, Florida.

Jobst stocking (garment) Elastic compression garments manufactured by the Jobst Institute, Inc., Toledo, Ohio. Used for the treatment of limb edema or orthostatic hypotension. Also used to prevent hypertrophic scarring.

Jones, Sir Robert A British orthopedic surgeon (1858–1933). He developed a cock-up wrist splint, a frame for mobilizing hip, a metatarsal bar and a spinal brace, all bearing his name.

Jordan, Henry H. German-born New York orthopedic surgeon (1897–1970). He developed a splint for congenital hip dislocation, a dynamic spinal orthosis, a cervical orthosis with two metal uprights (Jordan cement support), an ischial strap seat brace, and a shoulder abduction apparatus, all bearing his name.

KAFO Knee–ankle–foot orthosis. Orthosis encompassing the knee, ankle, and foot. Often called a long leg brace.

Kanavel splint One of several hand splints, mostly of the cock-up type, made of a variety of materials, for various conditions, devised by Chicago surgeon Allen B. Kanavel (1874–1938).[32]

Kinematics A biomechanical term used to describe motion without reference to the forces and masses involved.

Kinetics The analysis of the forces acting on a body that cause motion.

Klemick splint Hand orthosis (HdO) used in flexor tendon repair.

Klenzak brace An ankle–foot orthosis (AFO) to assist weak or absent dorsiflexors during gait. Comprised of Klenzak ankle joints (uprights) attached through a stirrup to a shoe.

Klenzak joint Mechanical ankle joint used in orthoses with an adjustable spring dorsiflexion assist and plantarflexion stop. Designed by J. Klenzak.

Knee lock The addition of a device to maintain the mechanical joint in a stable extended position. Knee locks come in various forms, droplocks use gravity to secure a metal ring around the joint to prevent flexion. Pawl locks such as the

Swiss, Bail, or French are easier to unlock when the patient wants to sit. These types connect medial and lateral sides of the joints through a lever located posterior to the knee.

Knee orthosis, rigid   Knee orthoses (KOs) without joints that are used to protect and immobilize all movement of the knee.

Knight spinal brace   A lumbosacral orthosis (LSO) consisting of a posterior padded aluminum frame of pelvic band, thoracic band, and lateral uprights. A corset front increases intra-abdominal pressure. Functions to reduce lumbar extension and restrict lateral trunk bending. Devised in 1874 by Maryland physician, James C. Knight (1810–1887). Commonly called a *chair back brace.*

Knight-Taylor brace   Hybrid style of thoracolumbosacral orthosis (TLSO), incorporating the increased lateral control from the Knight orthoses with the upper trunk control from the Taylor Orthoses. Restricts motion in the spine in the mediolateral and anteroposterior planes.

Knuckle bender   Dynamic hand–finger orthosis (HFO) applies a three-point pressure system to aid flexion of the metacarpal phalangeal joints. Rubber bands or springs are used to assist flexion.

KO   Knee orthosis. Orthosis encompassing the knee.

Kosair orthosis   A metal orthosis for scoliosis, developed at the Kosair Crippled Children's Hospital, Louisville, Kentucky.

Kydex   Acrylic polyvinyl chloride. A high-temperature thermoplastic used in various applications to fabricate orthoses.

Kyphosis   A normal anteroposterior thoracic curvature (convex posteriorly). Pathologic kyphosis is an abnormal amount of anteroposterior curvature in this region.

Last   Form on which a shoe is made. The term is sometimes used to describe the shape of a shoe. For example, a straight-last shoe is one without a medial inflare of the anterior part of the sole.

Legg-Calvé-Perthes orthosis   A knee–ankle–foot orthosis (KAFO) used to treat Legg-Calvé-Perthes disease. Most types allow ambulation while maintaining the hips in a stable position.

Lehneis spiral orthosis   Plastic ankle–foot orthosis (AFO) that wraps around the leg in a spiral fashion and cradles the heel. The foot part is applied inside the shoe. It is used in foot drop and similar conditions.[33,34]

Lenox Hill brace   Custom-made knee orthosis (KO) designed to provide mediolateral and anteroposterior control of the knee. Orthosis was developed by the Lenox Hill Brace Shop, Inc., New York.

Limited motion joint   Mechanical joint used to restrict the range of motion of an anatomic joint. Some are adjustable to allow controlled range of motion.

Lipscomb brace   Lumbosacral orthosis in which the lateral uprights are connected to the pelvic band by movable joints. Four straps hold an apron in place. Also called the Wilcox brace.[35]

Littler-Jones shoulder abduction splint   Light metal framework anchored to the pelvis by a webbing strap and extending halfway around the arm to support the humerus in abduction.[36,37]

Ljubljana FEPB (functional electronic peroneal brace)   A knee–ankle–foot orthosis (KAFO) combined with a system for electric stimulation. The latter includes a stimulator, electrodes inside an elastic stocking, and a switch on the shoe heel, which initiates a modulated train of electric impulses. Developed at the Rehabilitation Institute, Ljubljana, in the former Yugoslavia, published in 1966.[38]

Lofstrand crutch   Metal forearm crutch designed around 1944 by Adolf Lofstrand (ca. 1894–ca. 1974) in collaboration with George C.S. Woodward. In some areas called the *English cane.*

Long leg brace   Vernacular for knee–ankle–foot orthosis (KAFO) or a hip–knee–ankle–foot orthosis (HKAFO).

LSO   Lumbosacral orthoses.

LSU reciprocating gait orthosis   An HKAFO that uses cables to control hip flexion and extension designed at Louisiana State University. See *Reciprocating gait orthosis.*

MP extension stop   Metacarpal phalangeal extension stop applied to hand orthoses to limit the extension range of the metacarpal phalangeal joints.

MacAusland back brace   Thoracolumbosacral orthosis (TLSO) with clock-spring posterior uprights, a pelvic and thoracic band, and an apron kept in place by three straps attached to the back frame. Used mostly as a postural orthosis, allowing lateral motions. Designed by W. Russell MacAusland, Boston orthopedic surgeon (1882–1965).

Magnuson brace   Thoracolumbosacral orthosis (TLSO). Trunk support with large pelvic belt and a narrower thoracic band, the latter extending anteriorly and upward to end close to the manubrium sterni. The two transverse bands are connected by two pairs of rigid uprights, one in the back, one in the front.[35]

Mayo Clinic   In Rochester, Minnesota, where several orthotic devices have been developed and named: Mayo bar, a metatarsal bar; Mayo collar, a plastic cervical orthosis; Mayo sacroiliac belt.

McKibben muscle   Also called pneumatic, or artificial, muscle, this is an inflatable rubber tube in a woven nylon cover, used to supply external power to an orthosis. Developed in 1957 for his disabled daughter by Los Alamos physicist Joseph L. McKibben, in conjunction with Vernon L. Nickel, orthopedic surgeon.[39,40]

McNabb brace   A thoracolumbosacral orthosis (TLSO) consisting of two independently contoured frames. A posterior TLSO frame with corset front controls lumbar flexion and or extension while increasing intra-abdominal pressure. The second is a U-shaped anterior frame that applies a force through a sternal pad to prevent thoracic flexion.

MCP   Metacarpophalangeal joint.

Metatarsal bar   Tread material added to the external sole of a shoe proximal to the metatarsal heads. Reduces pressure on metatarsal heads by redirecting weight-bearing forces. A metatarsal bar secondarily functions as a rockered sole on the shoe to decrease flexion of the proximal interphalangeal joints of the foot during toe-off. Eponyms referring to different types include Denver, Jones, Mayo, and Hauser.

Metatarsal pads   Supportive pad(s) added to a foot orthosis or inside a shoe to support the transverse arch of the foot and reduce pressure on the metatarsal heads.

Midsagittal line   This line passes directly through the center of the body and divides it into equal left and right regions. It is sometimes referred to as the median plane, which is a vertical plane drawn from front to back of a body at right angles to the frontal and transverse planes.

Milwaukee brace   A cervicothoracolumbosacral orthosis (CTLSO) popularized in mid-1950s by Dr. Blount in Milwaukee, Wisconsin, for the conservative treatment of idiopathic scoliosis and/or kyphosis. Consists of a plastic or leather pelvic girdle foundation, metal uprights that are contoured and connected to a metal neck ring, and corrective pads.

Minerva brace Craniocervical orthosis (CCO) used to immobilize the head and cervical spine. Most Minerva orthoses have some extension to contain the occiput and the head. A Minerva jacket envelopes the trunk and extends down over the iliac crests. It is rarely used today. Minerva was the ancient Roman goddess of wisdom who is often depicted wearing armor and a helmet.

Molded to patient Orthoses made directly on the patient. Often, a low-temperature thermoplastic is heated then molded on the patient. When the plastic cools, the brace becomes more rigid. If the orthosis is made on top of a positive patient model, usually plaster of paris, it is termed *molded to patient model*.

Moment A moment is the turning tendency of a force, and a *moment of force* is the biomechanical term used to describe the force that causes or intends to cause rotation about an axis. It is measured in Newton-meters (Nm) and is the product of the force times the perpendicular of its line of action from the axis of rotation. Used in the practice of orthotics, moments are applied by orthoses to cause joints to be either stable or to be mobile. The forces applied are of great significance in the selection of orthotic materials to ensure sufficient strength.

Morton extension (pad), toe extension or shelf Metatarsal support extending an arch support medially to the distal phalanx of the first toe and laterally the fifth metatarsophanlangeal joint. The medial part elongates the short first metatarsal bone of a Morton toe.

Murray shoe The first type of so-called space shoes, it is molded directly over a cast of the individual foot. Used for various types of foot deformities. Developed around 1940 by Allan E. Murray, later manufactured by the Murray Space Shoe Company in Bridgeport, Connecticut.

Myo collar Occasionally—and wrongly—considered an eponymic term, *myo,* derived from Greek, denotes a relationship to muscle. The collar, a height-adjustable polyethylene support, was developed about 1959 by the Florida Brace Corporation, Winter Park, Florida.

Newington ambulation–abduction brace A bilateral knee–ankle–foot orthosis similar to the Toronto hip abduction orthosis, with a spreader bar at the level of the feet and a spreader device protecting the knees against valgus deformity.[41,42]

Newington brace for cerebral palsy Orthosis reaching from the lower trunk to both feet. It combines four separate sections: trunk, pelvis, lower limbs, and shoe assembly, allowing gradual withdrawal of the brace piece by piece as the child is being trained in controlling the respective body segment. A single upright is used for each limb.[43]

Nickel splint One of several splints such as a finger-driven flexor-hinge splint, a wrist-driven flexor-hinge splint, devised by Vernon L. Nickel, orthopedic surgeon at Rancho Los Amigos Hospital.[44]

Norton-Brown brace Thoracolumbosacral brace restricting flexion, extension, and lateral motions.[45]

Offset joint Mechanical knee joint in which the axis of rotation is placed posteriorly to the uprights. A force transmitted through the uprights causes the knee to extend, providing the patient with increased stability of the knee during the stance phase of gait. The offset joint may locate the mechanical axis more closely to the anatomic axis.

Oklahoma ankle joint A low-profile plastic single-axis ankle joint that can be formed into a plastic AFO to provide articulation at the ankle. Research into the development of this ankle joint was carried out in the Orthotic Section, University of Oklahoma's College of Medicine.

OOS See *Oregon Orthotic System.*

Oppenheimer splint A wrist–hand–finger orthosis (WHFO) used to provide wrist extension and functional thumb positioning.

Opponens splint A hand–finger orthosis (HFO) used to assist opposition by stabilizing the thumb and allowing a three jaw chuck prehension grip.

Oregon Orthotic System (OOS) Lower extremity orthotic system developed by Jean-Paul Nielsen, C.P., of Albany, Oregon. Consists of various carbon-fiber laminated AFOs, and KAFOs. The OOS philosophy involves emphasis on systematic treatment of pathomechanical deformities through bracing. Extensive assessment and test bracing of the patient are done before the final orthosis is fabricated. Orthoses are provided to the orthotist as a central fabrication service from Oregon Orthotic System, Inc., Albany, Oregon.

Orlau swivel walker A swivel walker, that is, a standing frame that allows a subject with paraplegia to stand and even to progress by motions of the trunk, without the use of the upper limbs. *Orlau* is an acronym referring to the Orthotic Research and Locomotor Assessment Unit at the Robert Jones and Angus Hunt Orthopaedic Hospital, Oswestry, England, where the device was developed in 1976.[46]

Orthopodium See *Standing frame.*

Orthosis An external orthopedic device using biomechanical forces to support or realign one or more body segments or to prevent or correct deformity. The origin of the term comes from the Greek *ortho* meaning "straight," "upright," "right," or "correct." The plural of *orthosis* is *orthoses.*

Orthotic technician An individual who assists the clinical orthotist in the fabrication of orthoses.

Orthotics The field of knowledge relating to orthoses and their use.

Orthotist A person trained in the practice of orthotics. A certified orthotist is an individual who has demonstrated a level of competence by passing an organized set of examinations, thus meeting a standard set by many countries in the ability to design, manufacture, and fit orthoses. See *Certified Orthotist.*

OTI Orthopedic Technology Incorporated. A company producing several knee orthoses called *OTI knee braces.*

Otto Bock German prosthetist, orthotist (1888–1953). Founded the corporation that continues to bear his name. The company designs and manufactures components used by orthotists and prosthetists in constructing orthoses and prostheses for the disabled.

Outflair shoe (boot) Shoe with a reverse outsole pattern used to apply pressure to the foot to maintain abduction of the metatarsals or reduce adduction. cf. *Inflare shoe.*

Oxford shoe A low quarter- or ankle-high shoe laced low in the front. Named for Oxford, England.

Palmar Refers to the volar, ventral, or grasping side of the hand.

Palmar flexion Flexion of the wrist in a palmar direction.

Parasagittal plane Any plane that is parallel to the sagittal plane.

Parapodium A thoracolumbosacral hip–knee–ankle–foot orthosis (TLSO-HKAFO). Variations are known as the Toronto or Rochester parapodium. Full-control frame used to help paraplegic children achieve a standing position. The Rochester parapodium differs from the Toronto parapodium by using independent locking orthotic joints at the hips and knees to facilitate easier sitting.

Paresis   Slight or incomplete paralysis.

Pavlic harness   Fabric hip abduction orthosis consisting of heel cups and medially directed shoulder straps to flex and abduct the hips. Used for the treatment of newborn hip dislocation, by keeping the femoral head in the most stable position in the acetabulum. Devised in 1944 by Czechoslovakian orthopedic surgeon Arnold Pavlic.

Pelvic band or belt   A pelvic band that serves as an anchor for hip joints when fabricating various hip orthoses and HKAFOs. It is also the posteroinferior segment of spinal braces needing attachments for uprights to make lumbosacral orthoses (LSO) or thoracolumbosacral orthoses (TLSO) such as the Knight spinal orthosis.

Pelvic girdle   A molded, plastic, leather, or cloth structure formed to fit on the pelvis. Uprights may be attached to it, as in the Milwaukee orthosis.

Perineal straps   Belt(s) of material used occasionally in spinal orthoses that pass from the posterior aspect of the brace under the groin (perineum) to the anterior aspect of the brace. It is used to prevent the orthosis from migrating superiorly on the patient. Generally not well tolerated by patients.

Perlstein orthosis   A single upright ankle orthosis with an off-center cam ankle joint for adjustment of the plantar flexion stop.

Phelps orthosis   A single upright round caliper adjustable AFO with a stop behind the upright that can be bent to adjust the degree of plantar flexion of the ankle.

Pes cavus   Abnormal structure of the foot with a higher than average longitudinal arch of the foot.

Pes planus   Common term used to describe a flatter than average medial longitudinal arch in the foot. Calcaneal valgus, pronation, lateral rotation, and abduction of the foot are often aspects of the deformity. cf. *Pes cavus.*

Philadelphia collar   A prefabricated semirigid plastazote (polyethylene foam) cervical orthosis consisting of a rear piece with occipital support and a front piece with chin support extending to the sternal area. It mostly limits flexion and extension of the cervical spine. Developed in 1971 and named by orthotist Anthony Calabrese, Charles Greiner & Co, Philadelphia, now at Philadelphia Cervical Collar Co in nearby Westville, New Jersey.

PIP   Proximal interphalangeal joint.

Plantar   The sole or ventral surface of the foot.

Plantar flexion   Flexion of the ankle joint in the direction of the plantar surface of the foot.

Plastazote   A cross-linked, closed cell polyethylene foam used frequently as padding for orthoses. Has a low molding temperature, so it can be formed directly on the patient.

Plastazote shoe   A custom shoe made from a soft flexible foam (Plastazote) that can be molded directly over an abnormally shaped foot to provide support and or protection.

Plaster of paris   The most widely used and inexpensive impression, molding, and casting material in orthotics and prosthetics. Chemically, it is calcinated gypsum (calcium sulfate). When mixed with water, it solidifies to provide a working model of the patient's affected part. It is easily shaped and molded. Plaster of paris bandage is a cloth impregnated with material and used for many years to immobilize fractures during healing. It was introduced in 1852 by Mathijesen and is extensively used today by orthotists to obtain a negative model of the patient's body part.

Polycentric joint   Mechanical joint used in orthotics. Action is in one plane with changing center of rotation. Most commonly used at the knee, with dual gears or sliding/pivoting mechanisms, these joints attempt to track more closely the complex motion of the anatomical knee joint.

Polyethylene   A common plastic used in the fabrication of orthoses. The high molding temperature 175°C (350°F) to mold this plastic requires the use of a model of the patient's limb to fabricate the orthosis. Polyethylene is a durable homopolymer plastic that can be flexible or rigid, depending on the molecular weight.

Polypropylene   A common plastic used in the fabrication of orthoses. The high moulding temperature 200°C (400°F) to mold this plastic requires the use of a model of the patient's limb to fabricate the orthosis. Polypropylene is a homopolymer plastic is durable, and depending on the molecular weight, can be flexible or rigid.

Posting   A wedge added to the outsole of a shoe or for foot orthosis. See *Extrinsic posting* and *Intrinsic posting.*

Pressure   A term frequently used in orthotics and defined as force per unit area. The formula P = F/A describes how much external force is applied in a given area. P = pressure, F = force, and A = area. Orthoses purposely apply pressure to achieve a desired effect. To avoid skin problems, applied pressure must be within the limits of skin tolerance. The force must either be distributed over a sufficient area of the skin or be reduced so that tissue trauma is avoided.

Pressure garments   Elastic compression garments used to control lymphedema or venous stasis or to prevent of deep vein thrombosis. Also used to reduce hypertrophic scarring after burns.

Pronation   When used in reference to the foot, relative to the leg, the term *pronation* describes a triplanar joint movement incorporating the combination of dorsiflexion, abduction, and eversion in the foot–ankle complex. When the term is used in reference to the hand with the elbow flexed, pronation is a movement in which the hand faces palm down through the movement of the radius around the ulna. In the anatomic position the hand, moves to face posteriorly.

PTB orthosis   Patellar tendon-bearing orthosis. An ankle–foot orthosis (AFO) used to unload axial forces from the tibia or ankle. A modification of an AFO named after patellar tendon weightbearing prosthesis. The patellar tendon-bearing shell redirects superimposed body weight to an area below the knee joint. The proximal socket redistributes the patient's weight on the surfaces of the patellar tendon, medial tibial flair, and the popliteal area. An external frame transmits the forces from this shell to the shoe during gait.

Quadrilateral brim   The shape of the proximal portion of a knee–ankle–foot orthosis (KAFO). Made from plastic, metal, or leather, roughly resembling a four-sided cylinder (quadrilateral), the shape redirects axial loading from the leg to the ischium and upper thigh.

Quarter   Posterior part of the upper portion of a shoe.

Queen-Anne collar   A plastic cervical orthosis that leaves the chin free while the posterior part rises to the occiput, thus restricting in particular cervical extension. Although the earliest use of the collar or the eponym, its originator, and the queen referred to are unknown, the collar is remindful of those seen on portraits of Princess Anne of Denmark, later Electress of Saxony (1532–1585), much less so of the collar worn by her contemporary, Queen Anne of Spain.[47]

Radial palsy splint   A dynamic wrist–hand orthosis (WHO) used to assist patients with radial nerve dysfunction. Because the radial nerve is primarily a nerve of extension in the hand, the orthosis provides dynamic extension assistance while allowing flexion. Elastics or spring wire are used to extend the joints.

Rancho Los Amigos splint, system, etc. Rancho Los Amigos Hospital, Downey, California. Several orthoses and orthotic components were devised there, including a system of upper limb orthotics. See *Nickel splint.*

Reciprocal WHO A wrist–hand orthosis (WHO) used to transmit wrist extension motion to create finger prehension. A mechanism from the wrist component is linked with the fingers to give a three jaw chuck grip on wrist extension. C5–C6 quadriplegics with wrist extension can benefit from this orthosis. See *Tenodesis splint.*

Reciprocating gait orthosis (RGO) Bilateral TLSO-HKAFO orthosis with linked hip joints so that flexion (or extension) of one hip sends an extension (or flexion) force to the contralateral side during gait. RGOs allow for a more normal bipedal gait.

Recurvatum Abnormal hyperextension of a joint.

Resist Descriptor of orthotic joint motion control to restrict or prevent motion. When prescribing an orthosis for a person with weak dorsiflexors, plantar flexion resist may be requested.

Resting splint An orthosis that is used to immobilize a limb segment in a desired position. Can be used at night to prevent contractures from forming.

Reverse knuckle bender A dynamic hand–finger orthosis (HFO) that applies a three-point pressure system to assist extension of the metacarpal phalangeal joints. Rubber bands or springs are used to assist extension.

RGO See *Reciprocating gait orthosis.*

Rochester parapodium See *Parapodium.*

Rocker sole An external shoe modification consisting of an elevation that tapers from full height to almost no elevation at the toe. This modification reduces rotational forces at the ankle joint and pressure on the metatarsal heads during the latter parts of stance phase. It is used to reduce pain when ranging the ankle joint is painful and to reduce breakage of orthoses resulting when a rigid orthotic ankle joint limits the ankle joint's range of motion. May be required bilaterally to avoid creating a leg length discrepancy. A full rocker bottom to the shoe reduces dorsiflexion and plantar flexion moments of force at the ankle during the stance phase of gait. A smoother rollover is achieved from heel strike to toe-off.

Rosen splint See *von Rosen splint.*

Rotation A motion in which a body part turns about an axis—angular displacement. cf. *Torque.*

Roylan hemi arm sling A sling devised to reduce pain and subluxation at the shoulder glenohumeral joint. The splint is made from a cuff and figure-eight harness.

SACH Solid ankle cushion heel. A modification to the heel of a shoe to incorporate a soft foam wedge in the heel. The effect cushions the forces at heel strike and secondarily provides a minor rocker effect to reduce the rotational forces on the ankle.

Sacroiliac belt A sacroiliac orthosis (SIO) that encircles the pelvis between the iliac crests and the trochanters. The function is to provide support to the sacroiliac and symphysis pubis joints.

Sagittal plane A vertical plane drawn from the front to the back of the body, at right angles to the frontal and coronal planes. The sagittal plane separates the body into right and left parts.

Scoliosis brace Any number of spinal orthoses (CTLSO, TLSO, or LSO) used for the conservative treatment of abnormal curvatures of the spine.

Scott-Craig orthosis A knee–ankle–foot orthosis (KAFO) used to stabilize the hip joint; for example in the treatment of Legg-Calvé-Perthes disease. Maintains the hip joints in their most stable position—abducted and internally rotated. Devised by B.A. Scott, orthotist at the Craig Rehabilitation Hospital, Englewood, Colorado.

Scottish Rite brace A hip orthosis (HpO) used to abduct the hips in children with Legg-Calvé-Perthes disease. A pelvic band is connected to plastic thigh cuffs by a free motion hip joint. A telescoping bar with swivel joints joins the thigh cuffs to maintain abduction while allowing hip flexion and permitting ambulation.

SEO Shoulder–elbow orthosis.

SEWHO Shoulder–elbow–wrist–hand orthosis. For control and containment of the complete arm including the shoulder joint.

Shoe buildup (shoe lift) Shoe sole material added to compensate for a leg length discrepancy.

Shoe horn brace Plastic ankle–foot orthosis (AFO) that fits inside a shoe and is closely contoured to fit the posterior aspect of the lower leg and sole of the foot. Used to assist weak or absent dorsiflexors. So named because when left in the shoe, the posterior aspect of the brace can act as a shoehorn to help the foot into the shoe.

Silesian bandage or belt Waist belt, usually made of cloth webbing, attached to a lower limb orthosis or prosthesis as a means of suspension.

Single-axis joint Any mechanical joint used on orthotics including ankle, knee, hip, that has a single axis of rotation. See *Polycentric joint.*

SIO Sacroiliac orthosis. A wide belt circling the pelvis between the iliac crests and the greater trochanters to exert a circumferential force on the sacroiliac joint.

Snook splint A dorsal wrist–hand orthosis designed to reduce hand spasticity by minimizing volar forearm and hand stimulation.

SO Shoulder orthosis.

Sole wedge External V-shaped sole material added to a shoe to apply a directive force to the foot or ankle during stance.

SOMI (brace, collar) Sternooccipital mandibular immobilizer. A prefabricated cervical orthosis used to reduce flexion and extension motions in the cervical spine. The anterior attachment points for the mandibular and occipital segments allow this orthosis to be donned and doffed by patients lying in bed.

Spasticity An increase in muscle tone with involuntary contractions. May be accompanied by heightened deep tendon reflexes and is usually associated with upper motor neuron lesions.

Spiral orthosis A molded ankle–foot orthosis (AFO) that corkscrews up the leg from the foot. Along with providing dorsiflexion assist during the swing phase of gait, the design can offer support for the medial side of the foot. See *Lehneis spiral orthosis.*

Splint Used interchangeably with the terms *brace* and *orthosis* in this text.

Spring-assist joint An articulated joint, usually at the ankle, that contains spring(s) to dynamically assist or resist motion in one direction.

Standing frame Various TLSO-HKAFO frame orthoses that allow children with neuromuscular deficits to ambulate and stand. Consists of a platform base with rigid tubes rising up to a knee stabilizer and extends to a corset to hold the trunk. Sometimes called an *orthopodium.*

Static orthosis Orthosis without articulation(s). Used to maintain a functional position of one or more joints, to prevent contractures, and to provide protection during burn or bone fracture healing.

Stax splint   Finger orthosis to immobilize distal interphalangeal joint after fractures or tendon repairs.

Steeper splint   Various orthoses manufactured by Hugh Steeper Ltd. in Roehampton, England.

Steindler, Arthur   Orthopedic surgeon, (1878 to 1959) from Iowa whose name was used to describe a TLSO back brace, a wrist–hand orthosis, and a heel modification using a pocket relief to remove pressure from painful plantar fasciitis.

Stirrup   Metal U-shaped base riveted to the sole of the shoe under the heel. Provides a distal attachment point for the medial and lateral metal uprights of the orthosis and generally incorporates an axis in the proximal end to receive an ankle joint. Various stirrup joint styles are available that allow for variations in ankle motion.

Stirrup, forked   The addition of an extra metal arm added to a stirrup (see above) to increase the base of support under the shoe and to restrict motion of the foot.

Stirrup, split   Metal base riveted to the sole of the shoe under the heel. The base has a channel to receive the medial and lateral uprights of the orthosis, hence the term *split*. This type of stirrup allows the upper part of the orthosis to be transferred to other shoes that also have a split stirrup attached.

Stop   Design feature of a mechanical joint used to prevent motion beyond a set point. May be adjustable or fixed. Ankle joints may have a posterior stop set to 90 degrees to prevent plantar flexion.

Strickland splint   A hand orthosis used in flexor tendon repair.

Supination   Supination of the foot, relative to the leg, is a triplanar joint movement incorporating a combination of plantar flexion, adduction and inversion in the foot–ankle complex. Supination of the hand with the elbow flexed, is a movement where the hand faces palm up through the movement of the radius around the ulna. In the anatomic position—to move to face anteriorly.

Surgical support   Historical term used to describe various types of adjustable soft cloth or canvas spinal orthoses. These orthoses are sometimes reinforced with metal stays. Often prescribed for low back pain or after abdominal surgery to support delicate tissues during healing. Many of these are prefabricated TLSOs and LSOs that fit a range of patient sizes. Being adjustable and prefabricated, they are quickly fit and dispensed to the patient.

Suspension slings   Elbow and wrist straps suspended by a bar, cables, and/or springs to an overhead frame to assist arm function when shoulder muscles are weak or nearly absent.

Swan neck splint   A proximal interphalangeal (finger) orthosis (FO) used to limit hyperextension of the proximal interphalangeal joint while allowing flexion.

Swanson orthosis   A postsurgical wrist–hand orthosis (WHO) used after Swanson's arthroplasty (joint replacement) to allow flexion and extension of the metacarpal phalangeal joints in one plane, while restricting lateral motion.

Swedish knee cage   A knee orthosis used to control mild knee hyperextension. Consists of medial and lateral uprights connected posteriorly by a semicircular horizontal bar and two webbing straps, above and below the knee. Designed in Sweden in 1966.

Swiss lock   See *Bail lock*.

Swivel walker An articulated base used by paraplegics using standing frames, parapodiums, and other HKAFOs to permit ambulation. When the patient shifts his center of gravity laterally, the swivel walker has a linkage mechanism that causes the contralateral side to pivot forward. This is repeated with a shift of weight to the other side to achieve a bipedal gait on level floors. cf. *Reciprocating gait orthosis.*

T-strap A padded leather strap in the shape of the letter T stitched on the side of a shoe. Used to pull a valgus or varus ankle joint into a corrected position.

Tachdjian orthosis A knee–ankle–foot orthosis (KAFO) used to abduct the hip in children with unilateral Legg-Calvé-Perthes disease. Consists of a proximal thigh brim for ischial weight bearing coupled to a single medial upright. The upright is attached to the sole of a shoe that has a medial outrigger in a wedge shape to keep the leg abducted. A drop-lock knee joint is used to keep the leg extended while walking, yet allows the knee to flex for sitting. Developed by Miran Tachdjian.

Taylor brace A thoracolumbosacral orthosis (TLSO). Made with a padded posterior metal frame with two paraspinal uprights extending from a pelvic band to the shoulders. Axillary straps prevent thoracic flexion. Corset front provides increased intra-abdominal pressure. Named for the brace's developer, Dr. Charles Fayatte Taylor, a New York orthopedic surgeon.

Taylor inflatable collar Inflatable soft cervical orthosis, consisting of a front section and a back section. Devised by Arabion N. Taylor, Alabama orthopedic surgeon.[48]

Tenodesis splint A dynamic wrist–hand orthosis (WHO) used in transmitting active wrist extension to achieve finger prehension. Used for spinal cord injury patients with residual wrist extension capabilities. The thumb is held in a functional position and the first two fingers are moved against it by the orthosis. Relaxing the wrist allows gravity to open the grip. Varieties have been given eponyms such as Rancho, Engen, and RIC (Rehabilitation Institute of Chicago).

Thomas heel Modified heel on a shoe that projects on the medial side anteriorly. It increases the base of support under the midfoot in cases of abnormally pronated subtalar joints or valgus ankles.

Thomas heel, reverse Modified heel on a shoe that projects anteriorly on the lateral side. It increases the base of support under the midfoot in cases of abnormally supinated subtalar joint or varus ankle.

Thomas splint, knee splint, or caliper Knee–ankle–foot orthosis (KAFO) consisting of two straight steel bars connected distally by a cross bar beyond the foot and proximally by a padded ring fitting tightly to the perineum and ischium. For emergency splinting, transportation, and traction in fractures of the thigh or leg. Weight bearing is transferred from the knee and foot to the pelvis.

Thomas, Hugh Owen Liverpool orthopedic surgeon (1834–1889). His name is associated with many orthoses including an arm abduction splint, a metatarsal bar, a collar, and special heels.

Three-point pressure Fundamental biomechanical principal used in orthotic treatment. A three-point pressure system applies two forces to a limb segment with a third counterforce between the two. Most orthoses apply force(s) to the body in such a way as to limit range of motion, prevent pain, or assist movement. Forces are usually distributed over a wide area instead of a point.

Three jaw chuck prehension A particular precision finger grasp where small objects are held between the thumb, index, and middle fingers.

Thumb post An orthosis that is often made from a low-temperature thermoplastic material or leather and used to provide stability to the thumb in a functional position and allow opposition prehension.

TIRR Abbreviation for Texas Institute for Rehabilitation and Research, Houston Texas, where several orthoses were developed.

TLSHKAFO Thoracolumbosacral hip–knee–ankle–foot orthosis. A group of full-control orthoses such as parapodiums and standing frames that assist paraplegics to obtain a standing position.

TLSO Thoracolumbosacral orthosis.

Toe box Reinforcement used in the construction of a shoe to retain the contours above the toes. Protects the toes against trauma or abrasion.

Toronto hip abduction orthosis A KAFO used for the management of hip dysplasia. Thigh cuffs are connected to shoe blocks (angled at 45 degrees) through a universal joint, while the orthosis abducts and internally rotates the hip joints. Hip joints are maintained in a stable position while allowing ambulation. Also known as the Toronto Legg-Perthes orthosis, developed at the Hospital for Sick Children, Toronto, Ontario, Canada.

Toronto parapodium See *Parapodium*.

Torque A force creating a turning tendency around a point, as in the action of a screwdriver.

Torque heel Special heel added to the shoe that forces the foot into external or internal rotation at heel strike.

Torticollis brace A cervical orthosis (CO) used for the treatment of torticollis by maintaining a three-point pressure system to laterally extend the cervical spine.

TRAFO Tone-reducing ankle–foot orthosis. Consists of posterior and anterior shells that are strapped together with a firm platform base. This orthosis was developed to assist the standing and walking of children with upper motor lesions, such as cerebral palsy. The rationale of these intimately fitting AFOs is to inhibit muscle tone through precise joint position and a stable base. Although the theory of the TRAFO's ability to reduce tone is controversial, there are advantages to the appropriate joint alignment and standing position they provide.

Translation In kinematics, *translation* describes motion where an object moves without rotation and results in linear displacement. cf. *Rotation*.

Transverse plane A plane drawn in cross section of a body and at right angles to both the frontal and sagittal planes and sometimes termed *horizontal plane*. A transverse plane divides the body into superior and inferior regions.

Tübingen orthosis A prefabricated hip abduction orthosis (HKAFO) that is used to abduct and flex the hips in pediatric patients with hip dysplasia. Named by the designer, Dr. Bernau, for the city in Germany where it was first devised, ca. 1990.

Twister cable(s) An external flexible shaft connecting the hip and foot and used to apply a torque to the unweighted leg during the swing phase of gait. Twister cables internally or externally rotate the hips through a preloaded torque to the cable running down the length of the leg. The proximal end is attached to a pelvic band, and the distal end is attached to an AFO or shoe. Also called a torsion control cable.

UCLA functional long leg brace University of California at Los Angeles knee–ankle–foot orthosis (KAFO) with plastic thigh and pretibial shells, double uprights, offset ball-bearing knee joints, and an ankle hydraulic cylinder control.[49]

UCBL   University of California at Berkeley Biomechanics Laboratory. Numerous orthoses have been developed here.

UCBL heel cup   A foot orthosis designed at University of California at Berkeley Biomechanics Laboratory to correct abnormal positioning of the hind foot. The term *UCBL* commonly refers to a thermoplastic foot orthosis with generous trim lines around the posterior aspect to better control the hindfoot.

Ulnar palsy splint   Various wrist–hand orthoses (WHOs) used for the treatment of ulnar nerve lesions. Generally, these lesions leave the patient with the inability to flex metacarpophalangeal joints and extend interphalangeal joints. These orthoses provide dynamic flexion of metacarpophalangeal and extension of the proximal interphalangeal joints through elastic bands or springs.

USMC   United States Manufacturing Company. American manufacturer and distributor of components used by Prosthetists and Orthotists, located in Pasadena, California.

Valgus   A frontal plane deformity of a joint in which the distal segment angulates away from the midline.

Vamp   The forepart of the upper portion of a shoe.

VAPC   Veterans Administration Prosthetics Center in New York, where various orthoses were developed.

Varus   A frontal plane deformity of a joint in which the distal segment angulates in the direction of the midline.

Velcro   A popular loop and hook fastening material used in the orthopedic and other fields. Velcro is a contraction of the French words *velour* and *crochet*. The concept was developed by Swiss engineer, George de Mestral in 1948, who noticed how the cockleburs clung to fabric. Noticing the shape of the tiny hooks and how they stuck to his clothing, he got the idea for a new kind of fastener. In 1956, a Swiss company was established to produce Velcro, and in 1959 the product was first produced by Velcro France. In 1977, Velcro France change its name to APLIX S.A., and development continues under this trademark.

Ventral   The front or face-up surface of the body. Also the downward surface, "The sole of the foot is ventral."

Volar   Palmar surface of the hand. cf. *Dorsal.*

von Rosen splint   A rigid pediatric hip abduction orthosis made from a metal or plastic frame in an H pattern for the positioning of hip joints in congenital dislocated hips (CDH). The top arms of the H curve over the shoulders. The bottom arms of the H curve up under the femurs and hold them in an abducted position. This allows the heads of the femurs to be maintained in a stable position in the acetabulums. Devised by S. von Rosen of Malmö, Sweden.

Wafer ankle   Metal single-axis ankle joint with a spring-assist and adjustable dorsiflexion stop. Formed into the AFO by moulding plastic on top of the joint. The joint is then integrated into the orthosis to provide articulation at the ankle. The Wafer ankle allows motion in one plane.

Warm Springs   The Warm Springs Foundation, formerly devoted to the treatment of poliomyelitis and located in Warm Springs Georgia. Several orthoses bear this name, including an upper limb orthosis, a crutch, spinal orthoses, and a foot orthosis.

Wheaton Brace   Prefabricated pediatric ankle–foot orthosis (AFO) used to apply corrective forces for the treatment of metatarsus adductus. Manufactured by the Wheaton Brace Company, Wheaton, Illinois.

WHFO Wrist–hand–finger orthosis. Orthosis that encompasses the wrist, hand, and one or more fingers.

WHO Wrist–hand orthosis. Orthosis that encompasses the wrist and hand.

Williams LSO A Thoracolumbosacral orthosis (TLSO) that is used to prevent lumbar extension and lateral trunk movement. Consists of thoracic and pelvic bands of padded aluminum connected by lateral uprights. A garment corset front increases intra-abdominal pressure. Devised by Dallas, Texas orthopedic surgeon Dr. P.L. Williams (1900–1978).

Wilson collar An orthosis for immobilization of the cervical spine, without chin piece, thus not interfering with the opening of the mouth. A large molded head piece embracing the forehead and the occipital area is connected by metal rods with a chest piece. An additional, removable chin piece may be used at night. Devised by C.L. Wilson, A.G. Hadjipavlou (orthopedic surgeons), and G. Barreta (orthotist) (all in Montreal).[50]

Wingfield-Morris shoulder abduction splint A modification of the Littler-Jones shoulder abduction orthosis.[8,37]

WO Wrist orthosis. Use of this term is not recommended, because to be biomechanically effective, a wrist orthosis in fact is a wrist–hand orthosis (WHO).

Wrist-driven prehension orthosis See *Tenodesis splint.*

Yale cervical orthosis A Philadelphia collar (q.v.) in which each of its two pieces (one anterior, one posterior) is prolonged downward by a solidly attached bib-like piece of molded fiberglass (Lightcast) further held in place by a strap around the lower part of the thorax. Designed to immobilize the cervical spine more than the collar bone alone by orthopedic surgeon Rollin M. Johnson, physical therapist Reivan Zelez-

nik, and others at Yale-New Haven Medical Center, New Haven Connecticut.[51] See *Philadelphia collar.*

Zimmer brace, splint, etc. Various prefabricated orthoses manufactured and distributed by the Zimmer Manufacturing Company, Warsaw, Indiana.

REFERENCES

1. Licht S, Kamenetz H: Orthotics Etcetera. Elizabeth Licht, New Haven, CT, 1966
2. Abouna JM: Splint for mallet finger. Br Med J 5432:444, 1965
3. Abouna JM, Brown H: The treatment of mallet finger. Br J Surg 55:653, 1968
4. American Academy of Orthopaedic Surgeons: Orthopaedic Appliances Atlas. Vol. 1. Braces, Splints, Shoe Alterations. JW Edwards, Ann Arbor, MI, 1952
5. Canty TJ: Functional full length leg brace. Am J Surg 81:474, 1951
6. Reed B: An evaluation of the C.A.R.S.U.B.C. knee orthosis. Orthotics Prosthet 33:25, 1979
7. Dorland's Illustrated Medical Dictionary. 26th Ed. WB Saunders, Philadelphia, 1981
8. Nangle EJ: Instruments and Apparatus in Orthopaedic Surgery. Blackwell, Oxford, England, 1951
9. Cloran AJ: Telescoping mouth instruments for severely handicapped patients. J Prosthet Dent 32:435, 1974
10. Muckart RD: p. 480. In Murdoch G (ed): Prosthetic and Orthotic Practice. London, 1970
11. Shands AR, Raney RB: Handbook of Orthopaedic Surgery. 7th Ed. CV Mosby, St. Louis, 1967
12. Cotrel Y: La technique de l'E.D.F. dans le traitment de la scoliose. Entretiens Bichat. Paris, Expansion Scientifique Francaise, 1962
13. Keim HA: Scoliosis. Ciba Clin Symp 21:21, 1972
14. Coughlin EJ, Jr: An abduction exercise splint for the shoulder. J Bone Joint Surg [Am] 31:438, 1949
15. An improved abduction exercise splint for the shoulder. J Bone Joint Surg [Am] 33:267, 1951
16. DeLorme TL et al: An adjustable lower-extremity brace. J Bone Joint Surg [Am] 43:205, 1961
17. Stauffer ES: Orthotics for spinal cord injuries. Clin Orthop 102:92, 1974
18. Jahss MH: p. 268. In American Academy of Orthopaedic Surgeons: Atlas of Orthotics. Biomechanical Principles and Application. CV Mosby, St. Louis, 1975

19. Anderson MH: A Manual of Lower Extremities Orthotics. Charles C Thomas, Springfield, IL, 1977

20. Milgram JE, Malcolm AJ: Footgear: therapeutic modifications of sole and heel. Orthop Rev 7:57, 1978

21. Engen TJ: Adjustable knee or elbow extension orthosis: a new orthotic development. Orthop Prosthet Appl J 45, 1961

22. Engen TJ: A modification of a reciprocal wrist extension, finger flexion orthosis. Orthop Prosthet Appl J 14:39, 1960

23. Jordan HH: Orthopedic Appliances. 2nd Ed. Charles C Thomas, Springfield, IL, 1963

24. Ewing MB: Long leg brace modification. Arch Phys Med Rehabil 44:656, 1963

25. Capener N: The hand in surgery. J Bone Joint Surg [Br] 38:128, 1956

26. Carlson JM, Winter R: The "Gillette" sitting support orthosis. Orthotics Prosthet 32(4):35, 1978

27. Glimcher MJ, Radin EL, Amrich MM: The design of a new style ischial weightbearing brace for use in the treatment of Legg-Perthes disease. Orthotics Prosthet 24(3):11, 1970

28. Burgess LG: The mechanism and use of abdominal supports and the treatment of pulmonary diseases. Am J Med Sci 187:692, 1934

29. Friddle WD, Brown LP: Greenville spinal orthosis—polypropylene. Inter-Clin Info Bull 15(9–10):7, 1976

30. Hartman JT: Cineradiography of the braced normal cervical spine. Clin Orthop 109:97, 1975

31. Ilfeld FW: The management of congenital dislocation and dysplasia of the hip by means of a special splint. J Bone Joint Surg [Am] 39:99, 1957

32. Kanavel AB: Splinting and physiotherapy in infections of the hand. JAMA 83:1984, 1924

33. Sarno JE, Lehneis HR: Prescription considerations for plastic below-knee orthoses. Arch Phys Med Rehabil 52:503, 1971

34. Lehneis HR: New developments in lower-limb orthotics through bioengineering. Arch Phys Med Rehabil 53:303, 1972

35. Thomas p. 213. In American Academy of Orthopaedic Surgeons: Orthopaedic Appliances Atlas Vol. 1. Braces, Splints, Shoe Alterations. JW Edwards, Ann Arbor, MI, 1952

36. Roaf R, Hodkinson LJ: Textbook for Orthopaedic Nurses. JB Lippincott, Philadelphia, 1964

37. Muckart RD: p. 475. In Murdoch G (ed): Prosthetic and Orthotic Practice. London, 1970

38. Gracanin F: Electrical stimulation as orthotic aid: experiences and prospects. p. 503. In Murdoch G (ed): Prosthetic and Orthotic Practice. London, 1970

39. Barber LM, Nickel VL: Carbon dioxide-powered arm and hand devices. Am J Occup Ther 23:215, 1969

40. Murphy, Burnstein p. 29. In American Academy of Orthopaedic Surgeons: Atlas of Orthotics. Biomechanical Principles and Application. CV Mosby, St. Louis, 1975

41. Curtis BH: Treatment for Legg-Perthes disease with the New-ington ambulation-abduction brace. J Bone Joint Surg [Am] 56:1135, 1974

42. Staros A, LeBlanc M: p. 229. In American Academy of Orthopaedic Surgeons: Atlas of Orthotics. Biomechanical Principles and Application. CV Mosby, St. Louis, 1975

43. Fuldner RV, Rosenberger J: The Newington brace for cerebral palsy. Clin Orthop 12:151, 1958

44. Nickel VL, Perry J, Garrett A: Development of useful function in the severely paralyzed hand. J Bone Joint Surg [Am] 45:933, 1963

45. Norton PL, Brown Thornton: The immobilizing efficiency of back braces: their effect on the posture and motion of the lumbosacral spine. J Bone Joint Surg [Am] 39:111–39, 220, 1957

46. Seymour RJ et al: Arch Phys Med Rehabil 63:490, 1982

47. Davenport M: The Book of Costumes. Vol. 1. Crown, New York, 1948

48. Taylor AN: An inflatable neck support. Clin Orthop 81:87, 1971

49. Strohm BR, Bray J, Colachis SC: The U.C.L.A. functional long leg brace: biomechanics and fabrication. J Am Phys Ther Assoc 43:713, 1963

50. Wilson CL, Hadjipavlou AG, Barreta G: A new non invasive halo orthosis for immobilization of the cervical spine. Orthotics Prosthet 32:16, 1978

51. Zeleznik R: Yale cervical orthosis. Fabrication. Phys Ther 58:861, 1978

SUGGESTED READINGS

Journals

American Journal of Medical Science
American Journal of Occupational Therapy
Archives of Physical Medicine and Rehabilitation
British Medical Journal
Bulletin of Prosthetics Research (U.S. Veterans Administration)
Clinical Orthopaedics and Related Research (the Association of Bone and Joint Surgeons)
Instructional Course Lectures (American Academy of Orthopaedic Surgeons)
Journal of Bone and Joint Surgery
Journal of Prosthetics and Orthotics
Journal of the American Medical Association
Journal of the American Physical Therapy Association
Prosthetics and Orthotics International

Books

American Academy of Orthopedic Surgeons: Atlas of Orthotics: Biomechanical Principles and Application. 2nd Ed. CV Mosby, St. Louis, 1985

American Orthotic and Prosthetic Association: An Illustrated Guide to Orthotics and Prosthetics. National Office of Orthotics and Prosthetics, Alexandria, VA, 1992

Anderson MH: A Manual of Lower Extremities Orthotics. Charles C Thomas, Springfield, IL, 1972

Bick EM: Source Book of Orthopaedics. 2nd Ed. Williams & Wilkins, Baltimore, MD, 1948; reprinted with additional references, 1968

Blauvelt CT, Nelson FRT: A Manual of Orthopedic Terminology. CV Mosby, St. Louis, 1981

Bloomberg MH: Orthopedic Braces. JB Lippincott, Philadelphia, 1964

Boyes JH: Bunnell's Surgery of the Hand. 4th Ed. JB Lippincott, Philadelphia, 1964

Bradford EH, Lovett RW: A Treatise on Orthopedic Surgery. William Wood & Co, New York, 1890

British Medical Dictionary. JB Lippincott, Philadelphia, 1963

Cailliet R: Hand Pain and Impairment. FA Davis, Philadelphia, 1982

Dahlschen E (ed): Orthotics and Prosthetics Digest Reference Manual. 2nd Ed. Edahl Productions, Ottawa, Canada, 1983

Inman VT, Ralston HJ, Todd F: Human Walking. Williams & Wilkins, Baltimore, MD, 1981

International Organization for Standardization: ISO 8549-3: Prosthetics and Orthotics Vocabulary. Part 3. Terms Relating to External Orthoses. International Organization for Standardization, Geneva, 1989

Licht S, Kamenetz H: Orthotics Etcetera. Elizabeth Licht, New Haven, CT, 1966

Redford JB (ed): Orthotics Etcetera. 2nd Ed. Williams & Wilkins, Baltimore, MD, 1980

Schuch CM (ed): Journal of Prosthetics and Orthotics. American Orthotic and Prosthetic Association, Alexandria, VA

Stedman's Medical Dictionary. 23rd Ed. Williams & Wilkins, Baltimore, MD, 1976

Turek SL: Orthopaedics: Principles and Their Application. 3rd Ed. JB Lippincott, Philadelphia, 1977

Weber DH (ed): Clinical Aspects of Lower Extremity Orthotics. Canadian Association of Prosthetists and Orthotists, Winnipeg, 1990

Major Manufacturers and Providers of Orthotic Equipment and Supplies

Ace Medical Co.
14105 S. Avalon Blvd.
Los Angeles, CA 90061-2691

Acor Orthopaedic Inc.
1850 S. Miles Parkway
Cleveland, OH 44128

AcroMed Corp. dba.
Bremer Medical Inc.
4801 Dawin Rd.
Jacksonville, FL 32207

Alimed Inc.
297 High St.
Dedham, MA 02026

Allied Resinous Products Inc.
Clark St. & Whitney Rd.
Conneaut, OH 44030-0620

Alps Corp.
Silicone Park
10 Plains Rd.
Malta, NY 12020

American Plastics Inc.
7451 Dogwood Park
Ft. Worth, TX 76118

Amfit Inc.
3004 Kifer Rd.
Santa Clara, CA 95051

Anatomical Concepts Inc.
930 Trailwood Dr.
Boardman, OH 44512

Apex Foot Health Industries
170 Wesley St.
South Hackensack, NJ 07606

Applied Composite Technology
192 E. 100 N.
P.O. Box 300585
Fayette, UT 84630

Atlanta International
P.O. Box 450864
Atlanta, GA 31145

Atlas International
4747 J St.
Sacramento, CA 95819-3937

Atlantic Rim Brace Manufacturing Corp.
13 Hampshire Dr.
Hudson, NH 03051

Becker Orthopedic Appliance Co.
635 Executive Dr.
Troy, MI 48083

Bell-Horn (Wm H. Horn & Bro. Inc.)
451 N. Third St.
Philadelphia, PA 19123-4197

Bledsoe Brace Systems
2601 Pinewood
Grand Prairie, TX 75051

Boston Brace International
20 Ledin Dr.
Avon, MA 02322-1156

Camp International Inc.
744 W. Michigan Ave.
Box 89
Jackson, MI 49204-0089

Cascade Orthopedic Supply Inc.
Hwy. 36 Chester Airport
P.O. Box 649
Chester, CA 96020

Center for Orthotics Design—The RGO Center
1629 Main St.
Redwood City, CA 94063

Central Orthopedic Brace Co.
7737 W. 96th Place
Hickory Hills, IL 60457

Century XXII Innovations Inc.
1339 Horton Rd.
P.O. Box 868
Jackson, MI 48026

Columbia Medical Mfg. Corp.
P.O. Box 633
Pacific Palisade, CA 90272

Comfort Products Inc.
705 Linton Ave.
Croydon, PA 19021

Convaid Product Inc.
P.O. Box 2458
Rancho Palos Cerdes, CA 90274

Daytona Plastix Inc.
1870 Mason Ave.
P.O. Box 9425
Daytona Beach, FL 32120

Dobi-Symplex Inc.
2360 Clark St.
P.O. Box 1070
Apopka, FL 32703-1070

Dynasplint Systems Inc.
645 Baltimore Annapolis Blvd., Suite 110
Severna Park, MD 21146-3923

DynOrthotics, LP
1200 Stirling Road, Suite 10
Dania, FL 33004

Fillauer Inc.
2710 Amnicola Hwy.
P.O. Box 5189
Chattanooga, TN 37406-0189

Florida Brace Corp.
601 Webster Ave.
P.O. Box 1299
Winter Park, FL 32789

Florida Manufacturing Corp.
FlaManCo International
501 Beville Rd.
Daytona Beach, FL 32119

Freeman Manufacturing Co.
900 W. Chicago Rd.
Drawer J
Sturgis, MI 49091

Friddle's Orthopedic
Appliances Inc.
Route 2, U.S. Highways 76 & 178
Honea Path, SC 29654

Gaffney Technology
P.O. Box 1018
Hillsboro, OR 97123

Generation II, USA Inc.
11818 N. Creek Parkway N., Suite 102
Bothell, WA 98011-8225

Hosmer Dorrance Corp.
561 Division St.
P.O. Box 37
Campbell, CA 95008

Innovation Sport Inc.
7 Chrysler
Irvine, CA 92718

IPOS North America Inc.
2045 Niagara Falls Blvd. 8
Niagara Falls, NY 14304

Jaeco Orthopedic Specialities Inc.
P.O. Box 75, 214 Drexel
Hot Springs, AR 71901

Johnson's Orthopedic Design Inc.
1920 E. Katella Ave. Suite G
Orange, CA 92667

JUZO—Juluis Zorn Inc.
80 Chart Rd.
P.O. Box 1088
Cuyahoga Falls, OH 44223

The Langer Biomechanics Group Inc.
450 Commack Rd.
Deer Park, NY 11729

Laurence Orthopedic Appliance Co.
3045 Telegraph Ave.
Oakland, CA 94609

Lenox Hill Brace Co.
11-20 43rd Rd.
Long Island City, NY 11101

Liberty Technology Prosthetics & Orthotics Group
71 Frankland Rd.
Hopkinton, MA 01748

Maramed Orthopedic Systems
2480 W. 82nd St.
Hialeah, FL 33016

Jerry Miller I.D. Shoe
3158 Main St.
P.O. Box 584
Buffalo, NY 14214

P.W. Minor Xtra Depth Shoes
3 Treadeasy Ave.
P.O. Box 678
Batavia, NY 14021-0678

National Orthotic Laboratories Inc.
P.O. Box 1939
Winter Haven, FL 33883-1939

OTS Corp.
735 N. Fork Rd.
P.O. Box 245
Barmardsville, NC 28709

Oregon Orthotic Systems Inc.
2280 Three Lakes Rd. S.E.
Albany, OR 97321

OrthoConcepts
285 Alpha Park
Cleveland, OH 44143

Ortho Systems Inc.
5150 N. 32nd St.
Milwaukee, WI 53209

Orthomedics Inc.
2950 E. Imperial Hwy.
Brea, CA 92622-2960

Orthomerica Products Inc.
Corporate Headquarters
505 Thirty-First St.
P.O. Box 2927
Newport Beach, CA 92663

Orthosis Corrective Systems Inc.
6554 44th St. N. Unit 1001
Pinellas Park, FL 34665

Orthotic Rehabilitation Product Inc.
7002 E. Broadway
Tampa, FL 33619

Otto Bock Orthopedic Industry Inc.
3000 Xenium Lane N.
Minneapolis, MN 55441

PEL Supply Co.
4666 Manufacturing Rd.
Cleveland, OH 44135

Pin Dot Products
6001 Gross Point Rd.
Niles, IL 60714-4027

PMT Corp.
1500 Park Rd.
Chanhassen, MN 55317

Precision O&P Components Inc.
P.O. Box 24556
Tempe, AZ 85285

Ralph Storrs Inc.
197 S. West Ave.
Kankakee, IL 60901

Raven Enterprises Inc.
241 E. Imperial Hwy. Suite 310
Fullerton, CA 92635

**Royalite Thermoplastics
Division of Uniroyal Tech Corp.**
312 N. Hill St.
Mishawaka, IN 46546

Scott Orthotic Labs Inc.
1831 E. Mulberry
Ft. Collins, CO 80524

Sigvaris Inc.
P.O. Box 570
32 Park Dr. E.
Branford, CT 06405

Smith & Nephew Donjoy Inc.
2777 Liker Ave. W., Suite 100
Carlbad, CA 92008-6601

Smithers Bio-Medical Systems
919 Marvin Ave.
P.O. Box 148
Kent, OH 44240

Spinal Technology Inc.
191 Mid Tech Dr.
West Yarmouth, MA 02673

TEC Interface Systems
510-8 25th Ave. N.
St. Cloud, MN 56303

Townsend Design
4630 Easton Drive, Suite 2
Bakersfield, CA 93309

Tribar Orthopedic Inc.
1403 Central Parkway
Cincinnati, OH 45214

Tru-Fit Shoes
49 Lawton St.
New Rochelle, NY 1801

Tru-Mold Shoes Inc.
49 Lasalle Ave.
Buffalo, NY 14217-1414

Truform Orthotics and Prosthetics
3960 Rosslyn Dr.
Cincinnati, OH 45209

UCO International
16 E. Piper Lane, Suite 120
Prospect Heights, IL 60070-1799

U.S. Manufacturing Co.
180 N. San Gabriel Blvd.
P.O. Box 5030
Pasadena, CA 91107

U.S. Orthotics Inc.
8605 Palm River Rd.
Tampa, FL 33619-4317

Wheaton Brace Co.
380 S. Schmale Rd.
Carol Stream, IL 60188

Yale Surgical—Yale Comfort Shoe
627-629 Chapel St.
New Haven, CT 06511

Index

Page numbers followed by f *indicate figures; those followed by* t *indicate tables.*

329